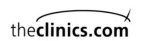

VETERINARY CLINICS
OF NORTH AMERICA

Small Animal Practice

The Thyroid

GUEST EDITOR
Cynthia R. Ward, VMD, PhD

July 2007 • Volume 37 • Number 4

SAUNDERS

An Imprint of Elsevier, Inc.
PHILADELPHIA   LONDON   TORONTO   MONTREAL   SYDNEY   TOKYO

W.B. SAUNDERS COMPANY
A Division of Elsevier Inc.

Elsevier, Inc., 1600 John F. Kennedy Blvd., Suite 1800, Philadelphia, PA 19103-2899

http://www.vetsmall.theclinics.com

VETERINARY CLINICS OF NORTH AMERICA:	**Volume 37, Number 4**
SMALL ANIMAL PRACTICE	**ISSN 0195-5616**
July 2007	**ISBN-13: 978-1-4160-5138-1**
Editor: John Vassallo; j.vassallo@elsevier.com	**ISBN-10: 1-4160-5138-4**

Veterinary Clinics of North America: Small Animal Practice (ISSN 0195-5616) is published bimonthly (For Post Office use only: volume 37 issue 4 of 6) by Elsevier Inc., 360 Park Avenue South, New York, NY 10010-1710. Months of issue are January, March, May, July, September, and November. Business and Editorial offices: 1600 John F. Kennedy Blvd., Suite 1800, Philadelphia, PA 19103-2899. Customer Service Office: 6277 Sea Harbor Drive, Orlando, FL 32887-4800. Periodicals postage paid at New York, NY and additional mailing offices. Subscription prices are $187.00 per year for US individuals, $297.00 per year for US institutions, $94.00 per year for US students and residents, $248.00 per year for Canadian individuals, $373.00 per year for Canadian institutions, $259.00 per year for international individuals, $373.00 per year for international institutions and $127.00 per year for Canadian and foreign students/residents. To receive student/resident rate, orders must be accompanied by name of affiliated institution, date of term, and the *signature* of program/residency coordinator on institution letterhead. Orders will be billed at individual rate until proof of status is received. Foreign air speed delivery is included in all *Clinics* subscription prices. All prices are subject to change without notice. **POSTMASTER**: Send address changes to *Veterinary Clinics of North America: Small Animal Practice*, Elsevier Periodicals Customer Service, 6277 Sea Harbor Drive, Orlando, FL 32887-4800, USA; phone: 1-800-654-2452 [toll free number for US customers], or (+1)(407) 345-4000 [customers outside US]; fax: (+1)(407) 363-1354; email: usjcs@elsevier.com.

Veterinary Clinics of North America: Small Animal Practice is also published in Japanese by Inter Zoo Publishing Co., Ltd., Aoyama Crystal-Bldg 5F, 3-5-12 Kitaaoyama, Minato-ku, Tokyo 107-0061, Japan.

Reprints: For copies of 100 or more, of articles in this publication, please contact the Commercial Reprints Department, Elsevier Inc., 360 Park Avenue South, New York, New York 10010-1710. Tel. (212) 633-3813 Fax: (212) 462-1935, email: reprints@elsevier.com.

Veterinary Clinics of North America: Small Animal Practice is covered in *Current Contents/Agriculture, Biology and Environmental Sciences, Science Citation Index, ASCA, Index Medicus, Excerpta Medica,* and *BIOSIS*.

Printed in the United States of America.

VETERINARY CLINICS
SMALL ANIMAL PRACTICE

The Thyroid

GUEST EDITOR

CYNTHIA R. WARD, VMD, PhD, Diplomate, American College of Veterinary Internal Medicine; Department of Small Animal Medicine, University of Georgia College of Veterinary Medicine, Athens, Georgia

CONTRIBUTORS

KARI L. ANDERSON, DVM, Department of Veterinary Clinical Sciences, College of Veterinary Medicine, University of Minnesota, St. Paul, Minnesota

LISA G. BARBER, DVM, Diplomate, American College of Veterinary Internal Medicine (Oncology); Assistant Professor, Department of Clinical Sciences, Cummings School of Veterinary Medicine, Tufts University, North Grafton, Massachusetts

DANIEL A. FEENEY, DVM, MS, Department of Veterinary Clinical Sciences, College of Veterinary Medicine, University of Minnesota, St. Paul, Minnesota

DUNCAN C. FERGUSON, VMD, PhD, Diplomate, American College of Veterinary Internal Medicine (Small Animal); Diplomate, American College of Veterinary Clinical Pharmacology; Department of Veterinary Biosciences, College of Veterinary Medicine, The University of Illinois at Urbana-Champaign, Urbana, Illinois

PETER A. GRAHAM, BVMS, PhD, CertVR, MRCVS, Diplomate, European College of Veterinary Clinical Pathology; Managing Director, NationWide Laboratories, Poulton-Le-Fylde, Lancashire, United Kingdom

CARMEL T. MOONEY, MVB, MPhil, PhD, Diplomate, European College of Veterinary Internal Medicine–Companion Animals; RCVS Specialist in Small Animal Medicine (Endocrinology); and Senior Lecturer in Small Animal Medicine, Small Animal Clinical Studies, School of Agriculture, Food Science and Veterinary Medicine, University College Dublin, Belfield, Dublin, Ireland

RAYMOND F. NACHREINER, DVM, PhD, Endocrinology Section, Diagnostic Center for Population and Animal Health, College of Veterinary Medicine, Michigan State University, East Lansing, Michigan

MARK E. PETERSON, DVM, Diplomate, American College of Veterinary Internal Medicine; Head, Department of Endocrinology; and Associate Director, The Caspary Institute; Director of Education, Institute for Postgraduate Education, The Animal Medical Center, New York, New York

MARYANN G. RADLINSKY, DVM, MS, Diplomate, American College of Veterinary Surgeons; Department of Small Animal Medicine and Surgery, University of Georgia College of Veterinary Medicine, Athens, Georgia

KENT R. REFSAL, DVM, PhD, Endocrinology Section, Diagnostic Center for Population and Animal Health, College of Veterinary Medicine, Michigan State University, East Lansing, Michigan

PATRICIA A. SCHENCK, DVM, PhD, Section Chief, Diagnostic Center for Population and Animal Health, Department of Pathobiology and Diagnostic Investigation, Endocrine Diagnostic Section; and Assistant Professor, Michigan State University, Lansing, Michigan

J. CATHARINE SCOTT-MONCRIEFF, MA, MS, Vet MB, MRCVS, Diplomate, American College of Veterinary Internal Medicine; Diplomate, European College of Veterinary Internal Medicine; Professor of Internal Medicine, Department of Veterinary Clinical Sciences, School of Veterinary Medicine, Purdue University, West Lafayette, Indiana

ROBERT E. SHIEL, MVB, Resident in Small Animal Medicine, Small Animal Clinical Studies, School of Agriculture, Food Science and Veterinary Medicine, University College Dublin, Belfield, Dublin, Ireland

HARRIET M. SYME, BSc, BVetMed, PhD, MRCVS, Diplomate, American College of Veterinary Internal Medicine; Diplomate, European College of Veterinary Internal Medicine; Senior Lecturer, Department of Veterinary Clinical Sciences, Royal Veterinary College, University of London, North Mymms, Hatfield, Hertfordshire, United Kingdom

LAUREN A. TREPANIER, DVM, PhD, Diplomate, American College of Veterinary Internal Medicine; Diplomate, American College of Veterinary Clinical Pharmacology; Associate Professor, Department of Medical Sciences, School of Veterinary Medicine; and Affiliate Professor, Department of Pharmaceutical Sciences, University of Wisconsin-Madison, Madison, Wisconsin

CYNTHIA R. WARD, VMD, PhD, Diplomate, American College of Veterinary Internal Medicine; Department of Small Animal Medicine, University of Georgia College of Veterinary Medicine, Athens, Georgia

The Thyroid

CONTENTS VOLUME 37 • NUMBER 4 • JULY 2007

The causes of canine hypothyroidism are varied, but most cases result
from irreversible acquired thyroid pathologic changes and only a small
proportion arise from congenital anomalies of the thyroid gland or
pituitary. Of primary thyroid failure, at least half is the result of immune-mediated thyroiditis. Recent research has focused on the genetics
and immunology of canine thyroid disease, adding to what is known
from experimental and human studies. Epidemiologic and diagnostic
laboratory studies continue to provide information on contributing factors and raise questions for future research directions. Serum antibodies
against thyroid components are common in thyroid pathologic conditions and dysfunction, and understanding their properties and frequency is important in the interpretation of thyroid diagnostic test
results.

None of the studies to date have isolated a single dominant factor that
could be incriminated in the development of hyperthyroidism in cats.
Rather, most of the studies provide further evidence of the widely
held view that hyperthyroidism is a multifactorial disease in this species.
At this time, the most likely candidates include one or more of the goitrogenic chemicals that have been shown to be present in cat food or the
cat's environment. In addition, mutations of the thyroid stimulating
hormone receptor gene or mutations of its associated G proteins seem
to play an important role in the pathogenesis of this disease.

Hypothyroidism is the most common endocrinopathy in the dog.
Rather than being a comprehensive review of all possible thyroid function tests, the focus in this article is on the logical progression of test
choice, highlighting total thyroxine, free thyroxine, triiodothyronine,
thyrotropin (TSH), and antithyroid antibodies. This article includes extensive discussion of the current status of the canine TSH assay and the
potential for improving this assay.

Hyperthyroidism remains a common endocrine disorder of cats. Although relatively easy to diagnose in classically presenting cats, the increased frequency of testing cats with early or mild disease has had significant implications for the diagnostic performance of many of the routine tests currently used. Further advances in the etiopathogenesis and earlier diagnosis are only likely with the advent of a species specific feline thyroid-stimulating hormone assay.

Hyperthyroidism is the most common endocrine disorder of cats, and hypothyroidism is the most common endocrine disorder of dogs. Little is known regarding the effects of hyperthyroidism, hypothyroidism, or treatment of these disorders on calcium metabolism in the dog or cat, however, especially any potential effects on bone. With better diagnostic tools, better treatments, and increased longevity of pets, the clinical impact of thyroid disorders on calcium metabolism and bone may be uncovered.

Canine hypothyroidism may present with a wide range of clinical signs. The most common clinical signs are those of a decreased metabolic rate and dermatologic manifestations; however, many other clinical signs have been associated with hypothyroidism. There is strong evidence for a causal relation between hypothyroidism and a variety of neurologic abnormalities; however, the association between hypothyroidism and other manifestations, such as reproductive dysfunction, clinical heart disease, and behavioral abnormalities, is less compelling. Further studies are necessary to determine the full spectrum of disorders caused by hypothyroidism.

In the simplest terms, hyperthyroidism is the clinical syndrome that results from an excess of thyroid hormones. This review considers the effects of hyperthyroidism on the cardiovascular and renal systems by reviewing the available literature on the clinical manifestations of this syndrome in the cat and also considering experimental studies and experience in other species, including human beings.

should be treated concurrently with atenolol, amlodipine, or an angiotensin-converting enzyme inhibitor.

Thyroid surgery is indicated for malignant and benign neoplasms or hyperplasia of the thyroid glands. A ventral midline cervical approach allows for bilateral thyroid exploration. Care should be taken to avoid the surrounding neurovascular structures and esophagus. Evaluation of both thyroids should be done before proceeding with partial or complete thyroidectomy. Complications of thyroid surgery include intraoperative hemorrhage and clinical signs associated with damage to the recurrent laryngeal nerves, parathyroid blood supply, or parathyroidectomy.

The indications, techniques, and expectations for radionuclide diagnostic studies on canine and feline thyroid glands are presented. In addition, the considerations surrounding radioiodine or external beam radiotherapy for benign and malignant thyroid disease are reviewed. The intent of this article is to familiarize primary care veterinarians with the utility of and outcome of the ionizing radiation-based diagnostic and therapeutic techniques for assessing and treating canine and feline thyroid disease.

FORTHCOMING ISSUES

RECENT ISSUES

Vet Clin Small Anim 37 (2007) xi–xii

VETERINARY CLINICS
SMALL ANIMAL PRACTICE

Preface

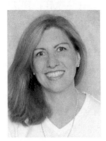

Cynthia R. Ward, VMD, PhD

Guest Editor

It has been an honor for me to be the guest editor for this edition of *Veterinary Clinics of North America: Small Animal Practice*, which is devoted to the thyroid. Since publication of the last issue on this topic more than 10 years ago, a great deal of knowledge has been realized and clarified in our understanding and recognition of thyroid disease. Detailed investigations into the etiopathology of thyroid diseases have increased our understanding of how these common endocrinopathies occur. Development of more accurate testing methodology has allowed the disease to be correctly diagnosed, and effective treatment regimes have resulted in better control of the disease. We have learned to recognize the wide range of concurrent clinical syndromes encompassing hyper- and hypothyroid disease in small animals. With the ability to identify subtle manifestations of thyroid disease, diagnosis and treatment can be given more quickly to benefit patients. Moreover, syndromes associated with thyroid disease can be more effectively managed.

I have organized this edition to take the reader through the whole spectrum of thyroid disease in, what is hopefully, an orderly fashion. The first two articles summarize our current understanding of the etiology of thyroid disease. The third and fourth articles are devoted to new testing modalities for hypo- and hyperthyroidism. The next five articles focus on the spectrum of electrolyte disorders and clinical syndromes occurring with thyroid disease, including manifestations of thyroid cancer. Finally, the last three articles conclude with current treatment modalities of thyroid disease, which include medicine, surgery, and radiation approaches.

It has truly been a pleasure to work with leaders in the field of thyroid medicine. I thank all the authors for taking the time to contribute their expertise

0195-5616/07/$ – see front matter
doi:10.1016/j.cvsm.2007.06.001

to this publication. I hope the reader will find the summation of this material interesting, enlightening, and helpful for everyday clinical practice.

Cynthia R. Ward, VMD, PhD
Department of Small Animal Medicine
University of Georgia College of Veterinary Medicine
501 DW Brooks Drive
Athens, GA 30602

E-mail address: cward@vet.uga.edu

Etiopathologic Findings of Canine Hypothyroidism

Peter A. Graham, BVMS, PhD CertVR MRCVS[a],*,
Kent R. Refsal, DVM, PhD[b],
Raymond F. Nachreiner, DVM, PhD[b]

[a]NationWide Laboratories, 23 Mains Lane, Poulton-Le-Fylde, Lancashire FY6 7LJ, UK
[b]Endocrinology Section, Diagnostic Center for Population and Animal Health,
College of Veterinary Medicine, Michigan State University, 4125 Beaumont Road,
East Lansing, MI 48910-8104, USA

I t is apparent that the generation of thyroid hormones and the control mechanisms for their production and effects in target tissues are governed by many complicated processes. Failure of any one of the multiple required steps in thyroid hormone production, loss of hormonal trophic support from the pituitary, or destruction of the thyroid glands can result in hypothyroidism.

Although a range of possible causes of canine hypothyroidism exists, most cases arise from irreversible acquired thyroid gland disease. Only a small proportion of hypothyroidism cases result from nutritional, congenital, pituitary, hypothalamic, or reversible conditions. Hypothyroidism arising from failure of the thyroid glands is described as primary, that arising from pituitary failure as secondary, and that arising from the hypothalamus as tertiary.

ADULT-ONSET HYPOTHYROIDISM

Almost all the naturally occurring hypothyroidism in adult dogs is attributable to irreversible destruction of the thyroid glands. Histologically, primary hypothyroidism is divided into two main pathologic categories: lymphocytic thyroiditis or idiopathic thyroid degeneration (idiopathic follicular atrophy). Most estimates indicate an approximately 1:1 ratio of these two types of thyroid pathologic findings as the origin of clinical hypothyroidism in dogs.

Lymphocytic thyroiditis, also referred to as autoimmune thyroiditis, is characterized by lymphocytic infiltration of the thyroid glands with progressive destruction of thyroid follicles. The presence of this thyroid inflammation can be detected in serum by the measurement of antibodies to thyroid components (usually antithyroglobulin antibodies [TgAAs]). The progression of this disease process is slow, and extensive pathologic changes have occurred before the appearance of clinical signs of hypothyroidism. This condition is recognized

*Corresponding author. E-mail address: pgraham@nwlabs.co.uk (P.A. Graham).

0195-5616/07/$ – see front matter
doi:10.1016/j.cvsm.2007.05.002

as a heritable trait [1–3]. Lymphocytic thyroiditis may sometimes present as a component of immune-mediated polyendocrinopathy [4,5].

Idiopathic thyroid degeneration is characterized by a loss of thyroid parenchyma, with replacement by adipose or fibrous tissue. The cause has not yet been defined, and it is likely that this category represents a collection of primary pathologic conditions, but there is evidence that at least a proportion of these cases represent an end-stage form of lymphocytic thyroiditis [5].

CONGENITAL HYPOTHYROIDISM

Congenital cases of hypothyroidism in the dog arise from defects in thyrotrophic support (absent or ineffective thyroid-stimulating hormone [TSH]), dyshormonogenesis of thyroid hormone, or thyroid gland development. In cases in which there is normal pituitary function, the failure of thyroid hormone production can be expected to result in goiter and histologic evidence of follicular hyperplasia. A nonsense mutation in the thyroperoxidase (TPO) gene causing hypothyroidism with goiter has been reported in Toy Fox Terries and related Rat Terriers [6,7]. Goiter is absent in most reports of congenital hypothyroidism. A lack of production of TSH is the suspected cause of juvenile hypothyroidism in Giant Schnauzer [8], Boxer [9], and Scottish Deerhound [10] dogs. Tertiary hypothyroidism has not been confirmed in dogs, although many reports of congenital hypothyroidism were published before the availability of the canine TSH assay, making the distinction between secondary and tertiary difficult to determine.

NATURAL HISTORY OF THYROID DISEASE

The pathway from completely healthy thyroid glands to glands that are sufficiently destroyed to result in such a degree of thyroid hormone deficiency that it becomes clinically apparent is probably not a short process in most circumstances of adult-onset hypothyroidism. The progression of lymphocytic thyroiditis from the earliest evidence of pathologic change to overt thyroid functional failure has been the subject of some study [5,11,12].

In the dog, the disease progresses through recognizable stages:

1. Subclinical (or silent) thyroiditis: the presence of focal and often peripheral lymphocytic infiltrates in the glands that have a normal histologic appearance otherwise; the only laboratory abnormality is TgAA in serum.
2. Antibody-positive subclinical hypothyroidism: if pathologic change encompasses more than 60% to 70% of the thyroid mass, we see a compensatory elevation of serum TSH concentration that stimulates the remaining portion of functional tissue to increase thyroid hormone production. Follicular epithelial cells demonstrate this stimulation histologically by a change from a cuboidal to columnar shape. Laboratory abnormalities in this stage include serum TgAA and increased TSH concentrations but normal concentrations of thyroxine (T_4) and triiodothyronine (T_3).

3. Antibody-positive overt hypothyroidism: when nearly all functional thyroid tissue has been destroyed by inflammation, T_4 production cannot be maintained and the classic laboratory pattern of decreased total T_4, increased TSH, and positive antibody is found. It may be sometime thereafter before physical clinical signs are documented. In experimental settings in which functionally overt hypothyroidism has been induced by surgery or radiation, clinical signs took some time to develop and were not clearly apparent until more than a year later [13].

4. Noninflammatory atrophic hypothyroidism: there is some evidence to suggest that there is eventually replacement of thyroid tissue by fibrous and adipose tissue, with disappearance of inflammatory cells leading to a noninflammatory and atrophic histologic appearance. The absence of inflammation is likely to result in the disappearance of antibodies from the circulation over time. What contribution this end-stage of thyroiditis makes to the 50% of canine hypothyroidism that is antibody-negative (idiopathic) has yet to be defined.

The progression of idiopathic follicular atrophy attributable to causes other than end-stage thyroiditis has not yet been studied, because there is not yet a diagnostic test for the subclinical form. It has to be assumed that the disease progresses through similar functional stages, but the time scale is unknown.

The progression of thyroiditis to functional hypothyroidism is supported by long-term follow-up of affected dogs [11,12,14] and database studies of age distributions of the different functional and pathologic stages (Fig. 1). Not all cases progress to overt disease, however, and there is limited or slow progression in some.

ETIOPATHOLOGIC FINDINGS OF CANINE INFLAMMATORY THYROID DISEASE

Little is known about the initiators of canine thyroid disease, although recent work has laid the groundwork for further study and epidemiologic surveys hope to give some direction for suitable areas of investigation. Most of what we understand about the initiation of canine thyroid disease comes from studies in other species, including human beings, although the canine disease has recently been the subject of further investigation.

The pathologic findings of thyroiditis are predominantly lymphocytic and consist of B- and T-cell components. Two forms of chronic autoimmune thyroiditis are recognized in human medicine: goitrous autoimmune thyroiditis (Hashimoto's disease), which does not occur in dogs, and atrophic autoimmune thyroiditis, which is more similar to the chronic autoimmune thyroiditis of dogs. The pathologic findings in these conditions are similar, with the exception of goitrous enlargement in the former, and include focal or diffuse lymphoplasmacytic infiltration with macrophages. Lymphoid germinal centers are often seen in moderate and severe cases, as is basement membrane disruption, including ultrastructural abnormalities consistent with antibody or antigen complex deposits. Enlarged, metaplastic, oxyphilic follicular epithelial

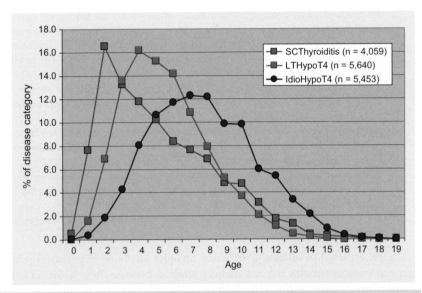

Fig. 1. Age distribution profiles for different categories of thyroid disease and dysfunction based on findings in 143,800 samples submitted for the investigation of thyroid disease in which an age was provided. IdioHypoT4, TgAA-negative hypothyroidism; LTHypoT4, TgAA-positive hypothyroidism; SC thyroiditis, subclinical TgAA-positive thyroiditis.

cells (Hürthle cells) with granular mitochondria-rich cytoplasm are also seen. In dogs, the pathologic findings of this condition have been described numerous times [11,15–23]. It is histologically identical to human chronic autoimmune thyroiditis, and histologic grading systems have been developed [15,23].

The immunologic and molecular pathogenesis of autoimmune thyroiditis in dogs has not yet been well characterized. Most of what is known about the condition has been learned from the induction of experimental disease and research of the human condition. Although thyroiditis has been studied in laboratory rodents and chickens and experimentally induced in dogs, it is not clear how well these models mimic naturally occurring disease. In human beings, the lymphocytic infiltrate contains B cells and mostly T cells. CD4 and cytotoxic CD8 T lymphocytes are present, and evidence exists for thyroid follicular cell destruction through antibody-dependent complement-mediated mechanisms and cytotoxic T cells [24]. Recent work has confirmed the proliferative responses of peripheral blood mononuclear cells to canine thyroglobulin in TgAA-positive hypothyroid dogs and suggests that a loss of self-tolerance in CD4+ cells is important in the pathologic findings of canine thyroiditis [25]. To what extent this immunologic phenomenon is an initiator rather than a consequence of the thyroid pathologic condition has yet to be understood.

Experimental thyroiditis and human autoimmune thyroiditis seem to be disorders of immunoregulation. Therefore, in the search for the underlying molecular abnormality in this condition, research effort has been focused on mechanisms of immunoregulation, particularly the contribution made by the human leukocyte antigen (HLA) complex. Some association has been documented between certain HLA subtypes and the presence of disease; however, to date, these associations have generally been weak. Work on the contributions of dog leukocyte antigen (DLA) subtypes to the disease in dogs is under investigation [26]. The genetics of the DLA have recently been investigated, and predisposing alleles have indeed been identified [27,28]. The DLA-DQA1*00101 allele seems to be particularly influential and is associated with an increased risk of hypothyroidism (overall odds ratio = 1.97; $P < .001$). Although especially prevalent in Doberman Pinschers, English Setters, and Rhodesian Ridgebacks (including unaffected individuals), this was not the case in other breeds, such as the Boxer. This is consistent with the predisposition associated with HLA subtypes.

In the investigation of potential nonimmunogenetic causes, such as mutations in the canine thyroglobulin gene or its promoter, no variations correlating with the presence of thyroiditis have been revealed [26], although canine thyroglobulin has now been cloned and sequenced [29], opening the possibility for further research in this area. The possibility that thyroiditis is induced in predisposed individuals by antigenic mimicry of thyroid antigens by viral or bacterial agents has been suggested. This possibility is supported by the protective effects of intestinal sterilization in experimental thyroiditis [30] and serologic evidence of recent infections in affected human patients [31,32]. *Yersinia enterocolitica* antibodies have been identified in human patients with Grave's disease [33] (a form of autoimmune thyroid disease in which anti-TSH receptor antibodies result in hyperthyroidism), and an increased frequency of antiretroviral antibodies has been found in human patients with autoimmune thyroiditis [34]. An alternative viral mechanism could be through the local induction of interferon-γ (IFNγ)–triggering H(D)LA expression by thyrocytes initiating an autoimmune process [34]. The contribution of immunoregulation in this disease is also inferred by the possible modulation of immunotolerance by oral feeding of thyroglobulin, after which some measures of thyroid autoimmunity can be ameliorated [35].

A protective effect of whole-body irradiation against familial lymphocytic thyroiditis in beagles, especially when administered at around 2 days of age, has been documented and was greatest in genetically predisposed dogs [1,2,36]. Whether this phenomenon is mediated through effects on the developing immune system or on thyroid gland structure or function requires further investigation.

The diversity of prevalence among breeds (Table 1) and several specific heritability studies [2,3,36,37] indicate the highly heritable nature of this condition, and further studies indicate that there is a breed influence on age and progression of the disease [5].

Table 1
Twenty breeds with the highest and 20 breeds with the lowest prevalence of thyroglobulin antibody in 140,821 serum samples submitted for investigation of thyroid disease

Name	Total sera	TgAA-positive	Prevalence
English Setter	585	184	31%
Old English Sheepdog	368	86	23%
Boxer	2642	496	19%
Giant Schnauzer	263	49	19%
American Pit Bull Terrier	345	64	19%
Beagle	2452	449	18%
Dalmatian	1372	246	18%
German Wirehaired Pointer	112	20	18%
Maltese Dog	594	105	18%
Rhodesian Ridgeback	626	107	17%
Siberian Husky	1129	164	15%
American Staffordshire Terrier	151	24	16%
Cocker Spaniel	8576	1305	15%
Chesapeake Bay Retriever	509	74	15%
Tibetan Terrier	106	15	14%
Shetland Sheepdog	5765	813	14%
Golden Retriever	17782	2397	13%
Borzoi	266	35	13%
Brittany Spaniel	556	71	13%
Dachshund	3612	115	3%
Basset Hound	699	22	3%
Cairn Terrier	590	18	3%
Schnauzer (unspecified)	1257	38	3%
Wirehaired Fox Terrier	170	5	3%
Cavalier King Charles Spaniel	274	8	3%
Welsh Corgi (undetermined)	457	13	3%
Yorkshire Terrier	1178	33	3%
Norwegian Elkhound	263	7	3%
Belgian Tervuren	235	6	3%
Chihuahua	611	15	2%
Greyhound	1409	32	2%
Pekingese	407	9	2%
Boston Terrier	500	11	2%
Pomeranian	1301	26	2%
Irish Wolfhound	210	4	2%
Whippet	114	2	2%
Soft-Coated Wheaten Terrier	214	3	1%
Bichon Frise	657	8	1%
Miniature Schnauzer	828	10	1%

Overall TgAA prevalence in this study was 10%.

There has been controversy in recent years concerning the possible contribution that routine vaccination might make to the origin of thyroiditis in dogs. In one study, it seemed that there might be support for vaccination as an initiator of thyroid pathologic change. Scott-Moncrief and colleagues [38,39] reported an increase in circulating antibodies that reacted with thyroglobulin after repeated vaccination; however, further research by the same group failed to demonstrate an increased prevalence of thyroiditis in vaccinated beagles postmortem after a 5.5-year follow-up study [40].

The research experience in other species and in related immune-mediated disease has shown that the origins of thyroiditis in an individual animal are likely to be multifactorial. Using a large research database containing the results of 143,000 serum thyroid investigations and questionnaire studies, researchers at Michigan State University have explored how candidate predisposing factors, including breed, seasonality, and geography, contribute to the initiation of thyroid pathologic change.

In addition to identifying the prevalence of TgAA (as a marker for the prevalence of thyroiditis) across a range of breeds, these researchers have also noted a wide variation in the relative proportions of antibody-positive (thyroiditis) and antibody-negative (idiopathic atrophy) hypothyroidism across breeds. The widely reported overall average of 50:50 holds true; however, in some breeds, the contribution of thyroiditis is much greater or much less. In English Setters, for example, more than 80% of cases diagnosed with hypothyroidism were TgAA-positive, whereas less than 30% of hypothyroid Doberman Pinschers were antibody-positive (Table 2). These findings suggest a different rate or type of progression of thyroiditis or breed differences in predisposition to non-inflammatory forms of thyroid disease.

Using age-distribution profiles similar to that in Fig. 1 on a breed-specific basis (Figs. 2 and 3), there is indeed some evidence to suggest that there may be different progression rates among breeds.

There may be a small contribution of season of the year to the occurrence of earliest evidence of thyroiditis. Of dogs with no laboratory evidence of thyroid dysfunction, the proportion with evidence of thyroiditis (positive TgAA) was highest in the summer (July, August, and September) and lowest in the fall (October, November, and December) (Table 3).

In a preliminary investigation of the influence of geography on the prevalence of thyroiditis in samples submitted to Michigan State University, some significant differences were observed. The prevalence of TgAA was significantly higher in samples submitted from North Dakota, Vermont, Wyoming, Minnesota, and Colorado compared with Michigan (range of odds ratios: 1.19–1.41; $P < .05$). The prevalence was significantly lower in samples from Massachusetts, Maryland, Virginia, North Carolina, Florida, South Carolina, Kentucky, Texas, West Virginia, Tennessee, and Alabama (range of odds ratios: 0.39–0.79; $P < .05$). There was no interaction with breed prevalence, but the underlying reasons (if any) for these observations have yet to be discovered.

Table 2
Proportion of TgAA-positive results by breed in 11,606 serum samples from dogs with laboratory results consistent with hypothyroidism (restricted to breeds with >40 cases)

Breed	TgAA-negative hypothyroidism	TgAA-positive hypothyroidism	Total hypothyroidism	Proportion TgAA-positive
English Setter	12	61	73	84%
Chesapeake Bay Retriever	15	36	51	71%
Golden Retriever	475	1050	1525	69%
Rhodesian Ridgeback	15	27	42	64%
Boxer	93	166	259	64%
Siberian Husky	45	74	119	62%
Irish Setter	16	26	42	62%
Cocker Spaniel	451	683	1134	60%
Border Collie	31	44	75	59%
Dalmatian	110	152	262	58%
Maltese Dog	39	52	91	57%
American Pit Bull Terrier	19	25	44	57%
Shetland Sheepdog	303	395	698	57%
Beagle	240	276	516	53%
Australian Shepherd	31	32	63	51%
Mixed breed	1249	1286	2535	51%
Akita	22	22	44	50%
Great Dane	30	29	59	49%
Brittany Spaniel	36	33	69	48%
Scottish Terrier	31	26	57	46%
Malamute	36	30	66	45%
Samoyed	30	23	53	43%
Labrador Retriever	577	376	953	39%
Rottweiler	102	60	162	37%
Chow Chow	53	28	81	35%
Springer Spaniel	75	38	113	34%
German Shepherd Dog	101	50	151	33%
Shih Tzu	31	14	45	31%
Keeshond	34	15	49	31%
Doberman Pinscher	392	135	527	26%
Poodle	68	22	90	24%
Collie	95	26	121	21%
Pomeranian	33	9	42	21%
Dachshund	68	13	81	16%
Grand total	5680	5926	11606	51%

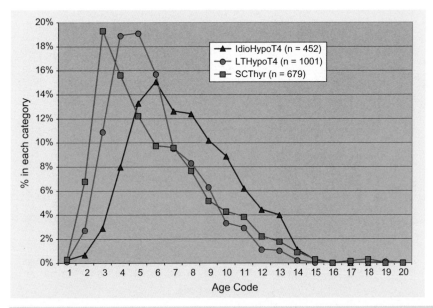

Fig. 2. Age distribution profiles for different categories of thyroid disease and dysfunction based on findings in 17,782 samples submitted from Golden Retrievers for the investigation of thyroid disease in which an age was provided. IdioHypoT$_4$, TgAA-negative hypothyroidism; LTHypoT$_4$, TgAA-positive hypothyroidism; SC thyroiditis, subclinical TgAA-positive thyroiditis.

LABORATORY DIAGNOSIS OF THYROIDITIS AND IMPLICATIONS FOR DIAGNOSIS OF HYPOTHYROIDISM

During the inflammatory process of lymphocytic thyroiditis, antibodies are released into the circulation. In the dog, these are predominantly reactive against thyroglobulin. In people, the most common antigen to which antibodies are detected in patients with thyroiditis is TPO. Studies of anti-TPO as part of the process of thyroiditis in dogs have yielded mixed results [14,41,42]. A recent report provides evidence that they may be part of the process [43], albeit that their presence is documented only in dogs that also have TgAA or thyroid hormone auto antibodies (THAAs). This study found that 17% of TgAA-positive serum samples also reacted with TPO.

The thyroglobulin molecule is large and complex and contains sites at which thyroid hormones are assembled, incorporated, and stored. The size and complexity of the thyroglobulin molecule is such that antibodies against it form a heterogenous group directed at several epitopic sites. Several different segments of the thyroglobulin molecule, including some hormonogenic sites, seem to have greater antigenicity than others [26,44], and a small number of tryptic peptides of canine thyroglobulin have been shown to react consistently with TgAA-positive serum samples from 10 hypothyroid dogs (43-, 32.5-, 31-, and possibly 25-kd fragments) [45], although other attempts have failed to find

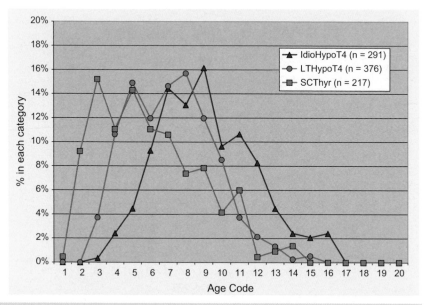

Fig. 3. Age distribution profiles for different categories of thyroid disease and dysfunction based on findings in 5765 samples submitted from Shetland Sheepdogs for the investigation of thyroid disease in which an age was provided. IdioHypoT$_4$, TgAA-negative hypothyroidism; LTHypoT$_4$, TgAA-positive hypothyroidism; SC thyroiditis, subclinical TgAA-positive thyroiditis. (*Data from* Michigan State University, East Lansing, Michigan, 2006.)

such fragment specificity in the dog [46]. Hormonogenic sites in canine thyroglobulin are conserved [29].

When an epitopic site includes a hormonogenic site, an antibody can be directed against a fragment that contains T_4 or T_3, creating an TgAA that cross-reacts with unbound T_3 or T_4. T_3 and T4 are not sufficiently large molecules to initiate an antibody themselves. The development of antibodies against epitopes that do not include hormonogenic areas results in TgAAs that do not

Table 3
Proportion of TgAA-positive results in 100,101 serum samples from euthyroid dogs by season

Season	Euthyroid TgAA-positive	Total euthyroid	Proportion TgAA-positive
January, February, March	850	19,345	4.39%
April, May, June	1084	23,722	4.57%
July, August, September	1465	29,885	4.90%
October, November, December	1072	27,149	3.95%
—	—	χ^2	31.19
—	—	P	.00000078

Table 4
Prevalence of thyroglobulin and thyroid hormone cross-reacting antibodies in different classes of serum from 143,800 samples submitted for investigation of thyroid disease

Category	Of 11,606 hypothyroid dogs	Of 5926 TgAA-positive hypothyroid dogs	Of 14,016 TgAA-positive dogs
TgAA	51%	100%	100%
Any THAA	30%	49%	39%
T_3AA	28%	46%	37%
T_4AA	8%	14%	11%
T_3AA and T_4AA	6%	11%	10%
TgAA but no THAA	26%	51%	61%
T_3AA but no T_4AA	21%	35%	27%
T_4AA but no T_3AA	2%	2%	2%
THAA but no TgAA	5%	—	—

cross-react with thyroid hormones. From Table 4, it can be seen that of dogs with circulating TgAAs, 37% have antibodies that cross-react with T_3 and 11% have antibodies that cross-react with T_4. Almost all dogs with anti-T_4 antibodies also have anti-T_3 antibodies, and approximately 50% of TgAA-positive serum samples do not react with thyroid hormones.

TgAAs that cross-react with free thyroid hormones (THAAs) are unlikely to have physiologic consequences in the circulation, given the tiny proportions of free (unbound) T_3 and free T_4. The presence of THAAs becomes important in the diagnostic laboratory when immunologic methods are used to measure serum concentrations of T_3 or T_4, however. Serum samples that contain TgAAs (THAAs) that cross-react with T_3 are described as T3 cross-reacting autoantibodies (T_3AA)-positive, and, similarly, those that cross-react with T_4 are T4 cross-reacting autoantibodies (T_4AA)-positive. Immunologic methods of thyroid hormone measurement depend on tightly controlled amounts of laboratory-derived antihormone antibody and labeled hormone. In the situation in which a patient sample brings it own antihormone antibodies to the reaction chamber, control of the reaction conditions is lost and false laboratory results are generated. In most assay systems, the effect of THAA is to cause a falsely higher measured concentration of the respective hormone. It is useful to note that this increase need not necessarily be greater than the laboratory reference range. In a few assay systems (eg, Michigan State University total T_3), a falsely lower value may be generated. The nature of the assay inaccuracy (falsely elevated versus falsely lowered) depends on the method used to separate radioligand bound to assay antibody from unbound radioligand, the so-called "separation step." If the dog's THAA becomes separated from the assay antibody, the calculated hormone concentration is falsely elevated. If the dog's

THAA remains with the assay antibody, the calculated result is falsely lowered. Assays like as the free T_4 by equilibrium dialysis method, which removes the patient antibody (by dialysis) before the immunoassay step, are free from THAA interference.

The high proportion of T_3AA in hypothyroid dogs is the underlying reason why serum total T_3 measurement has not been found to be a useful test in the diagnosis of canine hypothyroidism. When T_3AA-positive animals are excluded, the diagnostic performance of T_3 is similar to the other measures of thyroid function (total thyroxine [TT_4], TSH, and free T4 by equilibrium dialysis [FT_4d]).

The diagnostic implication of the prevalence of T_4AA in hypothyroid dogs is that a normal or high TT_4 alone cannot be used conclusively to rule out a diagnosis of hypothyroidism. The addition of T_4AA (or TgAA) to a panel gives an indication of whether a normal serum TT_4 result can be believed.

The diagnostic implication of TgAA in the absence of evidence of thyroid dysfunction is that around 1 in 5 cases has progressive dysfunction within a year and 1 in 20 cases is hypothyroid [12].

Several TgAA assays have been described in the literature [47–50], but many recent reports, including the data presented in this article, have used a commercially available canine TgAA ELISA (Oxford Biomedical Research, Oxford,

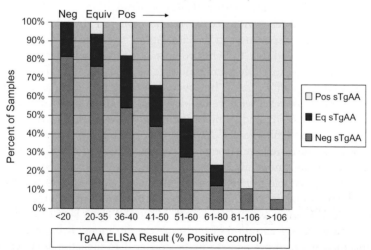

Fig. 4. Classification of direct thyroglobulin ELISA results with the outcome from adjustment for nonspecific binding in selected canine serum samples. Direct TgAA results are on the ordinate and expressed as the percentage of positive control (<20 is negative, 20–35 is equivocal, and >35 is positive). The vertical bars reflect the reclassification of the same samples after adjustment for nonspecific binding. (*Data from* Michigan State University, East Lansing, Michigan, 2006.)

Michigan). This assay has undergone development during recent years to re-duce the rate of false-positive and equivocal results. In the past, results from this assay were reported as patient optical density as a percentage of negative control optical density. Now, results can be expressed as percentage of a stan-dardized positive control, and nonspecific binding ELISA plates (which lack thyroglobulin in plate wells) are also now provided to reduce the effect of IgG titers unrelated to TgAA. Some of the initial concern about TgAA becom-ing borderline positive in the months after vaccination [38,39] may have been attributable to increased nonspecific IgG binding, and the modifications to the assay should have now improved the confidence in positive TgAA results. In the evolution of setting cutoff values for negative, equivocal, or positive TgAA results, it seems that current guidelines maximize diagnostic sensitivity of de-tecting positive autoantibodies. When the direct TgAA ELISA and the nonspe-cific binding modification are run on the same sample, discordant results most often occur in slightly increased direct ELISA results that become equivocal or negative when adjusted for nonspecific binding (Fig. 4).

Acknowledgments

The authors gratefully acknowledge Mark Bowman and Ryan Lundquist for their assistance in manipulating and interrogating the large data sets reported in the article. They also acknowledge the clients of the Diagnostic Center for Population and Animal Health for the provision of clinical samples and demo-graphic information with which epidemiologic studies are performed. Finally, they acknowledge the technical staff of the endocrine section for their expertise in performing the assays.

References

[1] Benjamin SA, Stephens LC, Hamilton BF, et al. Associations between lymphocytic thyroiditis, hypothyroidism, and thyroid neoplasia in beagles. Vet Pathol 1996;33:486–94.

[2] Benjamin SA, Lee AC, Angleton GM, et al. Mortality in beagles irradiated during prenatal and postnatal development. I. Contribution of non-neoplastic diseases. Radiat Res 1998; 150:316–29.

[3] Conaway DH, Padgett GA, Nachreiner RF. The familial occurrence of lymphocytic thyroid-itis in borzoi dogs. Am J Med Genet 1985;22:409–14.

[4] Feldman EC, Nelson RW. Hypothyroidism. In: Canine and feline endocrinology and repro-duction. 3rd edition. St Louis (MO): Saunders; 2004. p. 86–151.

[5] Graham PA, Nachreiner RF, Refsal KR, et al. Lymphocytic thyroiditis. Vet Clin North Am 2001;31(5):915–33.

[6] Fyfe JC, Kampschmidt K, Dang V, et al. Congenital hypothyroidism with goiter in toy fox ter-riers. J Vet Intern Med 2003;17:50–7.

[7] Pettigrew R, Fyfe JC, Gregory BL, et al. CNS hypomyelination in rat terrier dogs with congenital goiter and a mutation in the thyroid peroxidase gene. Vet Pathol 2007; 44(1):50–6.

[8] Greco DS, Feldman EC, Peterson ME, et al. Congenital hypothyroid dwarfism in a family of giant schnauzers. J Vet Intern Med 1991;5(2):57–65.

[9] Mooney CT, Anderson TJ. Congenital hypothyroidism in a boxer dog. J Small Anim Pract 1993;34:31–5.

[10] Robinson WF, Shaw SE, Stanley B, et al. Congenital hypothyroidism in Scottish deerhound puppies. Aust Vet J 1988;65(12):386–9.

[11] Conaway DH, Padgett GA, Bunton TE, et al. Clinical and histological features of primary progressive, familial thyroiditis in a colony of borzoi dogs. Vet Pathol 1985;22:439–46.

[12] Graham PA, Lundquist RB, Refsal KR, et al. 12-Month prospective study of 234 thyroglobulin antibody positive dogs which had no laboratory evidence of thyroid dysfunction [abstract]. J Vet Intern Med 2001;14:298.

[13] Johnson C, Olivier B, Nachreiner RF, et al. Effect of 131I-induced hypothyroidism on indices of reproductive function in adult male dogs. J Vet Intern Med 1999;13:104–10.

[14] Haines DM, Lording PM, Penhale WJ. The detection of canine autoantibodies to thyroid antigens by enzyme-linked immunosorbent assay, hemagglutination and indirect immunofluorescence. Can J Comp Med 1984;48:262–7.

[15] Beierwaltes WH, Nishiyama RH. Dog thyroiditis: occurrence and similarity to Hashimoto's struma. Endocrinology 1968;83:501–8.

[16] Fritz TE, Zeman RC, Zelle MR. Pathology and familial incidence of thyroiditis in a closed Beagle colony. Exp Mol Pathol 1970;12:14–30.

[17] Gosselin SJ, Capen CC, Martin SL. Histologic and ultrastructural evaluation of thyroid lesions associated with hypothyroidism in dogs. Vet Pathol 1981;18:299–309.

[18] Lucke VM, Gaskell CJ, Wotton PR. Thyroid pathology in canine hypothyroidism. J Comp Pathol 1983;93:415–21.

[19] Manning PJ. Thyroid gland and arterial lesions of Beagles with familial hypothyroidism and hyperlipoproteinemia. Am J Vet Res 1979;40:820–8.

[20] Mawdesley-Thomas LE. Lymphocytic thyroiditis in the dog. J Small Anim Pract 1968;9: 539–50.

[21] Mizejewski GJ, Baron J, Poissant G. Immunologic investigations of naturally occurring canine thyroiditis. J Immunol 1971;107:1152–60.

[22] Tucker WE. Thyroiditis in a group of laboratory dogs. Am J Clin Pathol 1962;38:70–4.

[23] Vajner L, Vortel V, Brejcha A. Lymphocytic thyroiditis in beagle dogs in a breeding colony: histological findings. Vet Med (Praha) 1997;42:43–9.

[24] Weetman AP. Chronic autoimmune thyroiditis. In: Braverman LE, Utiger RD, editors. Werner and Ingbar's the thyroid: a fundamental and clinical text. 8th edition. Philadelphia: Lippincott Williams and Wilkins; 2000. p. 721.

[25] Tani H, Nabetani T, Sasai K, et al. Proliferative responses to canine thyroglobulin of peripheral blood mononuclear cells from hypothyroid dogs. J Vet Med Sci 2005;67(4):363–8.

[26] Happ GM. Thyroiditis—a model canine autoimmune disease. Adv Vet Sci Comp Med 1995;39:97–139.

[27] Kennedy LJ, Huson HJ, Leonard J, et al. Association of hypothyroid disease in Doberman Pinscher dogs with a rare major histocompatibility complex DLA class II haplotype. Tissue Antigens 2006;67(1):53–6.

[28] Kennedy LJ, Quarmby S, Happ GM, et al. Association of canine hypothyroidism with a common major histocompatibility complex DLA class II allele. Tissue Antigens 2006;68(1): 82–6.

[29] Lee JY, Uzuka Y, Tanabe S, et al. Cloning and characterization of canine thyroglobulin complementary DNA. Domest Anim Endocrinol 2007;32:178–9.

[30] Penhale WJ, Young PR. The influence of microbial environment on susceptibility to experimental autoimmune thyroiditis. Clin Exp Immunol 1988;72:288–92.

[31] Tomer Y, Davies TF. Infection, thyroid disease, and autoimmunity. Endocr Rev 1993;14: 107–20.

[32] Valtonen VV, Ruutu P, Varis K, et al. Serological evidence for the role of bacterial infections in the pathogenesis of thyroid diseases. Acta Med Scand 1986;219:105–11.

[33] Wenzel BE, Heesemann J, Wenzel KW, et al. Antibodies to plasmid-encoded proteins of enteropathogenic Yersinia in patients with autoimmune thyroid disease. Lancet 1988; 1(8575–6):56.

[34] Dayan CM, Daniels GH. Chronic autoimmune thyroiditis. N Engl J Med 1996;335: 99–107.

[35] Lee S, Sherberg N, DeGroot LJ. Induction of oral tolerance in human autoimmune thyroid disease. Thyroid 1998;8:229–34.

[36] Benjamin SA, Saunders WJ, Lee AC, et al. Non-neoplastic and neoplastic thyroid disease in beagles irradiated during prenatal and postnatal development. Radiat Res 1997;147: 422–30.

[37] Musser E, Graham WR. Familial occurrence of thyroiditis in purebred Beagles. Lab Anim Care 1968;18:58–68.

[38] Hogenesch H, Azcona-Olivera J, Scott-Moncrieff C, et al. Vaccine-induced autoimmunity in the dog. Adv Vet Med 1999;41:733–47.

[39] Scott-Moncrieff JC, Azcona-Olivera J, Glickman NW, et al. Evaluation of antithyroglobulin antibodies after routine vaccination in pet and research dogs. J Am Vet Med Assoc 2002;221(4):515–21.

[40] Scott-Moncrieff JC, Glickman NW, Glickman LT, et al. Lack of association between repeated vaccination and thyroiditis in laboratory Beagles. J Vet Intern Med 2006;20(4):818–21.

[41] Thacker EL, Davis JM, Refsal KR, et al. Isolation of thyroid peroxidase and lack of autoantibodies to the enzyme in dogs with autoimmune thyroid disease. Am J Vet Res 1995;56: 34–8.

[42] Vajner L. Lymphocytic thyroiditis in beagle dogs in a breeding colony: findings of serum autoantibodies. Vet Med (Praha) 1997;42:333–8.

[43] Skopek E, Patzl M, Nachreiner RF. Detection of autoantibodies against thyroid peroxidase in serum samples of hypothyroid dogs. Am J Vet Res 2006;67(5):809–14.

[44] Henry M, Malthiery Y, Zanelli E, et al. Epitope mapping of human thyroglobulin. Heterogeneous recognition by thyroid pathologic sera. J Immunol 1990;145:3692–8.

[45] Lee JY, Uzuka Y, Tanabe S, et al. Tryptic peptides of canine thyroglobulin reactive with sera of patients with canine hypothyroidism caused by autoimmune thyroiditis. Vet Immunol Immunopathol 2004;101(3–4):271–6.

[46] Tani H, Shimizu R, Sasai K, et al. Recognition pattern of thyroglobulin autoantibody from hypothyroid dogs to tryptic peptides of canine thyroglobulin. J Vet Med Sci 2003; 65(10):1049–56.

[47] Beale K, Torres S. Thyroid pathology and serum antithyroglobulin antibodies in hypothyroid and healthy dogs. J Vet Intern Med 1991;5:128.

[48] Iversen L, Jensen AL, Hoier R, et al. Development and validation of an improved enzyme-linked immunosorbent assay for the detection of thyroglobulin autoantibodies in canine serum samples. Domest Anim Endocrinol 1998;15:525–36.

[49] Nachreiner RF, Refsal KR, Graham PA, et al. Prevalence of autoantibodies to thyroglobulin in dogs with nonthyroidal illness. Am J Vet Res 1998;59(8):951–5.

[50] Patzl M, Mostl E. Determination of autoantibodies to thyroglobulin, thyroxine and triiodothyronine in canine serum. J Vet Med A Physiol Pathol Clin Med 2003;50(2):72–8.

Etiopathologic Findings of Hyperthyroidism in Cats

Mark E. Peterson, DVM[a,b,*], Cynthia R. Ward, VMD, PhD[c]

[a]Department of Endocrinology, The Caspary Institute, New York, NY, USA
[b]Institute for Postgraduate Education, The Animal Medical Center, 510 East 62nd Street, New York, NY 10021, USA
[c]Department of Small Animal Medicine, University of Georgia College of Veterinary Medicine, 501 DW Brooks Drive, Athens, GA 300602, USA

H yperthyroidism (thyrotoxicosis) was first described in cats in 1979 and 1980 by investigators in New York City and Boston [1–3]. Over the past quarter century, it has emerged not only as the most common endocrine disorder of this species but as a disease frequently diagnosed in small animal practice throughout North America, Europe, Australia, New Zealand, and other parts of the world [4–7]. Although great strides have been made in the diagnosis and treatment of cats with hyperthyroidism, the underlying cause(s) of this disorder remains unknown. Because it is unlikely that improved diagnostic capabilities alone would account for such a dramatic increase in the prevalence of this disease, it is often suggested that hyperthyroidism may truly be a "new" disease of cats [8–10]. This theory is complicated by the increased awareness of the condition by practitioners and clients, a growing pet cat population, increased longevity of cats, or a combination of these factors.

THYROID PATHOLOGIC FINDINGS IN CATS WITH HYPERTHYROIDISM

Despite the fact that the underlying causes(s) of feline hyperthyroidism have not been clearly elucidated, the thyroid pathologic findings associated with hyperthyroidism have been well characterized. Functional thyroid adenomatous hyperplasia (or adenoma) involving one or both thyroid lobes is the most common pathologic abnormality associated with hyperthyroidism in cats [2,4,8,11]. Greater than 95% of cats have benign, adenomatous, or hyperplastic changes of the thyroid gland. In approximately 70% of hyperthyroid cats, both thyroid lobes are enlarged, whereas the remaining cats have involvement of only one lobe [3,8,12]. On histologic examination, such enlarged thyroid lobes contain one or more well-discernible foci of hyperplastic tissue, sometimes forming

*Corresponding author. Institute for Postgraduate Education, Animal Medical Center, 510 East 62nd Street, New York, NY 10021. E-mail address: mark.peterson@amcny.org (M.E. Peterson).

0195-5616/07/$ – see front matter
doi:10.1016/j.cvsm.2007.05.001

nodules ranging in diameter from less than 1 mm to 3 cm [2,4,11]. Thyroid carcinoma, the primary cause of hyperthyroidism in dogs, only rarely causes hyperthyroidism in cats, with a prevalence of less than 2% [13].

IS HYPERTHYROIDISM A NEW DISEASE OF CATS?

Until the late 1970s, few references pertaining to pathologic abnormalities of the feline thyroid gland had been reported. In a 1964 study by Lucke [14] and a 1976 study by Leav and coworkers [15], gross enlargement of the thyroid gland had been found at necropsy in cats and nodules were observed during histopathologic examinations; however, these abnormalities were relatively rare and were not associated with the clinical signs relating to hyperthyroidism. In the authors' review of approximately 7000 cats that had necropsies performed at The Animal Medical Center during the 14-year period from 1970 to 1984, an average of only 1.9 cats per year were found to have gross evidence of thyroid enlargement (caused by adenomatous hyperplasia, adenoma, or carcinoma) in the period before 1977, when the first cat with hyperthyroidism was diagnosed at that institution [16]. Since that time, the prevalence of thyroidal pathologic abnormalities and the associated clinical state of hyperthyroidism has been detected at an increasing frequency, with the incidence recently reported to be as high as 2% of all cats examined [17].

Based on these studies, it does seem that feline hyperthyroidism, if it did exist at all in cats before 1970, was extremely rare [14–16]. In addition, it is clear that the actual prevalence of this feline disorder has increased dramatically over the past 30 years, and some have even proposed that the increasing prevalence of feline hyperthyroidism is not solely the result of aging of the cat population [17].

CHARACTERISTICS OF THE ADENOMATOUS THYROID TISSUE IN HYPERTHYROID CATS

The time course of the functional and histopathologic progression of normal thymocytes to hyperfunctional adenomatous hyperplasia or adenoma is not known. It would likely take many months to years, however, inasmuch as hyperthyroidism is a disease that usually develops in elderly cats. This makes any prospective studies investigating the causative factors of hyperthyroidism in cats difficult. Over the past 30 years, a variety of potential etiologic factors have been proposed or studied but a single cause has yet to be identified.

Whatever pathogenesis of this disease is postulated, one must account for the following known facts concerning thyroid characteristics in these cats:

1. The pathologic changes in the thyroid glands of these cats are almost always benign, with adenomatous hyperplasia or adenoma reported in more than 98% of cats [4,11,16]. Less than 2% of cats have thyroid carcinoma, and it is possible that such malignant thyroid tumors could have a different pathogenesis than the typical benign lesions.
2. Once overt hyperthyroidism develops, the adenomatous hyperplastic thyroid tissue or nodules found in these cats function and secrete thyroid hormone in an autonomous fashion [8,11,18]. This autonomy of thyroid function, with

the resultant hypersecretion of thyroxine (T_4), suppresses thyrotropin (thyroid-stimulating hormone [TSH]) secretion. This can be demonstrated clinically by the lack of thyrotropin-releasing hormone (TRH) stimulation or triiodothyronine (T_3) suppression found in hyperthyroid cats, both of which are used as diagnostic tests for hyperthyroidism [19,20].

3. The feline thyroid gland normally contains a subpopulation of the follicular cells that have a high growth potential. In the thyroid gland eventually destined to develop adenomatous hyperplasia, this subpopulation of thyrocytes may replicate in an autonomous fashion. Once these rapidly dividing cells are present in sufficient numbers, they may continue to grow in the absence of extrathyroidal stimulation, such as TSH. Therefore, these thyroid adenomatous hyperplastic cells show autonomy of thyroid growth as well as the ability to function and secrete thyroid hormone in an autonomous fashion [8,11,18].

4. The individual thyroid adenomatous hyperplastic cells of cats with hyperthyroidism are heterogeneous with respect to function and growth potential. In primary cultures of thyroid adenomatous hyperplastic cells from cats and in cell lines from such tissues, we have learned to expect that heterogeneous responses are the rule rather than the exception [8,9].

5. A striking feature of this disease is that bilateral thyroid involvement is present in more than 70% of cats. This may be important in pathogenesis inasmuch as no physical connection exists between the two thyroid lobes in cats [3,12].

Based on these characteristics, investigators have proposed that immunologic factors (eg, immunoglobulins), nutritional factors (eg, iodine, goitrogens), environmental factors (eg, toxins, goitrogens), or genetic factors (eg, gene protein mutations) may interact to cause thyroid pathologic changes and, eventually, hyperthyroidism in the cat.

POSSIBLE FACTORS INVOLVED IN THE PATHOGENESIS OF HYPERTHYROIDISM IN CATS

Thyroid Autoimmunity and Circulating Stimulatory Factors

Initially, because of the prevalence of bilateral thyroid lobe involvement, early theories regarding the pathogenesis of feline hyperthyroidism revolved around it being similar to Graves' disease, the most common cause of hyperthyroidism in human patients. Graves' disease is an autoimmune disorder in which circulating antibodies (ie, thyroid-stimulating immunoglobulins [TSIs]) bind to the TSH receptor and mimic TSH, thereby promoting thyroid hormone production and secretion [21]. Because TSIs stimulate growth of all thyrocytes, diffuse hyperplasia of both thyroid lobes of the gland is a characteristic feature of Graves' disease [22].

In support of an autoimmune pathogenesis, early studies in hyperthyroid cats suggested that autoantibodies (ie, thyroid microsomal, antinuclear) were not uncommon and could be involved in the pathogenesis of the condition [23]. Of the 29 hyperthyroid cats studied, 34% had thyroid autoantibodies, as demonstrated by indirect immunofluorescence, and 14% were positive for antinuclear autoantibodies. These results could not be verified by the authors or by other investigators, however, greatly limiting the relevance of these findings in the etiology of feline hyperthyroidism.

Subsequent studies have also provided additional evidence against an autoimmune etiology for feline hyperthyroidism. To exclude high circulating levels of TSIs (specific autoantibody characteristic of Graves' disease) as the cause of feline hyperthyroidism, investigators measured the intracellular concentrations of cyclic adenosine monophosphate (cAMP) in functioning rat thyroid cells (the Fischer rat thyroid cell line [FTRL-5]) incubated with IgG extracted from the serum of hyperthyroid cats [24]. Because TSIs stimulate thyroid hormone secretion through activation of cAMP, their presence can be evidenced in vitro by generation of high cAMP concentrations in cultured thyroid cells. No significant difference was found in intracellular cAMP concentrations in FTRL-5 cells incubated with IgG from normal versus hyperthyroid cats [24]. In contrast, IgG from human patients with Graves' disease causes substantially more cAMP generation than normal human IgG or IgG from the cats of this study. Overall, these results indicate that feline hyperthyroidism does not result from high circulating concentration of TSIs and that, in this respect, it is not analogous to Graves' disease. Nevertheless, it should be noted that the study examined the effects of feline serum on a rat thyroid cell line, whereas potential cellular activators in the feline serum might only be active on feline cells.

Although circulating TSIs do not seem to play a role in feline hyperthyroidism, high titers of serum thyroid growth-stimulating immunoglobulins (TGIs) have been measured in cats with hyperthyroidism [25]. These autoantibodies, which act to promote thyroid growth but not to stimulate thyroid hormone secretion, also have been reported in human patients with toxic nodular goiter as well as in patients with Graves' disease, Hashimoto's thyroiditis, and euthyroid goiter [26]. Despite the presence of these autoantibodies, their clinical significance in human patients is unclear. Similarly, in cats, there is no correlation between thyroid function and TGI activity in vitro, and their role in the pathogenesis of hyperthyroidism is not known. It is highly unlikely, however, that TGIs or any other circulating autoantibody plays a role in the pathogenesis of the feline disease, given the overwhelming evidence that thyroid adenomatous tissue from hyperthyroid cats is autonomous in growth and function [8,11,18].

Further evidence against an autoimmune pathogenesis for feline hyperthyroidism was gained by transplanting thyroid tumor tissue collected from hyperthyroid cats at surgery into athymic nude mice [11]. After transplantation into the nude mice, the adenomatous thyroid tissue from hyperthyroid cats retains a histologic appearance identical to that of the donor tissue. This transplanted adenomatous tissue also continues to demonstrate hyperfunction (based on the ability to accumulate an increased fraction of radioiodine) and continues to grow (based on the demonstration of ^{3}H-thymidine incorporation into the adenomatous thyroid tissue). The ability of the thyroid adenomatous tissue to continue to grow and function when transplanted into nude mice confirms its autonomous nature [8,9,11].

These transplantation studies of feline hyperthyroid tissue into nude mice are similar to the results reported after transplantation of adenomatous thyroid tissue from human patients with toxic nodular goiter into nude mice [27]. After transplantation into the nude mice, the tissue from patients with toxic nodular goiter retains its histologic appearance and continues to function autonomously. In contrast, because circulating TSIs are responsible for the hyperthyroid state in human patients with Graves' disease, the associated hyperplastic thyroid changes normalize after transplantation into the nude mouse (an environment without abnormal circulating TSIs) [27]. These similarities between the feline disease and human toxic nodular goiter are not unexpected, inasmuch as the pathologic changes of adenomatous hyperplasia most closely resemble toxic nodular goiter in human beings, which is also caused by one or more hyperfunctioning adenomatous thyroid nodules [4,8,11].

Consistent with these transplantation studies, when adenomatous thyroid cells from hyperthyroid cats are cultured in TSH-free media, they also continue to grow and function autonomously [18]. These studies also strongly suggest that the intrinsic autonomy of thyroid follicular cells rather than extrathyroidal stimulating factors leads to the development of hyperplastic nodules and hyperthyroidism in the cat.

The most recent evidence against an autoimmune etiology was reported in a study in which the feline TSH receptor was cloned and transfected into an embryonic kidney cell line [28]. Purified serum IgG from human patients with Graves' disease activated the cAMP signal transduction system, as demonstrated by activation of cAMP-dependent luciferase activity in the cellular assay. To test the possibility that hyperthyroid cats develop antibodies to stimulate the autologous receptor, transfected cells were treated with sera or purified IgG obtained from the 16 hyperthyroid cats. There was no activation by the hyperthyroid cats' sera or IgG, again suggesting the absence of stimulatory autoantibodies.

Overall, these studies provide evidence against the presence of circulating thyroid stimulating factors as a mechanism underlying the pathogenesis of feline hyperthyroidism. In contrast, these studies support a model involving the intrinsic autonomy of thyroid follicular cell growth and function similar to that of human toxic nodular goiter [27].

Epidemiologic and Nutritional Risk Factors

Several epizootiologic studies have attempted to identify potential risk factors for feline hyperthyroidism, but a single dominant factor has not yet been isolated [7,17,29–31]. Genetic or hereditary factors, nutritional component(s) in cat food leading to metabolic thyroid dysfunction, or thyroid-disrupting compounds introduced into the environment or diet are the potential risk factors that have been most closely investigated.

Two genetically related breeds (Siamese and Himalayan) and purebred cats have been variably reported to be at decreased risk of developing hyperthyroidism [7,29,30]. This suggests a possible genetic or hereditary component, at least in some cat breeds. Although studies have reported no gender predilection for the disease, the two most recent studies have reported a male gender predilection [7,17].

Exposure to environmental chemicals (eg, pesticides, herbicides) is known to induce thyroid abnormalities in other species [32–34], and chemicals applied directly to a cat or to the cat's environment have been associated with increased risk of developing hyperthyroidism in some epidemiologic studies [7,29]. Regular exposure of cats to the topical flea control products was associated with an increased risk of developing hyperthyroidism in previous studies. None of these studies, however, was able to identify a specific commercial antiflea product or ingredient associated with the risk.

In one study, an association was found between the use of cat litter and the development of hyperthyroidism [30]. Moreover, because litter use is a marker for indoor cats [29], those findings complement the finding that hyperthyroidism in cats predominantly occurs in indoor cats rather than outdoor cats. Litter may contain chemicals (eg, goitrogenic compounds) that exert a biologic effect on the thyroid gland. No difference in risk was found among brands of litter [30], however, suggesting that any toxin or goitrogenic present in cat litter is common to most brands. In the absence of a clear explanation of the relation between litter use and hyperthyroidism, use of cat litter simply may be a marker for cats that live primarily indoors, receive better than average care, enjoy longer lives, and are more likely to reach the age at which cats develop hyperthyroidism.

All epidemiologic studies reported to date have identified that an increased risk of hyperthyroidism occurs with feeding an increased proportion of canned cat food in the diet [7,17,29–31]. One of these studies incriminated particular flavors of canned food (fish, liver, and giblets), and another incriminated cans with plastic linings in easy-open (pop-top) lids [17].

Because of this dietary association, several studies have attempted to implicate iodine in the cause or progression of the disease. The iodine content of cat food is extremely variable and often up to 10 times the recommended level [35,36]. The foods exceeding the recommended iodine level were products derived from the liver, kidney, beef byproducts, and marine fish. It has been postulated that wide swings in daily iodine intake may contribute to the development of thyroid disease in cats. Although circulating free T_4 concentrations are acutely affected by varying iodine intake, more prolonged ingestion of high- or low-iodine diets has no apparent effect [37,38]. Therefore, the role that iodine plays in the development of this disease remains unknown. Dietary iodide may have a modulatory effect on circulating thyroid hormone concentrations; however, neither iodine excess nor deficiency can explain the development of thyroid adenomatous hyperplasia or the autonomous nature of hyperthyroidism in cats. Finally, although perhaps not relevant to the causation of hyperthyroidism, one study showed that feeding a low-iodine diet to cats with preexisting hyperthyroidism failed to affect their high circulating thyroid hormone concentrations [16].

Like iodine, selenium plays an important role in the regulation of thyroid function in many species. Although the significance is unclear, circulating values seem to be high in cats, possibly through increased intake [6]. Like iodine, however, selenium status alone does not seem to affect the incidence of hyperthyroidism in cats.

In addition to iodine or selenium, there are many other goitrogenic materials that cats may be exposed to through their diet or the environment that could contribute to the development of thyroid adenomatous hyperplasia and hyperthyroidism [32–34]. Such agents generally cause goiter by acting directly on the thyroid gland to reduce thyroid hormone synthesis; the resultant low circulating T_4 concentrations lead to increased pituitary TSH secretion, which, in turn, leads to thyroidal enlargement. Other goitrogens, however, act indirectly to alter the regulatory mechanisms of the thyroid gland or the peripheral metabolism and excretion of thyroid hormones.

Most commercial cat foods contain relatively high levels of goitrogenic compounds (eg, phthalates), and cats can be exposed to many other goitrogens (eg, resorcinol, polyphenols, polychlorinated biphenyls, isoflavones) in the environment or through their diets. Many of these goitrogenic compounds may be of greater importance in the cat because they are metabolized by glucuronidation, a particularly slow metabolic pathway in the cat. For example, the polyphenolic compound bisphenol A (BPA), a plasticizer used as a food can liner, has been detected in 15 canned cats foods [39]. BPA is a possible thyroid receptor antagonist that might act at the pituitary level to increase TSH secretion [40]. Polyphenolic soy isoflavones, in particular, genistein and daidzein, have also been identified in almost 60% of the cat foods tested [41]. Virtually all dry and semimoist foods containing soy protein had high isoflavone content in concentrations adequate to interfere with thyroid function. Soy isoflavones inhibit 5′-deiodinase activity, the enzymes that convert total T_4 into the biologically active T_3 [42]. In a feeding study in clinically normal cats, cats receiving the soy diet had higher total T_4 and free T_4 concentrations, but total T_3 concentrations remained unchanged [43]. Detectable urinary concentrations of the isoflavone genistein were found in 10 of the 18 cats in the study, suggesting that cats may have clinically significant body burdens of this goitrogen [43].

Overall, these studies suggest that numerous nutritional and environmental factors might be involved in the pathogenesis of hyperthyroidism in cats. These goitrogens may have dose-, time-, and age-dependent cumulative effects on the feline pituitary-thyroid axis, resulting in chronic stimulation of TSH. This may lead to the pathologic abnormalities of nodular adenomatous hyperplasia of the thyroid gland and, eventually, the clinical state of hyperthyroidism.

Molecular Biology and Genetic Factors

In human patients with toxic multinodular goiter, recent investigation into the pathogenesis of this disease has centered around the signal transduction system of the thyroid cell. Normally, secretion of thyroid hormones is directly regulated by TSH, which is released by the pituitary gland. The interaction of TSH with its receptor on the surface of thyroid cells results in activation of receptor-coupled guanosine triphosphate–binding proteins (G proteins) that control cAMP concentrations in the thyroid cells [44]. The thyroid cell is unique, because cell proliferation and hormone production are controlled by TSH receptor–G protein–cAMP signaling. Because the division and functional activity of the thyroid cells are increased with disregard to normal cellular activation, abnormalities at any step of this signal transduction system could result in disease. Therefore, each component of this TSH receptor–G protein–cAMP pathway has been examined for abnormalities that could result in human toxic nodular goiter.

In normal thyroid cells, after the TSH receptor is activated by TSH, G proteins are activated that control the initiation of adenylyl cyclase activation and cAMP levels. G proteins couple to the TSH receptor and can be stimulatory (Gs), resulting in an increase in cAMP, or inhibitory (Gi), resulting in a decrease in cAMP. The relative amounts of Gs and Gi proteins determine the ultimate levels of cAMP in the cell. If the balance is altered in favor of Gs, by overexpression of Gs or underexpression of Gi, it results in overproduction of cAMP and overactivation of the thyroid cell. Investigations in cases of human toxic nodular goiter have demonstrated just such imbalances. Overexpression of Gs and underexpression of Gi have been demonstrated in some cases of human toxic nodular goiter [45–47]. These data suggest that abnormal G protein expression is responsible for some cases of human toxic nodular goiter.

Other studies looking at this same pathway of the TSH receptor–G protein–cAMP system in human toxic nodular goiter cells focused on mutations of the TSH receptor or G proteins that would result in autonomous or constitutive activation of these proteins. Mutations of the genes encoding for the α-subunit of Gs have been identified in human beings. The altered genes produce a mutated protein that cannot be turned off by normal cellular regulatory proteins [48,49]. Because Gs remains active, the relative activation of Gs and Gi proteins is tipped in favor of Gs. This causes increases of cAMP levels without regard to cellular negative feedback. The cellular result is the unregulated mitogenic and functional activation of the thyroid cell that is seen in human toxic nodular goiter.

Activating mutations of the TSH receptor have also been identified in human toxic nodular goiter [50–55]. These mutations produce a cellular response similar to that seen with Gs mutations. The TSH receptor is and remains activated without ligand (ie, TSH). This results in activation of Gs and resultant unregulated cAMP elevations. TSH receptor mutations seem to be more prevalent than Gs mutations in human toxic nodular goiter [52]. More than 25 different point mutations in the TSH receptor gene have been identified. They occur most often within exon 10 of the TSH receptor, which encodes for the transmembrane domain of the TSH receptor protein [56].

After the research into the pathogenesis of human toxic nodular goiter, similar approaches have been used to attempt to identify Gs and TSH receptor mutations as part of the pathogenesis of hyperthyroidism in cats. Pearce and colleagues [57] examined codons 480 to 640 of the feline TSH receptor gene, the area corresponding to exon 10, the area of the human TSH receptor having the most point mutations. Primers designed from homologous areas of the human, bovine, and canine TSH receptor were used to amplify DNA isolated from thyroids from 13 hyperthyroid and 2 normal cats by polymerase chain reaction (PCR). These products were compared with amplified genomic DNA from peripheral leukocytes using the same primers. These investigators were unable to identify any mutations in the TSH receptor gene in the hyperthyroid cats. This study was repeated for a larger part of the TSH receptor gene, codons 66 to 530, in 10 hyperthyroid cats and 1 euthyroid cat, with no TSH receptor mutation being identified [58]. Further mutational analysis of the α-subunit of the Gs gene from the same cats revealed a point mutation in one of two regions in 4 of 10 hyperthyroid cats [58].

Further experimentation examined PCR amplification products covering codons 386 to 698, also within exon 10 of the feline TSH receptor [59]. Instead of using DNA from the whole thyroid gland, these investigators isolated hyperplastic nodules from the normal paranodular tissue for DNA extraction as a means of concentrating any potential mutagen. They also increased the number of cats studied and isolated the hyperplastic nodules from the thyroids of 50 cats. Using these methods, they identified 10 different TSH receptor mutations in 28 of the 50 cats examined. In most feline thyroids in which more than one hyperplastic nodule was examined, there were multiple mutations. These data suggest that activating mutations of TSH receptor may be part of the pathogenesis of feline hyperthyroidism in some cats. There have been no studies to date that demonstrate any increased activity associated with the TSH receptor or Gs mutated proteins, however. Therefore, the importance of these mutations has yet to be established.

The authors' laboratory has also been interested in abnormalities of the TSH receptor–G protein–cAMP signal transduction cascade that may result in feline hyperthyroidism. The authors' group has focused on abnormalities in Gs and Gi protein expression that favor unregulated cAMP elevation. They obtained membrane-enriched preparations from eight hyperthyroid cats and four age-matched euthyroid cats and examined them for Gs and Gi protein expression. Although Gs expression was identical in the hyperthyroid cats as compared with the euthyroid cats, Gi expression was significantly decreased in the hyperthyroid cats [60]. Furthermore, the authors' group examined these tissues more specifically for Gi protein subtype expression and determined that Gi2 was specifically decreased in the hyperthyroid tissue, whereas Gi1 and Gi3 expression was not different than in tissues from euthyroid cats [61,62]. These results indicate that like human toxic nodular goiter, abnormalities of G protein expression regulating cellular cAMP levels play a role in the pathogenesis of feline hyperthyroidism.

Abnormal oncogene expression has also been theorized to have a potential role in the pathogenesis of feline hyperthyroidism. Proto-oncogenes are found in normal cells, and overexpression could eventually lead to autonomous function. One study using immunohistochemistry on formalin-fixed thyroid tissue from 18 hyperthyroid cats revealed overexpression of the c-Ras protein, which is coded for by the oncogene *c-ras* [63]. Products of the oncogenes of *bcl2* and the tumor suppressor gene *p53* did not reveal staining. The trigger for stimulating the increase in expression of the oncogene *c-ras* remains to be elucidated, and its significance remains unknown. Although c-Ras may be overexpressed, this could be a function of a mitogenically active cell population and not particular to feline hyperthyroidism.

SUMMARY

None of the studies to date have isolated a single dominant factor that could be incriminated in the development of hyperthyroidism in cats. Rather, most of the studies provide further evidence of the widely held view that hyperthyroidism is a multifactorial disease in this species. Autoimmune or circulating factors do not seem to have a causative role in the feline disease. Likewise, although nutritional factors may be important in the pathogenesis of hyperthyroidism in cats, dietary iodine content does not seem to play an important causative role. At this time, the most likely candidates include one or more of the goitrogenic chemicals that have been shown to be present in cat food or the cat's environment. In addition, mutations of the TSH receptor gene or mutations of its associated G proteins seem to play an important role in the pathogenesis of this disease.

References

[1] Peterson ME, Johnson JG, Andrews LK. Spontaneous hyperthyroidism in the cat. Scientific Proceedings of the American College of Veterinary Internal Medicine; 1979:108.

[2] Holzworth J, Theran P, Carpenter JL, et al. Hyperthyroidism in the cat: ten cases. J Am Vet Med Assoc 1980;176:345–53.

[3] Peterson ME, Kintzer PP, Cavanagh PG, et al. Feline hyperthyroidism: pretreatment clinical and laboratory evaluation of 131 cases. J Am Vet Med Assoc 1981;183:103–10.

[4] Hoenig M, Goldschmidt MH, Ferguson DC, et al. Toxic nodular goitre in the cat. J Small Anim Pract 1982;23:1–12.

[5] Thoday KL, Mooney CT. Historical, clinical and laboratory features of 126 hyperthyroid cats. Vet Rec 1992;19(131):257–64.

[6] Foster DJ, Thoday KL, Arthur JR, et al. Selenium status of cats in four regions of the world and comparison with reported incidence of hyperthyroidism in cats in those regions. Am J Vet Res 2001;62:934–7.

[7] Olczak J, Jones BR, Pfeiffer DU, et al. Multivariate analysis of risk factors for feline hyperthyroidism in New Zealand. N Z Vet J 2005;53:53–8.

[8] Gerber H, Peter H, Ferguson DC, et al. Etiopathology of feline toxic nodular goiter. Vet Clin North Am Small Anim Pract 1994;24:541–65.

[9] Ferguson DC. Pathogenesis of hyperthyroidism. In: August JR, editor. Consultations in feline internal medicine, vol. 2. Philadelphia: W.B. Saunders; 1994. p. 133–42.

[10] Mooney CT. Pathogenesis of hyperthyroidism. The Journal of Feline Medicine and Surgery 2002;4:167–9.

[11] Peter HJ, Gerber H, Studer H, et al. Autonomy of growth and of iodine metabolism in hyperthyroid feline goiters transplanted onto nude mice. J Clin Invest 1987;80:491–8.

[12] Birchard SJ, Peterson ME, Jacobson A. Surgical treatment of feline hyperthyroidism: results of 85 cases. J Am Anim Hosp Assoc 1984;20:705–9.

[13] Turrel JM, Feldman EC, Nelson RW, et al. Thyroid carcinoma causing hyperthyroidism in cats: 14 cases (1981–1986). J Am Vet Med Assoc 1988;193:359–64.

[14] Lucke VM. A histological study of thyroid abnormalities in the domestic cat. J Small Anim Pract 1964;5:351–8.

[15] Leav I, Schiller AL, Rijnberk A, et al. Adenomas and carcinomas of the canine and feline thyroid. Am J Pathol 1976;83:61–122.

[16] Peterson ME, Randolph JF, Mooney CT. Endocrine diseases. In: Sherding RG, editor. The cat: diseases and clinical management, vol. 2. 2nd edition. New York: Churchill Livingstone; 1994. p. 1403–506.

[17] Edinboro CH, Scott-Moncrieff JC, Janovitz E, et al. Epidemiologic study of relationships between consumption of commercial canned food and risk of hyperthyroidism in cats. J Am Vet Med Assoc 2004;224:879–86.

[18] Peter HJ, Gerber H, Studer H, et al. Autonomous growth and function of cultured thyroid follicles from cats with spontaneous hyperthyroidism. Thyroid 1991;1:331–8.

[19] Peterson ME, Graves TK, Gamble DA. Triiodothyronine (T$_3$) suppression test: an aid in the diagnosis of mild hyperthyroidism in cats. J Vet Intern Med 1990;4:233–8.

[20] Peterson ME, Broussard J, Gamble DA. Use of the thyrotropin releasing hormone stimulation test to diagnose mild hyperthyroidism in cats. J Vet Intern Med 1994;8:279–86.

[21] Saravanan P, Dayan CM. Thyroid autoantibodies. Endocrinol Metab Clin North Am 2001;30:315–37, viii.

[22] Belfiore A, Russo D, Vigneri R, et al. Graves' disease, thyroid nodules and thyroid cancer. Clin Endocrinol (Oxf) 2001;55:711–8.

[23] Kennedy RL, Thoday KL. Autoantibodies in feline hyperthyroidism. Res Vet Sci 1988;45:300–6.

[24] Peterson ME, Livingston P, Brown RS. Lack of circulating thyroid-stimulating immunoglobulins in cats with hyperthyroidism. Vet Immunol Immunopathol 1987;16:277–82.

[25] Brown RS, Keating P, Livingston PG, et al. Thyroid growth immunoglobulins in feline hyperthyroidism. Thyroid 1992;2:125–30.

[26] Brown RS. Immunoglobulins affecting thyroid growth: a continuing controversy. J Clin Endocrinol Metab 1995;80:1506–8.

[27] Peter HJ, Gerber H, Studer H. Pathogenesis of heterogeneity in human multinodular goiter: a study on growth and function of thyroid tissue transplanted onto nude mice. J Clin Invest 1985;76:1992–2002.

[28] Nguyen LQ, Arseven OK, Gerber H, et al. Cloning of the cat TSH receptor and evidence against an autoimmune etiology of feline hyperthyroidism. Endocrinology 2002;143:395–402.

[29] Scarlett JM, Moise NS, Ravl J. Feline hyperthyroidism: goitrogens descriptive and case-control study. Prev Vet Med 1988;6:295–309.

[30] Kass PH, Peterson ME, Levy J, et al. Evaluation of environmental, nutritional, and host factors in cats with hyperthyroidism. J Vet Inten Med 1999;13:323–9.

[31] Martin KM, Rossing MA, Ryland LM, et al. Evaluation of dietary and environmental risk factors for feline hyperthyroidism. J Am Vet Med Assoc 2000;217:853–6.

[32] Gaitan E. Goitrogens in food and water. Annu Rev Nutr 1990;10:21–39.

[33] Brucker-Davis F. Effects of environmental synthetic chemicals on thyroid function. Thyroid 1998;8:827–56.

[34] Boas M, Feldt-Rasmussen U, Skakkebaek NE, et al. Environmental chemicals and thyroid function. Eur J Endocrinol 2006;154:599–611.

[35] Mumma RO, Rashid KA, Shane BS, et al. Toxic and protective constituents in pet foods. Am J Vet Res 1986;47:1633–7.

[36] Johnson LA, Ford HC, Tarttelin MF, et al. Iodine content of commercially-prepared cat foods. N Z Vet J 1992;40:18–20.

[37] Tarttelin MF, Johnson LA, Cooke RR. Serum free thyroxine levels respond inversely to changes in levels of dietary iodine in the domestic cat. N Z Vet J 1992;40:66–8.

[38] Kyle AH, Tarttelin MF, Cooke RR, et al. Serum free thyroxine levels in cats maintained on diets relatively high or low in iodine. N Z Vet J 1994;42:101–3.

[39] Moriyama K, Tagami T, Akamizu T, et al. Thyroid hormone action is disrupted by bisphenol A as an antagonist. J Clin Endocrinol Metab 2002;87:5185–90.

[40] Kang JH, Kondo F. Determination of bisphenol A in canned pet foods. Res Vet Sci 2002;73:177–82.

[41] Court MH, Freeman LM. Identification and concentration of soy isoflavones in commercial cat foods. Am J of Vet Res 2002;63:181–5.

[42] Doerge DR, Sheehan DM. Goitrogenic and estrogenic activity of soy isoflavones. Environ Health Perspect 2002;110(Suppl 3):349–53.

[43] White HL, Freeman LM, Mahony O, et al. Effect of dietary soy on serum thyroid hormone concentrations in healthy adult cats. Am J Vet Res 2004;65(5):586–91.

[44] Kohn LD, Shimura H, Shimura Y, et al. The thyrotropin receptor. Vitam Horm 1995;50:287–384.

[45] Derwahl M, Hamacher C, Papageorgiou G. Alterations of the stimulatory G protein (Gs)-adenylate cyclase cascade in thyroid carcinomas: evidence for up regulation of inhibitory G protein. Thyroid 1995;5(Suppl 1):S-3.

[46] Delemer B, Dib K, Patey M, et al. Modification of the amounts of G proteins and of the activity of adenylyl cyclase in human benign thyroid tumours. J Endocrinol 1992;132:477–85.

[47] Selzer E, Wilfing A, Schiferer A, et al. Stimulation of human thyroid growth via the inhibitory guanine nucleotide binding (G) protein Gi: constitutive expression of the G protein alpha subunit Gi alpha-1 in autonomous adenoma. Proc Natl Acad Sci U S A 1993;90:1609–13.

[48] Horie H, Yokogoshi Y, Tsuyuguchi M, et al. Point mutations of ras and Gs alpha subunit genes in thyroid tumors. Jpn J Cancer Res 1995;86:737–42.

[49] Matsuo K, Friedman E, Gejman PV, et al. The thyrotropin receptor (TSH-R) is not an onco-gene for thyroid tumors: structural studies of the TSH-R and the alpha-subunit of Gs in human thyroid neoplasms. J Clin Endocrinol Metab 1993;76:1446–51.

[50] Parma J, Duprev L, Van Sande J, et al. Somatic mutations in the thyrotropin receptor gene cause hyperfunctioning thyroid adenomas. Nature 1993;365:649–51.

[51] Parma J, Duprez L, Van Sande J, et al. Diversity and prevalence of somatic mutations in the thyrotropin receptor and Gs alpha genes as a cause of toxic thyroid adenomas. J Clin Endocrinol Metab 1997;82:2695–701.

[52] Parma J, Van Sande J, Swillens S, et al. Somatic mutations causing constitutive activity of the thyrotropin receptor are the major cause of hyperfunctioning thyroid adenomas: identification of additional mutations activating both the cyclic adenosine 3′,5′-mono-phosphate and inositol phosphate-Ca2+ cascades. Mol Endocrinol 1995;9:725–33.

[53] Fuhrer D, Holzapfel HP, Wonerow P, et al. Somatic mutations in the thyrotropin receptor gene and not in the Gs alpha protein gene in 31 toxic thyroid nodules. J Clin Endocrinol Metab 1997;82:3885–91.

[54] Holzapfel HP, Fuhrer D, Wonerow P, et al. Identification of constitutively activating somatic thyrotropin receptor mutations in a subset of toxic multinodular goiters. J Clin Endocrinol Metab 1997;82:4229–33.

[55] Russo D, Arturi F, Suarez HG, et al. Thyrotropin receptor gene alterations in thyroid hyper-functioning adenomas. J Clin Endocrinol Metab 1996;81:1548–51.

[56] Kopp P. The TSH receptor and its role in thyroid disease. Cell Mol Life Sci 2001;58:1301–22.

[57] Pearce SHS, Foster DJ, Imrie H, et al. Mutational analysis of the thyrotropin receptor gene in sporadic and familial feline thyrotoxicosis. Thyroid 1997;7:923–7.

[58] Peeters ME, Timmermans-Sprang EP, Mol JA. Feline thyroid adenomas are in part associated with mutations in the G (s alpha) gene and not with polymorphisms found in the thyrotropin receptor. Thyroid 2002;12:571–5.

[59] Watson SG, Radford AD, Kipar A, et al. Somatic mutations of the thyroid-stimulating hor-mone receptor gene in feline hyperthyroidism: parallels with human hyperthyroidism. J Endocrinol 2005;186:523–37.

[60] Hammer KB, Holt DE, Ward CR. Altered expression of G proteins in thyroid gland adeno-mas obtained from hyperthyroid cats. Am J Vet Res 2000;61:874–9.

[61] Ward CR, Achenbach SE, Peterson ME. The inhibitory G protein Gi2 shows decreased expression in adenomatous thyroid tissue from hyperthyroid cats. J Vet Intern Med 2001;15:298.

[62] Ward CR, Achenbach SE, Peterson ME, et al. Expression of inhibitory G proteins in adenomatous thyroid glands obtained from hyperthyroid cats. Am J Vet Res 2005;66:1478–82.

[63] Merryman JI, Buckles EL, Bowers G, et al. Overexpression of c-Ras in hyperplasia and adenomas of the feline thyroid gland: an immunohistochemical analysis of 34 cases. Vet Pathol 1999;36:117–24.

Testing for Hypothyroidism in Dogs

Duncan C. Ferguson, VMD, PhD

Department of Veterinary Biosciences, College of Veterinary Medicine, The University of Illinois at Urbana-Champaign, 2001 South Lincoln Avenue, Urbana, IL 61802, USA

Hypothyroidism is the most common endocrinopathy in the dog. The author has had the opportunity to review this subject for *Veterinary Clinics of North America Small Animal Practice* previously in 1984 and 1994 [1,2]. The principles of thyroid physiology outlined in those articles have obviously not changed. The status of diagnostic tests in 1994 led this author to propose a still appropriate but highly complicated diagnostic flow chart for diagnosis. The point then was to compare the state of diagnostic tests with the situation in human medicine, in which a single blood test was and is used today to measure an index of free thyroxine (FT_4) and to measure thyrotropin (TSH). Technology applied to diagnostic testing since then has resulted in enhancement of the diagnostic capabilities for the dog. By way of example, in 1984, the most definitive diagnostic test suggested was the TSH stimulation test. In 1994, the direct dialysis measurement of FT_4 (FT_4D) had just been introduced by the Nichols Institute (currently Antech Diagnostics, Lake Success, New York) and was providing promising results, and this promise has been borne out by many subsequent studies. The loss of pharmaceutic bovine TSH came after concerns with bovine spongiform encephalopathy (BSE) and the development of recombinant human TSH (rhTSH). Today, we have 10 years of experience with largely one commercial endogenous canine TSH assay, but this assay has diagnostic limitations. Since then, canine TSH has been cloned, sequenced, and expressed, opening up the possibility of further improvement of immunodiagnostic reagents and the possibility of a defined standard. The inherited autoimmune etiology of primary hypothyroidism in the dog has been highlighted with development of the antithyroglobulin autoantibody (TgAA) ELISA; however, this assay has opened up questions over the diagnostic and therapeutic dilemma associated with preclinical and subclinical disease. With the enhanced set of diagnostic tests, we have seen conscientious dog breeders seeking to identify early disease with a single serum sample. The recent cloning of the canine genome should put the profession on the verge of genetic tests; however, much work remains to identify genetic changes that might lead to clinical disease.

E-mail address: dcf@uiuc.edu

0195-5616/07/$ – see front matter
doi:10.1016/j.cvsm.2007.05.015

Rather than being a comprehensive review of all possible thyroid function tests, the focus in this article is on the logical progression of test choice, highlighting total thyroxine (TT_4), FT_4, triiodothyronine (T_3), TSH, and antithyroid antibodies. The re-emerging role of the use of rhTSH for TSH stimulation tests is also discussed. A review of the perspective of an endocrine diagnostic laboratory was presented in an issue of this publication in 2004 [3].

UNDERSTANDING THE BASIS OF THYROID FUNCTION TESTING

Comparative Aspects of the Hypothalamic-Pituitary-Thyroid-Extrathyroid Axis

Physicians have measured serum TSH concentrations diagnostically for more than 30 years, and these values have been used in canine thyroid diagnostics for approximately 10 years. The negative feedback effect of thyroid hormones (in the free or unbound form) is the primary mechanism regulating TSH secretion, although tonic stimulation of thyrotropin-releasing hormone (TRH) has a permissive role in TSH secretion. The pituitary thyrotrope cell completely deiodinates thyroxine (T_4; derived from the plasma) to T_3, which then inhibits TSH. There is now also some direct evidence that thyroid hormones may have a direct negative feedback effect on the hypothalamus to inhibit the release of TRH [4,5].

Comparative Aspects of Serum Thyroid Hormone Binding

Most evidence suggests that the free hormone fraction predicts the amount of hormone that is available to tissues at equilibrium. Plasma proteins buffer hormone delivery into tissue and provide a hormone reservoir. The overall affinity of the thyroid hormone–binding proteins for T_4 is lower in dogs than in human beings. Partly as a result of this weaker protein binding, TT_4 concentrations are lower (and the unbound or free fraction of circulating T_4 is higher [~0.1% versus ~0.03%]) [1]. This binding relation may change in response to drugs or illness. In significant part, this is because the dog has approximately 15% of the concentration of circulating thyroxine-binding globulin (TBG) seen in human beings. Circulating T_4 and T_3 bind to other plasma proteins as well, most notably transthyretin (thyroid hormone–binding prealbumin) [6].

Extrathyroidal Metabolism of Thyroid Hormone in Dogs Versus Human Beings

In dogs, approximately 40% to 60% of T_3 is derived from extrathyroidal enzymatic 5'-deiodination of T_4. In people, approximately 80% of T_3 is derived extrathyroidally [7–9]. Therefore, although it also has intrinsic metabolic activity, T_4 has been called a prohormone, with activation by deiodination to T_3 being a step regulated individually by peripheral tissues. Although its circulating levels largely depend on tissue T_4 uptake and deiodination, the isolated measurement of serum free triiodothyronine (FT_3) or total triiodothyronine (TT_3) concentrations is a less meaningful estimate of thyroid function than is the measurement of serum FT_4 or TT_4 concentration.

ETIOPATHOGENESIS OF CANINE HYPOTHYROIDISM
Autoimmune Thyroiditis Dominates

Despite the addition of the TSH assay to the diagnostic tools, the picture remains one of primary thyroid failure in approximately 95% of cases. Hypothyroidism may also result rarely from an impaired ability of the pituitary gland to synthesize and secrete TSH, resulting in secondary thyroid follicular atrophy. Secondary hypothyroidism can be caused by pituitary tumors, a congenital pituitary malformation, isolated TSH deficiency, or pituitary trauma or surgery, and it accounts for less than 5% of clinical cases of hypothyroidism. Other rare forms of canine hypothyroidism include iatrogenic conditions, neoplastic destruction of thyroid tissue, and congenital (or juvenile-onset) hypothyroidism (cretinism) [10–12].

For many years, it was stated that approximately 50% of all canine cases with hypothyroidism were caused by autoimmune thyroiditis and the other 50% were caused by idiopathic atrophy. The picture has now emerged of idiopathic atrophy (peak age for diminished T_4 and negative thyroglobulin autoantibodies (TgAA) titers is 8 years old) being a late stage of earlier autoimmune damage (peak age of 4 years). A Michigan State University Animal Health Diagnostic Laboratory study of more than 16,000 thyroid profiles and 1093 hypothyroid dogs revealed an incidence of the following autoantibodies in hypothyroid patients. TgAA was positive in 50% to 60% of the cases, supporting the idea that this percentage of patients is experiencing thyroid autoimmunity. Of animals with only the abnormality of TgAA positivity, approximately 20% progress within a year to additional clinical or laboratory abnormalities consistent with hypothyroidism. In fact, animals with a positive TgAA status but no other laboratory abnormalities, if followed sequentially with repeat TSH measurements, show a highly statistically significant increase in serum TSH concentration, even if the values remain within the normal range. More discussion on the value of TSH and TgAA as diagnostic tests is found elsewhere in this article. Hypothyroidism is also most highly associated with breeds with the highest incidence of thyroiditis and TgAA positivity. Breeds with the highest prevalence of hypothyroidism are the English Setter, Dalmatian, Basenji, Rhodesian Ridgeback, Old English Sheepdog, Boxer, Maltese Dog, Chesapeake Bay Retriever, Beagle, Cocker Spaniel, Shetland Sheepdog, Siberian Husky, Border Collie, Husky, Akita, and Golden Retriever [13–16].

Although the autoimmune nature of primary hypothyroidism lends itself to studies of early disease, and even genetic testing, it has also led to speculation regarding the triggers of autoimmunity. For example, hypotheses without a peer-reviewed evidentiary basis have been forwarded, suggesting that vaccination against infectious diseases resulted in an increase in autoimmune thyroiditis. Although one study demonstrated an apparent increase in TgAA titers, there was concern that the effect was a nonspecific increase in immunoglobulins, which increase the assay blank [17]. As a result of this observation, the commercial assay (Oxford Laboratories, Oxford, Michigan) has been modified since then to include the option for a nonspecific blank. It seems to this author that all ELISA assays should be properly blanked for nonspecific matrix effects. At the least, a positive result should be repeated with appropriate blank subtraction. A follow-up prospective study in healthy laboratory Beagles re-evaluated vaccination with the multivalent vaccine, rabies vaccine, or both com-pared with unvaccinated controls. Serum was collected for thyroid function tests, including TgAA; the dogs were euthanized at 5.5 years of age, and a thy-roid histopathologic examination was performed. Although no association was seen between vaccination and thyroiditis at postmortem examination, there was an overall rate of thyroiditis of 40% and abnormal thyroid function test results were observed in 25% of these dogs [18]. Essentially, these studies confirmed the known high genetic background for thyroiditis in Beagles and suggested that a larger group of animals might be necessary to prove the lack of significant difference. The hypothesis of a cause-effect relation between vaccination or vac-cination frequency is supported by no published evidence at this time, however.

CLINICAL FINDINGS LEADING TO A SUSPICION OF HYPOTHYROIDISM

The purpose of this review is not to reiterate the multiple and variable clinical signs of hypothyroidism. The clinical presentation of hypothyroidism has been reviewed previously elsewhere [11,19]. In 2002, the Society for Comparative Endocrinology (SCE) was asked by American College of Veterinary Internal Medicine (ACVIM) to draft a consensus statement on recommendations for tests for the diagnosis of hypothyroidism in the dog. The recommendations were presented at the 2002 ACVIM meeting and in greater detail at the 2003 meeting [20]. It is useful to note that there was agreement that thyroid function test results should not be interpreted in a clinical vacuum; that is, the diagnostic performance and predictive value of thyroid function tests are greatly enhanced when they are used to confirm a clinician's suspicion of dis-ease based on suggestive history and clinical signs as well as on the results of general medical diagnostic tests. Other conditions or confounding therapies should be ruled out first or resolved. The choice and timing of tests result from full consideration of the potential complicating factors, such as drug ther-apy or nonthyroidal illness (NTI). These confounding factors are discussed elsewhere in this article. Symptoms of classic cases of adult-onset hypothyroid-ism include lethargy and weakness and dullness of mental attitude. Dermato-logic findings may include nonpruritic bilateral symmetric alopecia or recurrent skin infections after a reasonable course of antimicrobial therapy. Hypothyroidism may not present in a "classic" appearance, however, manifest-ing only generalized neuropathy or myopathy [21,22]. Irrespective of the organ system(s) apparently involved on clinical presentation, hypothyroidism should be recognized to be a multisystemic disorder, and all cases merit a general med-ical workup, including but not limited to a complete blood cell count, biochem-ical screen, and urinalysis. Of clinicopathologic evaluations, the most consistent observation is a mild nonregenerative anemia and an elevated serum cholesterol level [19,23].

SPECIFIC THYROID FUNCTION TESTS

First, the reader should realize that the application of thyroid diagnostic tests does not always lead to a definitive diagnosis. Early stages of thyroid dysfunction may often be associated with discordant or confusing results. Furthermore, although not widely available, the ideal is to interpret laboratory tests against breed-specific normal ranges, particularly in the sighthounds, in which TT_4 and FT_4 can be much lower than in other breeds but TT_3 concentrations are similar to those of other breeds.

Serum Total Thyroxine Concentrations

The sole determination of serum TT_4 concentration by radioimmunoassay (RIA) is only diagnostic if the value is normal or elevated. This is significant, however, because hypothyroidism may be essentially ruled out by the observation of a normal value. It is true that dogs with hypothyroidism can, in most cases, be distinguished from normal dogs on the basis of a low resting serum T_4 concentration. The use of in-hospital test kits for measurement of TT_4 should be applied with caution and care with respect to quality control [24]. Nonthyroidal conditions on the list of differential diagnoses, certain drugs, and even the time of day may also lower baseline serum T_4 and T_3 concentrations, however [20,25–28].

Effect of Nonthyroidal Illness on Total Thyroxine

Of additional concern, many NTIs and certain drugs may lower baseline serum T_4 or T_3 concentrations in the dog, reducing the diagnostic specificity of a low value. The lowering of TT_4 may not be accompanied by a low FT_4 concentration; however, in some cases, FT_4 concentrations may also be depressed. The effects of NTI on thyroid hormone metabolism (ie, the euthyroid sick syndrome) are less well characterized in dogs than in human beings. A lowering of serum TT_3 concentration alone (the low T3 syndrome) is less likely to be observed than is the lowering of TT_4 and TT3 concentrations (the low T_4 state of medical illness). In people, these changes have been labeled as protective phenomena associated with the body's response to illness and nutritional state. Reductions in serum TT_4 concentration in severe medical illness in human beings, dogs, and cats correlate with higher mortality. Therefore, serum T_4 concentrations may prove to have important prognostic value in serious illness [30].

Is the Low Thyroxine State of Medical Illness to be Treated with Thyroid Hormone Therapy?

In most species, reductions in thyroid hormone concentrations in NTI seem to serve to protect against the catabolism of illness. It is thus probably inappropriate to intervene to "correct" these low thyroid values through thyroid hormone therapy. In fact, inappropriate thyroid hormone therapy may actually induce a state of relative hyperthyroidism in some tissues.

Principle 1 is as follows: approximately 10% of hypothyroid dogs are missed if you rely on TT_4 alone for screening. A normal TT_4 measurement can be observed in only 10% of hypothyroid patients. Most of these would seem to be attributable to the presence of anti-T_4 autoantibodies (T_4AA), however (see section on antithyroid antibodies).

Serum Total Triiodothyronine Concentrations

T_3 is the most potent thyroid hormone at the cellular level; however, in the dog, a large proportion (40%–50%) is not made in the thyroid gland and is not the predominant circulating thyroid hormone. As can be seen in Table 1 [29,30], the sensitivity and accuracy of a serum TT_3 measurement for the diagnosis of hypothyroidism are low. Likewise, immunoassays claiming to measure FT_3 provide little diagnostic value. The reader is referred to the section on nondialysis assays for FT_4 to understand the argument against using similar assays to measure FT_3. In sighthounds (eg, Greyhounds, Afghans Hounds, Salukis, Whippets), the normal range for serum T_3 concentrations, although not generally provided on a breed-specific basis by most laboratories, is generally similar to T_3 concentrations in other breeds [31].

Principle 2 is as follows: TT_3 measurements are generally poor screening tests for hypothyroidism. In sighthounds, however, because TT_4 and FT_4D are lower than in other breeds but TT_3 is not, there may be confirmatory value in documenting a low TT_3 level.

Diagnostic criteria are as follows:

- Sensitivity is the fraction of cases actually positive that are labeled as positive by the test.
- Specificity is the fraction of euthyroid dogs that have values in the reference range.
- Accuracy is the fraction of cases that are neither falsely positive nor falsely negative.

Free Thyroxine Concentrations

Measuring FT_4 (unbound) provides an in vitro assessment of the concentration of hormone available to tissues, and FT_4 has been shown to correlate highly with the clinical state of the animal. Accurate measurement, although

Table 1
Thyroid diagnostic test comparisons in the dog

Test	Low TT_4	Low TT_3	Low FT_4D	High TSH	Low TT_4/high TSH	Low FT_4D/high TSH
Sensitivity	0.89/1[a]	0.10	0.98/0.80	0.76/0.87	0.67/0.87[a]	0.74/0.80[a]
Specificity	0.82/0.75	0.92	0.93/0.94	0.93/0.82	0.98/0.92[a]	0.98/0.97[a]
Accuracy	0.85	0.55	0.95	0.84	0.82	0.86

[a] Positive anti-T_4AA cases removed [39].
Data from Kantrowitz LB, Peterson ME, Melian C, et al. Serum total thyroxine, total triiodothyronine, free thyroxine, and thyrotropin concentrations in dogs with nonthyroidal disease. J Am Vet Med Assoc 2001;219:765–9; and Dixon RM, Mooney CT. Evaluation of serum free thyroxine and thyrotropin concentrations in the diagnosis of canine hypothyroidism. J Small Anim Pract 1999;40:72–8.

technically more difficult, is key to distinguishing conditions with disturbances of serum thyroid hormone binding caused by illness or drugs. The types of assays being performed by veterinary diagnostic laboratories are briefly reviewed. A more extended discussion of the technical aspects of the procedures and the clinical value of accurate measurement of FT_4 is provided in a previous review by the author [32].

Direct Dialysis

Equilibrium dialysis is the "gold standard" procedure for the measurement of FT_4. For domestic animal sera, with less TBG, the lower affinity-binding proteins contribute proportionally more to binding thyroid hormone in serum, and the higher FT_4 fraction and lower TT_4 concentration are a result [32]. At the present time, direct dialysis systems, including one commercially available assay from Antech Diagnostics (previously owned by Nichols Institute), seem to measure FT_4 concentrations accurately. These assays are not as rapid and are more expensive to purchase and run than the analog immunoassays for FT_4. Across a wide variety of medical conditions, including the presence of drugs and the presence of T_4AA, the FT_4D assay showed a diagnostic accuracy of 95%, with a specificity of 93%, representing the highest values associated with any single thyroid function test (see Table 1) [29,30]. Most studies indicate that only the dialysis methods for FT_4 measurement provide the additional information needed to distinguish animals with low TT_4 concentrations attributable to nonthyroidal conditions from those with hypothyroidism.

Nondialysis Immunoassays for Measurement of Free Thyroid Hormones

Commercial FT_4 assays designed to measure the FT_4 concentration directly by RIA have also been used by veterinary diagnostic laboratories. Unfortunately, these assays contain reagents optimized for human serum. Although more rapid and practical than equilibrium dialysis, these assays depend on the dominance of hormone binding by TBG as observed in human serum [6] and are not accurate in animals. Kits that use an analog method have been seriously questioned, because the labeled analogue of T_4 binds to serum albumin and results are subject to variation with serum albumin and nonesterified free fatty acid concentrations. A study compared the results of FT_4 analog RIAs with those of standard (tracer) equilibrium dialysis (SED) and modified equilibrium dialysis (MED; also called direct dialysis). Thirty health dogs, 10 dogs with hypothyroidism, and 31 dogs with NTI were studied. With analog RIAs, the values were consistently lower than with the dialysis procedures, a result that would overestimate hypothyroidism. Of greatest concern for misdiagnosis, the RIAs produced the highest number of low FT_4 results in dogs with NTI [33].

Furthering the concern about FT_4 immunoassays, a recent study compared the Coat-a-Count's (Diagnostic Products Corporation, Los Angeles, California) analogue-based FT_4 immunoassay with its TT_4 immunoassay kit. Each assay was applied to the fractions of serum T_4 obtained by ultrafiltration and equilibrium dialysis. Both were applied to serum-based solutions in which FT_4, T_4-binding proteins, protein-bound T_4, and TT_4 were systematically varied. The analogue-based FT_4 assay did not detect dialyzable or ultrafilterable serum T_4. Both assays measured the T_4 retained with serum proteins. The analogue-based FT_4 assay, like TT_4 results, was unresponsive to a 500-fold variation in dialyzable T_4 concentrations [34]. An excellent review of the problems with measuring FT_4 using nondialysis assays was written by Nelson and coworkers [35].

Principle 3 is as follows: FT_4D is the single test with the highest combination of sensitivity, specificity, and accuracy, and it correlates best with the clinical thyroid status of the animal.

SERUM THYROTROPIN CONCENTRATIONS

The development of a commercial canine species-specific immunoassay for TSH (Diagnostic Products Corporation) in 1997 opened up the possibility of improving understanding of the canine pituitary-thyroid axis. A goal for the canine TSH assay would be its use as a screening test for hypothyroidism as it is used in human medicine. A test approaching 100% sensitivity would be required, however. Several studies have raised questions about the diagnostic sensitivity of the assay, because approximately one fourth of hypothyroid dogs had normal TSH values [29,30,36,37]. More recent studies have shown TSH concentrations in the normal range in dogs with abnormal TSH stimulation test results or thyroid biopsies [38]. Using a different assay now offered by Alpco Diagnostics (Windham, New Hampshire), Ramsey and coworkers [36] showed that three of nine confirmed hypothyroid cases had normal serum TSH concentrations. Most studies have been conducted with the Diagnostic Products Corporation (DPC) chemiluminescence or immunoradiometric assay. The following discussion reviews the diagnostic performance of the TSH assay and the possible reasons associated with its reduced diagnostic sensitivity and suggests strategies for improving the assay.

Available Commercial Canine Thyrotropin Assays

There are three formats of the DPC assay: immunoradiometric, chemiluminescent, and ELISA. The reagents are identical except for the manner in which the detection antibody in the "sandwich" antibody is labeled. The chemiluminescent format (Immulite Canine TSH) showed the best precision and certainly has the potential for the greatest sensitivity [39]. The assays correlated less well when values were less than 0.1 ng/mL, with better correlation when values were in the range seen in hypothyroidism (>0.5 ng/mL). Another ELISA assay is also available from Alpco Diagnostics [36]. Both assay formats claim diagnostic sensitivity of 0.01 ng/mL, but most independent investigators consistently report sensitivity to 0.03 ng/mL. At times, the Michigan State Endocrinology Diagnostic Laboratory has offered a canine TSH assay developed in-house, and results from this assay are recognizable by its use of standards in bioassay units of mU/L (μU/mL). Currently, this diagnostic laboratory is using this assay for dog and cat samples but has not reported comparisons between that assay and the DPC assay. The normal range for TSH listed by this laboratory for the dog is less than 37 mU/L, which would translate to less than 3.3 ng/mL using the accepted conversions for the TSH bioactivity of highly purified standards (vide infra). This suggests that the standard used for this assay is of much lower specific activity than that for the DPC assay or the recombinant canine TSH produced in the author's laboratory. As a single-antibody assay using a polyclonal antibody, this assay may also have reduced sensitivity compared with the sandwich assays. Indeed, the first-generation human TSH assays were less sensitive than second- and third-generation assays.

Most clinical studies have been performed with the DPC assay in some format. Today, most laboratories are using the Immulite format of the DPC assay because of its precision and sensitivity relative to the immunoradiometric assay and because the reagent shelf life is longer. The functional sensitivity of human TSH immunoassays is defined by whether the limit of functional sensitivity is based on the National Hormone and Peptide Program (NHPP) cadaver-source pituitary standard. Canine TSH standards are highly immunoaffinity purified and are provided according to weight (ng/mL) by the manufacturer. Highly purified or recombinant TSH has bioactivity of approximately 0.09 ng/μU. The Immulite DPC immunoassay has been described as having, in its most chemiluminescent-sensitive format, a detection limit of somewhere between 0.01 and 0.03 ng/mL, approximately the sensitivity of a second-generation assay. Many laboratories using the immunoradiometric assay (IRMA) form of the assay do not report a lower limit of sensitivity of the assay. The clinical conclusion is that one cannot reliably distinguish a normal TSH value from a low one unless possibly comparing paired samples from the same animal.

Recombinant Canine Thyrotropin as an Assay Standard

In the literature provided with the DPC and Alpco Diagnostics assays, it is stated that the cross-reactivity to other pituitary glycoproteins is negligible. No data are provided, however, other than to mention that peptides like luteinizing hormone (LH), follicle-stimulating hormone (FSH), and human chorionic gonadotropin (hCG) were examined. It is not clear why a human glycoprotein's cross-reactivity would be clinically relevant to the canine assay. Using a highly purified canine LH standard from the NHPP, the author's laboratory has determined that TSH immunoreactivity can be detected in canine LH. Aside from cross-reactivity, it is possible that there is significant contamination of the LH preparation with TSH, which has a similar molecular weight and shares an identical α-subunit structure. As an example, early preparations of TSH developed by the NHPP in the late 1970s were stated to be only 1% pure. Independent studies simultaneously measuring LH and TSH in the same dog suggest that the cross-reactivity maximally could be approximately 4% [40]. Regardless of the actual cross-contamination, this uncertainty highlights the potential value of using highly purified recombinant TSH devoid of other pituitary glycoproteins.

In the author's laboratory, researchers have developed a recombinant standard for canine TSH, with quantification in a protein assay using pure bovine

TSH as a standard and correcting for purity using silver-stained polyacrylamide gel electrophoresis. Recombinant canine TSH was detected with approximately 73% efficiency by the DPC assay. It suggests that the DPC TSH standard is of high purity [41–44].

Diagnostic Sensitivity and Specificity

The biggest concern regarding the DPC TSH assay is that a significant proportion of hypothyroid dogs do not have elevated TSH. In Table 1, the individual measurement of TSH and its combination with TT_4 and FT_4 by dialysis (FT_4D) is assessed for diagnostic sensitivity, specificity, and accuracy [35,45]. In general, because elevated TSH is a rarity in euthyroid dogs, except perhaps during recovery from NTI, elevated TSH is highly specific for primary hypothyroidism. The overall significance of these observations is that the use of TSH alone is not justified as a screening procedure for primary hypothyroidism as it is in human patients. TSH does add specificity to the observation of a low T_4 or FT_4 determination, however [29,30,46].

Potential Contributions to Low Diagnostic Sensitivity

Biologic variation

It has been hypothesized that pulsatile ultradian release of TSH might account for poor sensitivity of a baseline TSH value. Pulsatile release has been confirmed in hypothyroid but not euthyroid dogs, and there was no overlap in values of these two groups in experimental dogs, suggesting that only in cases of mild hypothyroidism might there be inconclusive results. TSH may not be elevated in a large percentage of confirmed cases, however [47].

Pituitary exhaustion

It been proposed that with prolonged hypothyroidism, there might be pituitary "exhaustion," with a decrease in previously high TSH values in dogs with hypothyroidism. This phenomenon has rarely been described in other species. It might be consistent with the observation that TRH does not release TSH further (vide infra), however, suggesting that it has reached a maximal secretory rate.

Glycosylation pattern

The oligosaccharide chains on TSH have been shown to be important in biosynthesis, subunit association, secretion, immunoreactivity, and bioactivity. Microheterogeneity of the carbohydrate constituents of human TSH causes heterogeneity in affinity for the receptor and in metabolic clearance of the hormone. Immunoreactivity has also been shown to be affected by this heterogeneity. In the author's laboratory, deglycosylated feline TSH showed immunologic parallelism to pituitary-source canine TSH standards and to untreated recombinant feline TSH. Because an ideal immunoassay standard's recognition would be glycosylation independent, this study supports the possibility that recombinant feline TSH, and presumably canine TSH, standardized for purity and protein content, could be used as an immunoassay standard

[41,42]. Indeed, recent studies have demonstrated greater immunologic consistency of rhTSH preparations and have even proposed that enzymatic "remodeling" of rhTSH produced much better correlation to serum TSH than did pituitary-source human TSH calibrators [48].

Does Stimulating Thyrotropin with Thyroid-Releasing Hormone Increase Diagnostic Sensitivity and Specificity?

The evaluation of TRH-stimulated TSH has generally not enhanced the sensitivity of diagnosis, because it seems that TSH is already maximally stimulated in most canine patients [5,49]. In human patients, an increased response of TSH to TRH generally demonstrated an enhanced response in early or mild primary hypothyroidism.

Potential for Improvement of Thyrotropin Assays

Improvement of the canine TSH assay and its interpretation might result from accomplishing any or all of the following steps:

1. Develop a universal canine TSH standard with known purity or bioactivity. The author proposes that recombinant canine TSH expressed in a mammalian cell line would be ideal.
2. Identify anticanine TSH antibodies with higher affinity. Sandwich assays of two carefully screened monoclonal antibodies are probably necessary to improve sensitivity.
3. Improve detection technology.
4. Understand the relevance of glycosylation patterns, particularly as they might relate to disease states.

Principle 4 is as follows: TSH measurement is a poor screening test for primary hypothyroidism, but a high value adds considerable specificity for the disease when low TT_4 or FT_4D is measured concurrently.

TESTS OF THYROID AUTOIMMUNITY
Antithyroglobulin Antibodies

Although discussed previously in the context of the etiopathology of hypothyroidism, it is worth noting again that positive TgAA results are worth noting because they are almost always associated with underlying thyroiditis. Recently, antibodies against another major thyroid protein, thyroid peroxidase, have also been identified in dogs with lymphocytic thyroiditis. This assay is not commercially available, however, and no systematic comparison of its value with that of the TgAA assay has been performed [50]. The fact that thyroid gland antibodies may become negative is now believed to be associated with progression to a later phase of disease. Despite the association with lymphocytic thyroiditis, dogs with only positive TgAA and normal T_4, FT_4, and TSH values should be scheduled for more frequent follow-up monitoring (perhaps once every 6 months) rather than being considered candidates for treatment. These animals are not considered candidates for immunosuppression, because the side effects of immunosuppressant drugs are much more severe than simply replacing levothyroxine (L-T_4), and L-T_4 is only necessary when clinical signs or diagnostic tests suggest thyroid hormone insufficiency.

Antitriiodothyronine and Antithyroxine Antibodies

Thyroglobulin, which carries T_3 and T_4 covalently linked to its structure, occasionally acts as a hapten to immunize the animal against these hormones. When high autoantibody titers are reached, the antibodies may interfere with the hormone immunoassay measurements. High serum T_3 or, occasionally, T_4 concentrations in the face of clinical signs of hypothyroidism should alert the clinician to this possibility. Apparent elevations in serum thyroid hormones are usually seen, but in certain assays, the antibodies may cause an "undetectable" or extremely low result. An animal with an undetectable serum T_3 concentration despite a normal T_4 concentration (before or after L-T_4 treatment) is not an animal with 5'-deiodinase enzyme deficiency as has been suggested; in these cases, anti-T_3 autoantibodies (T_3AA) have resulted in an artifactually low result. The true serum T_3 concentration may actually be normal.

After several large studies of this phenomenon in dog sera, the investigators at Michigan State University recognize other diagnostic criteria for dogs with hypothyroidism (low FT$_4$D, high TSH, or low FT$_4$D/TSH ratio); 35% of these dogs have T_3AA and 14% have T_4AA. All dogs with T_3AA or T_4AA also have positive TgAA; thus, positive results are evidence of thyroid autoimmunity. The 10 breeds with the highest prevalence of thyroid hormone antibodies (THAA), many of those with a propensity for autoimmune thyroiditis, were the Pointer, English Setter, English Pointer, Skye Terrier, German Wirehaired Pointer, Old English Sheepdog, Boxer, Maltese, Kuvasz, and Petit Basset Griffon Vendeen. In large part of the T_3AA incidence, which invalidates the results of the T_3 immunoassay in most laboratories, it may explain poor diagnostic accuracy of T_3 measurements. Subdividing the dogs with T_4AA with respect to the impact of the autoantibodies on TT$_4$ immunoassay results, approximately 1% result in a high TT$_4$ value, 5% result in a low TT$_4$ value, and 8% to 9% result in an artificially "normal" TT$_4$ result. The high and normal results explain most of the diagnostic false-negative results in interpreting the significance of TT$_4$. The observation of a low TT$_4$ value is the result of the presence of T_4AA. When patients with T_4AA are removed from consideration, the diagnostic sensitivity of a normal T_4 value in identifying a euthyroid patient rises essentially to 100% [30]. It is important to recognize that these antibodies have no influence on the choice of thyroid medication, because the capacity of the antibodies to bind thyroid hormone is relatively small and can be saturated with administered thyroid hormone [15,16,51].

Principle 5 is as follows: the presence of TgAA seems to be the earliest known indicator of thyroid pathologic change. Although positivity for TgAA is highly suggestive of later development of clinical hypothyroidism, it does not clarify the odds of the animal having hypothyroid offspring.

THYROTROPIN STIMULATION TESTS

The bovine TSH stimulation test was the definitive test when this author reviewed the topic in 1984 [1]. The principle behind this test is the evaluation of the increment of TT_4 concentration after administration of TSH as a pharmaceutic agent. The test evaluates an animal's thyroid "functional reserve," and it has been stated that approximately 75% of the thyroid gland must be destroyed before thyroid hormone production is diminished. This test has been touted as the noninvasive gold standard for thyroid function. A normal response has been interpreted as an increase in TT_4 to a value greater than the normal "resting" range or as an adequate multiple of the resting (pre-TSH) value. Both criteria tend to be problematic with significant alterations of serum thyroid hormone binding.

The pharmaceutic product of bovine TSH has been replaced in human medicine by rhTSH (Thyrogen [TM]; Genzyme Corporation, Cambridge, Massachusetts). The bioactivity of this product is 4 to 12 IU/mg, and each vial contains 1.1 mg of rhTSH. Several studies have recently evaluated the use of rhTSH for the TSH stimulation test in dogs. The first study, a dose-ranging study in 6 healthy Beagles, determined an optimal dose of rhTSH to be 50 µg, with a peak response at 6 hours after intravenous administration. Using this dose, the post-TSH serum T_4 concentration increased by more than 24 nmol/L (1.9 µg/dL), exceeding 45 nmol/L (3.5 µg/dL) in 5 of the 6 dogs. Intramuscular or subcutaneous administration resulted in a less consistent response. Of course, the absolute values for a normal response should be established individually for each laboratory [52,53]. A subsequent study evaluated the effect of subdividing a vial of rhTSH and storing the dose. Twelve euthyroid Beagles were studied in a crossover trial. A 91.5-µg dose of rhTSH was administered after 3 different storage protocols: fresh reconstitution, refrigerated at 40°C for 4 weeks, and frozen at −20°C for 8 weeks. There was no significant difference in TT_4 or FT_4 concentration after stimulation with fresh, refrigerated, and frozen rhTSH [4]. Another study compared rhTSH with bovine TSH in 18 Beagles and 20 healthy client-owned dogs weighing more than 20 kg. The dose of rhTSH (75 µg) was compared with a 1-U dose of bovine TSH in a crossover design. As might be expected from the bioactivity of rhTSH, the two treatments resulted in an identical response of serum TT_4. In this study, no difference was seen between intravenous and intramuscular routes for rhTSH. The authors used a less stringent criterion for a normal post-TSH response, however—greater than 32 nmol/L (2.5 µg/dL) and at least 1.5 times the pre-TSH value [53].

Despite the re-emergence of the TSH stimulation test out of frustration over the limitations of the current endogenous canine TSH assay, one study examined the accuracy of diagnosis in dogs with low TT_4 concentrations. Animals were separated into 14 dogs with primary hypothyroidism and 13 with NTI by thyroid biopsy results. The authors compared static tests with dynamic tests, such as the TSH response to TRH, the rhTSH stimulation test, and quantitative pertechnetate uptake. The only test that reliably discriminated the two groups was pertechnetate uptake. The authors questioned the gold standard status of the TSH stimulation test. Such testing, although not invasive, is expensive, requires anesthesia, and is limited only to research institutions, however [5].

THYROID ULTRASONOGRAPHY

High-resolution ultrasonic probes are also now being applied to evaluate thyroid volume and echogenicity. In a study of 87 healthy control dogs (26 dogs with NTI, 30 TgAA-positive hypothyroid dogs, and 23 TgAA-negative dogs), significant differences between euthyroid and hypothyroid dogs were identified in thyroid volume and mean cross-sectional surface area (MCSA), whereas no significant differences in thyroid size were detected between healthy euthyroid dogs and dogs with euthyroid sick syndrome. In euthyroid and euthyroid sick dogs, the parenchymal echotexture was homogeneous and hyperechoic, whereas the relative thyroid echogenicity of TgAA-positive and TgAA-negative hypothyroid dogs was less. In particular, the thyroid volume was found to have a highly specific predictive value for hypothyroidism. It seems that, carefully interpreted, thyroid ultrasound may prove to be a useful noninvasive indicator of thyroid pathologic conditions [54].

GENETIC SCREENING FOR HYPOTHYROIDISM

For the purposes of advising breeders, it would be desirable to have thyroid function tests that would predict the future development of hypothyroidism. Early detection of a genetically inherited trait is a desirable goal. Although some diagnostic laboratories now include basal serum T_4 measurement for health screens of dogs and cats, no presently available test can detect thyroid insufficiency before it is present. Additionally, because most dogs do not develop hypothyroidism until the age of 3 years of age or later, most of the suspect animals are already involved in active breeding programs. It has been proposed that an animal should have a serum T_4 or T_3 concentration greater than a certain value within the normal range before recommending that the animal be bred. There is no objective or logical basis on which to justify this approach. Pedigree analyses of the incidence of TgAA indicate that thyroiditis is hereditary, however. With completion of the recent sequencing of the canine genome, it seems likely that identification of the genetic locus or loci would eventually allow identification of dogs carrying the tendency to develop hypothyroidism before they enter a breeding program. In fact, a recent study has determined an association between canine hypothyroidism and a rare major histocompatibility complex (MHC) DLA haplotype allele in Doberman Pinschers. Other candidate genes are under investigation [55].

PUTTING IT TOGETHER

Focusing on the most common static single-sample tests, two key comprehensive studies contributed to develop the summary in Table 1 [29,30]. Both of the studies reviewed a large number of clinical cases, with confirmation of hypothyroidism by use of the older TSH stimulation test or response to therapy or by presuming that a FT_4D/TSH ratio greater than 7.5 was tantamount to a definitive diagnosis. Of course, the appropriate cutoff number for this ratio should be determined for each laboratory. The second study eliminated from consideration any cases involving confirmed anti-T_4AAs. Excellent screening tests are those with a high sensitivity. A value in the normal range would exclude hypothyroidism with the certainty shown. In Table 1, values of 1 would indicate a perfect prediction. Excellent confirmation tests are those that have a high specificity and accuracy.

COMPLICATING FACTORS: EFFECTS OF DRUGS AND DISEASE

Older studies of the effect of NTI have been previously reviewed [25]. A major diagnostic dilemma is associated with reduced T4 and T3 hyperadrenocorticism [56,57]. Newer insights from recent studies are reviewed here. In general terms, NTI results in a depression in TT_4 and TT_3, with a reduction in FT_4D being observed only in the most severe illnesses. An endotoxin model has demonstrated the thyroid-suppressive effects of an acute illness: TT_3 and TT_4 concentrations decreased significantly, whereas the reverse T_3 (rT_3) concentration increased significantly within 8 hours. The TT_4 value then returned to the reference range and again decreased significantly on days 6 to 12 and days 16 to 20. Of great interest, the FT_4D concentration increased significantly at 12, 24, and 48 hours after cessation of endotoxin treatment, compared with baseline values. These results confirm the screening value of FT_4D in the context of acute NTI [12.58,59].

How Is Nonthyroidal Illness Distinguished from Hypothyroidism?

The clinician's first tool is the clinical assessment of the animal. Most of the time, a careful history, physical examination, laboratory screening tests, and common sense allow one to distinguish NTI from hypothyroidism. It is therefore inappropriate to institute thyroid hormone therapy based on the sole observation of a low serum T_4 concentration in an animal without clinical signs consistent with hypothyroidism. To date, most studies have not shown a clear picture of the response of TSH as an assessment of thyroid status in assessing NTI, and it may depend on the phase of the disease. For example, the TSH concentration may be normal or low during the illness phase and increased during the recovery phase. Conversely, a normal or high FT_4D value helps to rule out hypothyroidism. A high FT_4D value should not elicit suspicion of hyperthyroidism in most dogs [26]. The stress of extreme exercise (eg, sled dog racing) has also been demonstrated to suppress TT_4 and FT_4 and to increase TSH in a manner that might be confused with primary hypothyroidism [60]. In summary, when an acute reversible condition occurs, it is most logical to delay thyroid function testing if possible.

Effect of Obesity and Weight Loss

In one study, thyroid function tests, including an rhTSH stimulation test, were evaluated in 12 lean and 12 obese dogs and obesity resulted in a significant increase in TT_3 and TT_4 concentrations. It is not clear why FT_4D was not increased, because the results imply that the percentage of T_4 binding in serum fell in obesity. In 8 obese dogs, however, the impact of weight loss demonstrated a fall in TT_3 and TSH [45].

Effect of Drugs

Veterinarians and clinical pathologists should be aware of the potential drugs that may influence thyroid function test results. Some of the more common interactions that have been studied in dogs are listed here. More detail is provided in two review articles [61,62]. The only drugs that may induce true hypothyroidism are the sulfa antimicrobials, which essentially act as antithyroid drugs, [63–67] and, possibly, phenobarbital, which enhances biliary clearance of thyroid hormones [68–70]. In both cases, large dosages lead to lower FT_4 and elevated TSH levels.

The effect of a 3-week course of phenobarbital on TT_4, FT_4D, and TSH was assessed, and no significant alteration of these values was observed over this time frame. Another study dissected out the effects of phenobarbital, documenting TT_4 and TSH values in 78 dogs receiving phenobarbital and comparing them with those of 48 untreated epileptic dogs. Of the dogs on phenobarbital, 40% had low TT_4 and 7% had elevated TSH, whereas only 8% of untreated dogs had low TT_4 and none had elevated TSH. Of the latter group, only dogs with recent seizure activity had low TT_4 values. The investigators found no effect of phenobarbital on serum binding of T_4. The mean serum TT_4 value was significantly lower and mean serum TSH level was significantly higher in the phenobarbital-treated group. As with the subacute study, there did not seem to be a correlation between phenobarbital dosage or duration of treatment and the serum TT_4 and TSH concentrations [68–70]. Great care should be taken in interpreting the results of thyroid function tests in dogs with seizure disorders. The proximity of sampling to seizure activity and the frequency of such activity were shown to depress TT_4 concentrations just as in other NTIs [71].

Previous studies had shown that the effect of prednisone on serum TT_4, FT_4D, and T_3 was largely dosage dependent, with an anti-inflammatory dose of prednisone of 0.5 mg/kg administered every 12 hours suppressing serum T_3 but not T_4 concentrations, whereas an immunosuppressive dose of 1 to 2 mg/kg administered every 12 hours suppressed TT_4 concentrations as well. A recent study added new information that serum TSH concentrations do not seem to change significantly with glucocorticoid administration. It has been postulated that the pituitary production of TSH would be suppressed by glucocorticoids. As the authors discuss, however, detection of TSH suppression may be an issue of lack of assay sensitivity within the normal range for the dog [38,72–74].

Table 2 summarizes the current status of the impact of drugs on thyroid function test results as described in detail in a previous review article [61].

Table 2
Drug effects on thyroid function tests

Drugs	TT_4	FT_4	TSH
Glucocorticoids	↓ or =	↓ or =	= or ↓
Phenobarbital	↓ or =	↓ or =	= or ↓
Sulfonamides	↓	↓	↑
Propranolol	=	=	=
Potassium bromide	=	=	=
Clomipramine	↓	↓	=
Aspirin	↓	=	=
Ketoprofen	↓	=	=
Carprofen	↓ or =	↓ or =	↓ or =

Data from Refs. [59,62–71,73–78].

Dealing with Discordant Results

Discordant results of TT_4 or FT_4D measurement with TSH and TgAA may reflect intermediate stages of thyroid pathologic conditions, such as progressive development of autoimmune thyroiditis. One of the most common situations is the observation of a normal TSH concentration in the face of low TT_4 or FT_4D. It should be recognized that a significant proportion (15%–40%) of hypothyroid dogs may have a normal TSH concentration. Also, a normal TSH concentration with a "low" TT_4 or FT_4D value may be associated with the sighthound breeds. In these patients, in euthyroidism, TT_3 is often in the normal range. Although not yet completely studied, by analogy to human patients, we might also expect discordance of diagnostic test results when the animal is recovering from an illness.

THERAPEUTIC TRIALS

In some cases, diagnostic tests are equivocal, and it may make sense to proceed to a therapeutic trial with L-T_4 therapy. It is important to recognize that a positive clinical response to L-T_4 treatment is a crucial confirmation of abnormal diagnostic test results, however. Therapeutic trials should be considered only when clinical signs are supportive, when there are no other significant illnesses that might be treated successfully before retesting, and only if there is a clinical sign or lesion that can be monitored objectively during therapy. A therapeutic trial should be considered only if there is one of the following results in diagnostic testing:

1. Low TT_4
2. Normal TT_4 and positive T_4AA
3. Normal TT_4 and high TSH

Of course, the strongest evidence is gained by the observation of a response to L-T_4 and then a relapse when the medication is removed. The clinician should be aware that there may also be pharmacologic effects of L-T_4 (ie, a "T_4-responsive" condition) even in patients with no diagnostic evidence of hypothyroidism. Conditions specifically shown to be T_4-responsive include poor coat quality, seasonal flank alopecia, and polyneuropathies [20].

Occasionally, when the clinical suspicion for hypothyroidism is high and available thyroid function tests are not performed or give equivocal results, therapy is started without a definitive diagnosis. From the animal's standpoint, if the animal is otherwise healthy, there is little medical risk to administering L-T_4 at replacement dosages. If the thyroid gland is normal, exogenous L-T_4 suppresses endogenous TSH and the normal thyroid gland atrophies. Therapeutic trials are often defended as being cost-effective for the owner; however, it is important to recognize that replacement therapy is generally necessary for the remainder of the animal's life. Therefore, an incorrect diagnosis can also be quite expensive, a delayed diagnosis of another disease could be detrimental, and definitive diagnostic procedures can be quite difficult to interpret after a therapeutic trial. It is recommended to wait 6 to 8 weeks after discontinuation of replacement therapy before thyroid function testing is attempted.

MONITORING TREATMENT

In almost every case, the treatment of hypothyroidism should be with L-T_4 preparations (0.02 mg/kg administered orally twice daily to start and 0.02–0.04 mg/kg given once daily or, if necessary, divided twice daily to maintain), because they constitute the most physiologic compound for providing thyroid hormone to tissues. Therapeutic success should be judged first on clinical grounds and, if necessary, corroborated with measurements of serum T_4 after achievement of steady-state concentrations (generally within 1 week after initiation of treatment). The most valuable sampling time for "postpill" serum T_4 measurement is just before a dose. Iatrogenic hyperthyroidism is rare in dogs but is more common in large-breed dogs dosed on a per body weight dosage regimen. The dosage protocol of 0.5 mg/m^2 of body surface area generally allows for more hormone for small dogs and less for large dogs on a body weight basis. Most dogs, once clinical signs have resolved, should be tried on once-daily L-T_4 to see if this more convenient protocol adequately maintains clinical euthyroidism. It is now apparent that endogenous canine TSH concentrations normalize within a week of instituting replacement T_4 therapy given at 0.02 mg/kg only once daily and may indicate that the common dosing schemes deliver pharmacologic quantities of thyroid hormone [79](Fig. 1). Given that some euthyroid dogs seem to increase fatty acid turnover in the skin in response to similar dosages, a beneficial response to L-T_4 may not necessarily provide a definitive diagnosis of hypothyroidism [80] (see Fig. 1).

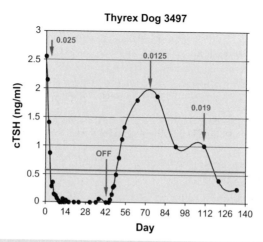

Thyrex Dog 3497

Fig. 1. Effect of titrating an oral dosage of L-T$_4$ on a single thyroidectomized dog over 19 weeks. The number represents the daily dose of L-T$_4$ (mg/kg). The horizontal bar represents the upper level of the normal range for TSH (0.6 ng/mL). (*Data from* Ferguson DC, Hoenig M. Re-examination of dosage regimens for L-thyroxine in the dog: bioavailability and persistence of TSH suppression. Presented at the Proceedings of the American College of Veterinary Internal Medicine. May 1997).

SUMMARY AND RECOMMENDATIONS FOR OPTIMAL TEST SEQUENCE

In looking for the most utilitarian set of thyroid diagnostic tests, consider the following conclusions regarding currently available thyroid function tests for the dog:

1. Normal FT$_4$D and TSH values almost always identify a euthyroid animal. Some laboratories have established the FT$_4$D/TSH ratio as a valuable discriminator.
2. Low TT$_4$ or FT$_4$D, together with high TSH, confirms hypothyroidism in most cases.
3. Demonstration of positive TgAA is most valuable to support abnormal TT$_4$, FT$_4$D, or TSH values. When other test results are normal, its predictive value in a given patient remains to be determined.
4. Low TT$_3$ is probably only of diagnostic value to support the diagnosis of hypothyroidism in sighthounds.

References

[1] Ferguson DC. Thyroid function tests in the dog. Vet Clin North Am Small Anim Pract 1984;14:783–808.
[2] Ferguson DC. Update on the diagnosis of canine hypothyroidism. Vet Clin North Am 1994;24(3):515–40.
[3] Kemppainen RJ, Behrend EN. Diagnosis of canine hypothyroidism. Perspectives from a testing laboratory. Vet Clin North Am Small Anim Pract 2004;31(5):951–62.

[4] De Roover K, Duchateau L, Carmichael N, et al. Effect of storage of reconstituted recombinant human thyroid-stimulating hormone (rhTSH) on thyroid-stimulating hormone (TSH) response testing in euthyroid dogs. J Vet Intern Med 2006;20(4):812–7.

[5] Diaz-Espineira MM, Mol JA, Peeters ME, et al. Assessment of thyroid function in dogs with low plasma thyroxine concentration. J Vet Intern Med 2007;21:25–32.

[6] Larsson M, Pettersson T, Carlstrom A. Thyroid hormone binding in serum of 15 vertebrate species: isolation of thyroxine-binding globulin and prealbumin analogs. Gen Comp Endocrinol 1985;58:360–75.

[7] Kaptein EM, Hoopes MT, Ferguson DC, et al. Comparison of reverse triiodothyronine distribution and metabolism in normal dogs and humans. Endocrinology 1990;126: 2003–14.

[8] Kaptein EM, Moore GE, Ferguson DC, et al. Effects of prednisone on thyroxine and 3;5;3'-triiodothyronine metabolism in normal dogs. Endocrinology 1992;130: 1669–79.

[9] Kaptein EM, Moore GE, Ferguson DC, et al. Thyroxine and triiodothyronine distribution and metabolism in thyroxine-replaced athyreotic dogs and normal humans. Am J Phys (Endocrinol Metab 27) 1993;264:E90–100.

[10] Kemppainen RJ, Clark TP. Etiopathogenesis of canine hypothyroidism. Vet Clin North Am 1994;24(3):467–76.

[11] Scott-Moncrieff CR, Guptill-Yoran L. Hypothyroidism. In: Ettinger SJ, Feldman EC, editors. Textbook of veterinary internal medicine. 5th edition; 2000. p. 1419–29.

[12] Peterson ME, Ferguson DC. Thyroid diseases. In: Ettinger SJ, editor. Textbook of veterinary internal medicine, vol. 27. Philadelphia: WB Saunders and Co; 1990. p. 1632–75.

[13] Graham PA, Lundquist RB, Refsal KR, et al. Clinical history and presentation associated with serum thyroglobulin autoantibody in dogs. Presented at the American College of Veterinary INternal Medicine Forum Proceedings, 2002.

[14] Nachreiner RF, Refsal KR, Graham PA, et al. Prevalence of autoantibodies to thyroglobulin in dogs with nonthyroidal illness. Am J Vet Res 1998;59(8):951–5.

[15] Nachreiner RF, Refsal KR, Graham PA, et al. Prevalence of serum thyroid hormone autoantibodies in dogs with clinical signs of hypothyroidism. J Am Vet Med Assoc 2002;220(4): 466–71.

[16] Nachreiner RF, Refsal KR, Thacker EL, et al. Incidence of T3 and T4 autoantibodies in dogs using a sensitive binding assay. J Vet Intern Med 1990;4(2):114.

[17] Scott-Moncrieff JC, Azcona-Olivera J, Glickman NW, et al. Evaluation of antithyroglobulin antibodies after routine vaccination in pet and research dogs. J Am Vet Med Assoc 2002;221(4):515–21.

[18] Scott-Moncrieff JC, Glickman NW, Glickman JT, et al. Lack of association between repeated vaccination and thyroiditis in laboratory Beagles. J Vet Intern Med 2006;20(4):818–21.

[19] Ferguson DC, Hoenig ME. Canine hypothyroidism. In: Allen DG, editor. Small animal medicine. Philadelphia: J.B.Lippincott Co; 1991. p. 845–65.

[20] Ferguson DC, Graham P, Kintzer P, et al. Thyroid function tests in the dog: SCE consensus refined and defined. Presented at the American College of Veterinary INternal Medicine Forum Proceedings. Charlotte (NC), May 2003.

[21] Jaggy A, Oliver JE. Neurological manifestations of thyroid disease. Vet Clin North Am 1994;24(3):487–94.

[22] Jaggy A, Oliver JE, Ferguson DC, et al. Neurological manifestations of hypothyroidism: a retrospective study of 29 dogs. J Vet Intern Med 1994;8(5):328–36.

[23] Ferguson DC, Hoenig M. Endocrine system. In: Latimer KS, Mahaffey EA, Prasse KW, editors. Duncan and Prasse's veterinary laboratory medicine: clinical pathology. 4th edition. Ames (IA): Iowa State Press; 2003. p. 270–303.

[24] Lurye JC, Behrend EN, Kemppainen RJ. Evaluation of an in-house enzyme-linked immuno-sorbent assay for quantitative measurement of serum total thyroxine concentrations in dogs and cats. J Am Vet Med Assoc 2002;221(2):243–9.

[25] Ferguson DC. Effect of nonthyroidal factors on thyroid function tests in the dog. Compendium for Continuing Education (Small Animal) 1988;10(12):1365–77.

[26] Kantrowitz LB, Peterson ME, Melian C, et al. Serum total thyroxine, total triiodothyronine, free thyroxine, and thyrotropin concentrations in dogs with nonthyroidal disease. J Am Vet Med Assoc 2001;219:765–9.

[27] Kantrowitz LB, Peterson ME, Trepanier LA, et al. Serum total thyroxine, total triiodothyronine, free thyroxine, and thyrotropin concentrations in epileptic dogs treated with anticonvulsants. J Am Vet Med Assoc 1999;214:1804–8.

[28] Kaptein EM, Hays MT, Ferguson DC. Thyroid hormone metabolism: a comparative evaluation. Vet Clin North Am 1994;24(3):431–66.

[29] Peterson ME, Melian C, Nichols R. Measurement of serum total thyroxine, triiodothyronine, free thyroxine, and thyrotropin concentrations for diagnosis of hypothyroidism in dogs. J Am Vet Med Assoc 1997;211:1396–402.

[30] Dixon RM, Mooney CT. Evaluation of serum free thyroxine and thyrotropin concentrations in the diagnosis of canine hypothyroidism. J Small Anim Pract 1999;40:72–8.

[31] Hill RC, Fox LE, Lewis DD, et al. Effects of racing and training on serum thyroid hormone concentrations in racing greyhounds. Am J Vet Res 2001;62:1969–72.

[32] Ferguson DC. Free thyroid hormone measurements in the diagnosis of thyroid disease. In: Bonagura J, Kirk RW, editors. Current veterinary therapy XII. Philadelphia: WB Saunders; 1995. p. 360–63.

[33] Schachter S, Nelson RW, Scott-Moncrieff C, et al. Comparison of serum free thyroxine concentration determined by standard equilibrium dialysis, modified equilibrium dialysis, and five radioimmunoassays in dogs. J Vet Intern Med 2004;18:259–64.

[34] Fritz KS, Wilcox RB, Nelson JC. A direct free thyroxine (T4) immunoassay with the characteristics of a total T4 immunoassay. Clin Chem 2007;53:911–5.

[35] Nelson JC, Wang R, Asher DT, et al. The nature of analogue-based free thyroxine estimates. Thyroid 2004;14(12):1030–6.

[36] Ramsey IK, Evans H. Herrtage. Thyroid-stimulating hormone and total thyroxine concentrations in euthyroid, sick euthyroid and hypothyroid dogs. J Small Anim Pract 1997;38(12): 540–5.

[37] Reese S, Breyer U, Deeg C, et al. Thyroid sonography as an effective tool to discriminate between euthyroid sick and hypothyroid dogs. J Vet Intern Med 2005;19(4):491–8.

[38] Torres SMF, Feeney DA, Lekcharoensuk C, et al. Morphology and function of the thyroid in severe sickness. J Am Vet Med Assoc 2003;222:1079–85.

[39] Marca MC, Loste A, Orden I, et al. Evaluation of canine serum thyrotropin (TSH) concentration: comparison of three analytical procedures. J Vet Diagn Invest 2001;13:106–10.

[40] Meij BP, Mol JA, Rijnberk A. Thyroid-stimulating hormone responses after single administration of thyrotropin-releasing hormone and combined administration of four hypothalamic releasing hormones in Beagle dogs. Domest Anim Endocrinol 1996;13(5):465–8.

[41] Rayalam S, Eizenstat LD, Davis RR, et al. Expression and purification of feline thyrotropin (fTSH): immunological detection and bioactivity of heterodimeric and yoked glycoproteins. Domest Anim Endocrinol 2006;30:185–202.

[42] Rayalam S, Eizenstat LD, Hoenig M, et al. Cloning and sequencing of feline thyrotropin (fTSH): heterodimeric and yoked constructs. Domest Anim Endocrinol 2006;30:203–17.

[43] Yang X, McGraw RA, Su X, et al. Canine thyrotropin β-subunit gene: cloning and expression in *Escherichia coli*, generation of monoclonal antibodies, and transient expression in the Chinese Hamster ovary cells. Domest Anim Endocrinol 2000;18(4):363–78.

[44] Yang X, McGraw RA, Ferguson DC. cDNA cloning of canine common α gene and its Co-expression with canine thyrotropin β gene in baculovirus expression system. Domest Anim Endocrinol 2000;18(4):379–93.

[45] Daminet S, Jeusette I, Duchateau L, et al. Evaluation of thyroid function in obese dogs and in dogs undergoing a weight loss protocol. J Vet Med A Physiol Pathol Clin Med 2003;50(4): 213–8.

[46] Scott-Moncrieff CR, Nelson RW, Bruner JM, et al. Comparison of serum concentrations of thyroid-stimulating hormone in healthy dogs, hypothyroid dogs, and euthyroid dogs with concurrent disease. J Am Vet Med Assoc 1998;212:387–91.

[47] Kooistra HS, Diaz-Espineira M, Mol JA, et al. Secretion pattern of thyroid-stimulating hormone in dogs during euthyroidism and hypothyroidism. Domest Anim Endocrinol 2000; 18(1):19–29.

[48] Rafferty B, Das RG. Comparison of pituitary and recombinant thyroid-stimulating hormone (rhTSH) in a multicenter collaborative study: establishment of the first World Health Organization reference standard for rhTSH. Clin Chem 1999;45(12):2207–15.

[49] Hoenig M, Ferguson DC. Comparison of TRH-stimulated thyrotropin (cTSH) to TRH- and TSH-stimulated T4 in euthyroid, hypothyroid, and sick dogs. Presentated at the American College of Veterinary INternal Medicine Forum Proceedings. May 1997.

[50] Skopek E, Patzl M, Nachreiner RF. Detection of autoantibodies against thyroid peroxidase in serum samples of hypothyroid dogs. Am J Vet Res 2006;67(5):809–14.

[51] Refsal KR, Nachreiner RF. Thyroid hormone autoantibodies in the dog: their association with serum concentrations of iodothyronines and thyrotropin and distribution by age, sex, and breed of dog. Canine Pract 1997;22(1):16–7.

[52] Suave F, Paradis M. Use of recombinant human thyroid-stimulating hormone for thyrotropin stimulation test in euthyroid dogs. Can Vet J 2000;41:215–9.

[53] Boretti FS, Sieber-Ruckstuhl NS, Willi B, et al. Comparison of the biological activity of recombinant human thyroid-stimulating hormone with bovine thyroid-stimulating hormone and evaluation of recombinant human thyroid-stimulating hormone in healthy dogs of different breeds. Am J Vet Res 2006;67(7):1169–72.

[54] Broemel C, Pollard RE, Kass PH, et al. Ultrasonographic evaluation of the thyroid gland in healthy, hypothyroid, and euthyroid golden retrievers with nonthyroidal illness. J Vet Intern Med 2005;19(4):499–506.

[55] Kennedy LJ, Quarmby Happ SGM, Barnes A, et al. WER: association of canine hypothyroidism with a common major histocompatibility complex DLA class II allele. Tissue Antigens 2006;68(1):82–6.

[56] Ferguson DC, Peterson ME. Serum free and total iodothyronine concentrations in dogs with hyperadrenocorticism. Am J Vet Res 1992;53:1636–40.

[57] Peterson ME, Ferguson DC, Kintzer PP, et al. Effects of spontaneous hyperadrenocorticism on serum thyroid hormone concentrations in the dog. Am J Vet Res 1984;45(10): 2034–8.

[58] Panciera DL, Ritchey JW, Ward DL. Endotoxin-induced nonthyroidal illness in dogs. Am J Vet Res 2003;64(2):229–34.

[59] Paull LC, Scott-Moncrieff JCR, DeNicola DB, et al. Potassium bromide effects on thyroid function and morphology. J Am Anim Hosp Assoc 2003;39:193–202, 2003.

[60] Panciera DL, Hinchcliff KW, Olson J, et al. Plasma thyroid hormone concentrations in dogs competing in a long-distance sled dog race. J Vet Intern Med 2003;17(4):593–6.

[61] Daminet S, Ferguson DC. Influence of drugs on thyroid function in dogs. J Vet Intern Med 2003;17:463–72.

[62] Gulikers KP, Panciera DL. Evaluation of the effects of clomipramine on canine thyroid function tests. J Vet Intern Med 2003;17(1):44–9.

[63] Gookin JL, Trepanier LA, Bunch SE. Clinical hypothyroidism associated with trimethoprim-sulfadiazine administration in a dog. J Am Vet Med Assoc 1999;214:1028–31.

[64] Hall IA, Campbell KL, Chambers MD, et al. Effect of trimethoprim/sulfamethoxazole on thyroid function in dogs with pyoderma. J Am Vet Med Assoc 1993;202:1959–62.

[65] Panciera DL, Post K. Effect of oral administration of sulfadiazine and trimethoprim in combination on thyroid function in dogs. Can J Vet Res 1992;56:349–52.

[66] Post K, Panciera DL, Clark EG. Lack of effect of trimethoprim and sulfadiazine in combination in mid- to late gestation on thyroid function in neonatal dogs. J Reprod Fertil 1993; 47(Suppl):477–82.

[67] Williamson NL, Frank LA, Hnilica KA. Trimethoprim-sulfamethoxazole effects on thyroid function. J Am Vet Med Assoc 2002;221:802–6.

[68] Gaskill CL, Burton SA, Gelens HCJ, et al. Effects of phenobarbital treatment on serum thyroxine and thyroid-stimulating hormone concentrations in epileptic dogs. Am Vet Med Assoc 1999;215(4):489–96.

[69] Gieger TL, Hosgood J, Taboada J, et al. Thyroid function and serum hepatic enzyme activity in dogs after phenobarbital administration. J Vet Intern Med 2000;14:277–81.

[70] Müller PB, Wolfsheimer KJ, Tabaoda J, et al. Effects of long-term phenobarbital treatment on the thyroid and adrenal axis and adrenal function tests in dogs. J Vet Intern Med 2000;14: 157–64.

[71] Von Klopmann T, Boettcher IC, Annett Rotermund A, et al. Euthyroid sick syndrome in dogs with idiopathic epilepsy before treatment with anticonvulsant drugs. J Vet Intern Med 2006;20(3):516–22.

[72] Daminet S, Paradis M, Refsal KR, et al. Short term influence of prednisone and phenobarbital on thyroid function in euthyroid dogs. Can Vet J 1999;40:411–5.

[73] Moore GE, Ferguson DC, Hoenig M. Effects of oral administration of anti-inflammatory doses of prednisone on thyroid hormone response to thyrotropin-releasing hormone and thyrotropin in clinically normal dogs. Am J Vet Res 1993;54:130–5.

[74] Torres S, McKeever PJ, Johnston SD. Effects of oral administration of prednisolone on thyroid function in dogs. Am J Vet Res 1991;52:416–21.

[75] Ferguson DC, Moore GE, Hoenig M. Carprofen lowers total T4 and TSH but not free T4 concentrations in the dog. J Vet Intern Med 1999;13:243.

[76] Suave F, Paradis M, Refsal KR, et al. Effects of oral administration of meloxicam, carprofen, and a nutraceutical on thyroid function in dogs with osteoarthritis. Can Vet J 2003;44: 474–9.

[77] Center SA, Mitchell J, Nachreiner RF, et al. Effects of propranolol on thyroid function in dogs. Am J Vet Res 1984;45:109–11.

[78] Daminet S, Croubels S, Duchateau L, et al. Influence of acetylsalicylic acid and ketoprofen on canine thyroid function tests. Vet J 2003;166:224–32.

[79] Ferguson DC, Hoenig M. Re-examination of dosage regimens for L-thyroxine in the dog: bioavailability and persistence of TSH suppression. Presented at the American College of Veterinary INternal Medicine Forum Proceedings. May 1997.

[80] Campbell KL, Davis CA. Effects of thyroid hormones on serum and cutaneous fatty acid concentrations in dogs. Am J Vet Res 1990;51(5):752–6.

Testing for Hyperthyroidism in Cats

Robert E. Shiel, MVB*, Carmel T. Mooney, MVB, MPhil, PhD

Small Animal Clinical Studies, School of Agriculture, Food Science and Veterinary Medicine, University College Dublin, Belfield, Dublin 4, Ireland

F eline hyperthyroidism was first recognized as a distinct clinical entity in 1979. Since then, it has become an extremely important and common disorder of older cats. The clinical syndrome results from excessive circulating concentrations of the active thyroid hormones thyroxine (T_4), and triiodothyronine (T_3) produced by an abnormally functioning thyroid lobe. The underlying pathologic finding in more than 98% of cases is benign adenomatous hyperplasia (adenoma); as such, the disease carries a favorable prognosis with effective therapy. Thyroid carcinoma is a rare cause of hyperthyroidism in cats. Hyperthyroidism has also been described in a young kitten, but this likely represents a separate disease entity that remains extremely rare [1].

The clinical features of feline hyperthyroidism have by now been well described. Because of the multisystemic effects of thyroid hormones, a wide variety of clinical signs are possible; however, today, presumably because of increased awareness and earlier diagnosis, cats are far less symptomatic than previously [2,3]. There has been a change in emphasis from simply confirming a diagnosis in a cat presenting with classic clinical signs to diagnosing hyperthyroidism in cats with few, if any, signs or ruling it out in cats presenting with varied problems that may or may not be related to hyperthyroidism. This has an impact on the efficacy of the diagnostic tests used, because the changes induced by hyperthyroidism become more subtle and the possibility of occult hyperthyroidism with or without a concurrent disease becomes greater. This article reviews those routine clinicopathologic and endocrinologic changes typically associated with hyperthyroidism and highlights recent advances in the diagnostic tests used to support and confirm a diagnosis of hyperthyroidism in cats.

SCREENING LABORATORY TESTS

A complete blood cell count, serum biochemistry, and urinalysis are often performed in the investigation of hyperthyroidism, and such results may prove

*Corresponding author. E-mail address: robert.shiel@ucd.ie (R.E. Shiel).

0195-5616/07/$ – see front matter
doi:10.1016/j.cvsm.2007.03.006

useful in supporting a diagnosis or eliminating other diseases with similar clinical signs.

Hematologic Analyses

In early reports of hyperthyroidism, mild to moderate erythrocytosis and macrocytosis were common. In one study of 131 hyperthyroid cats, an increased packed cell volume (PCV), mean corpuscular volume (MCV), red blood cell (RBC) count, and hemoglobin concentration were reported in 47%, 44%, 21%, and 17% of cases, respectively, and the prevalence of such changes remained as high 10 years later [2,3]. Such changes may reflect increased erythropoietin production resulting from increased oxygen consumption or direct thyroid hormone–mediated β-adrenergic stimulation of erythroid marrow. In a similar study of 57 cats in the United Kingdom, however, there were minimal changes in RBC parameters and macrocytes were rare [4]. Anemia seems to be rare and usually associated with severe hyperthyroidism, and it may result from bone marrow exhaustion or iron or other micronutrient deficiency [4]. A significantly higher incidence of Heinz body formation has been reported in cats with hyperthyroidism compared with healthy cats, although with fewer and smaller bodies than typically seen in diabetic cats [5]. Hyperthyroid cats also seem to have a higher mean platelet size than healthy cats, but the significance of this remains unclear [6].

Changes in white blood cell parameters are not unusual in hyperthyroidism but are relatively nonspecific. The most frequent changes include leukocytosis, mature neutrophilia, lymphopenia, and eosinopenia presumably reflecting a stress response [2–4]. Eosinophilia and lymphocytosis may occur in a small number of cats, however, and potentially result from a relative decrease in available cortisol because of excess circulating thyroid hormone concentrations [4].

It is important to note that apart from the rare cases of thyrotoxic anemia, the hematologic abnormalities are subtle in hyperthyroid cats and are not clinically significant. In some affected cases, hematologic parameters may not be altered, and in hyperthyroid cats with concurrent illness, the abnormalities present may reflect the latter rather than the former disease.

Biochemical Analyses

The most striking biochemical abnormalities are elevations in the liver enzymes, alanine aminotransferase (ALT), alkaline phosphatase (ALKP), lactate dehydrogenase (LDH), and aspartate aminotransferase (AST). At least one of these enzymes is elevated in more than 90% of hyperthyroid cats [2–4]. The elevations in these enzymes can be dramatic (>500 IU/L each, respectively), but at least in one study, serum ALKP and total T_4 concentrations were significantly correlated [7]. As such, the degree of elevation is more subtle, if present at all, in early cases of hyperthyroidism. In addition, liver enzyme concentrations decrease to within the reference range with successful management of hyperthyroidism [8]. If marked elevations in liver enzymes are observed in cats with mildly elevated thyroid hormone concentrations or if such elevations persist despite successful treatment of the hyperthyroidism, concurrent hepatic disease should be considered and investigated.

Despite the marked elevations in hepatic enzymes, histologic examination of the liver of hyperthyroid cats has revealed only modest and nonspecific changes, including increased pigment within hepatocytes, aggregates of mixed inflammatory cells in the portal regions, and focal areas of fatty degeneration [9]. In more severe cases, centrilobular fatty infiltration may occur together with patchy portal fibrosis, lymphocytic infiltration, and proliferation of bile ducts [3,9]. Suggested explanations for such abnormalities have included malnutrition, congestive cardiac failure, infections, hepatic anoxia, and direct toxic effects of thyroid hormones on the liver. Several reports have examined the possibility of other sources of these enzymes, however, and have shown that the liver and bone contribute to increased ALKP activity in hyperthyroid cats [7,10,11]. In one of these studies, the bone isoenzyme contributed up to 80% of the total ALKP activity [10].

Hyperphosphatemia, in the absence of azotemia, was originally reported in approximately 20% of cases and was more recently reported in a higher percentage (36%–43%) of hyperthyroid cats, particularly when compared with an age-matched control group [3,10,12]. This, together with the elevation in the bone isoenzyme of ALKP, is consistent with altered bone metabolism in hyperthyroidism. Certainly, in human thyrotoxic patients, there is an increased risk of osteoporosis because of a direct effect of thyroid hormone on bone. The net bone loss leads to the release of calcium and a tendency toward hypercalcemia, hyperphosphatemia, hypoparathyroidism, and reduced concentrations of activated vitamin D. Studies in hyperthyroid cats have demonstrated significant differences compared with people, however. Circulating osteocalcin concentration, used as a measure of osteoblastic activity and bone remodeling, although variable, was elevated (mean $\pm$ SD: 0.32 $\pm$ 0.3, range: 0–1.7 ng/mL) in 16 (44%) of 36 hyperthyroid cats compared with values from 10 healthy cats (range: 0–0.25 ng/mL) [10]. In a further preliminary study, osteocalcin, the bone isoenzyme of ALKP, the carboxy-terminal propeptide of type I collagen (PICP), the carboxy terminal telopeptide of type I collagen (ICTP), serum cross-linked carboxy-terminal collagen telopeptide (CTx), and deoxypyridinoline (Dpd) concentrations were measured in 4 healthy and hyperthyroid cats before and after radioactive iodine treatment. All concentrations were increased in the hyperthyroid cats and decreased after successful therapy, suggesting thyrotoxic-induced increased bone turnover [13]. Early reports of feline hyperthyroidism suggested that the circulating calcium concentration was largely unaffected by hyperthyroidism, but only total calcium was measured. In two separate studies, 18 (50%) of 36 [10] and 4 (27%) of 15 [12] hyperthyroid cats had serum ionized calcium concentrations lower than the reference range. In addition, hyperparathyroidism seems to be common in hyperthyroid cats [12]. In 30 hyperthyroid cats, the circulating parathyroid hormone (PTH) concentration was elevated in 23 (77%) cases (mean $\pm$ SEM: 85.0 $\pm$ 17.2, range: 33.1–120.3 pg/mL [reference range: 2.9–26.3 pg/mL]), with values approaching up to 19 times the upper limit of the reference range. Of 8 hyperthyroid cats in which the plasma 1,25 vitamin D concentration was measured, three values were higher than the reference range rather than suppressed as in human beings, but there was no overall significant difference between this group and 20 healthy cats [12]. The etiology of hyperparathyroidism, hyperphosphatemia, ionized hypocalcemia, and elevated bone marker concentrations in cats remains unclear and warrants further study. These abnormalities have not typically been associated with any specific clinical signs. There has been at least one report of a hyperphosphatemic hyperthyroid cat with calcification of multiple paws that resolved with induction of euthyroidism, however [14]. There has also been some suggestion that the altered bone marker concentrations may provide a sensitive method for monitoring treatment in hyperthyroid cats, but further studies are required. Although not typically associated with human hyperthyroidism, concurrent hyperparathyroidism has recently been diagnosed in 13 of 96 patients [15], and the cat may prove to be a suitable model for further investigations in this field.

In early reports of hyperthyroidism, mild to moderate azotemia seemed to be common, occurring in 25% to 70% of cases [3,4]. Current figures suggest that just more than 10% of hyperthyroid cats are azotemic. Although azotemia is not unexpected in a group of aged cats, it could be exacerbated by the increased protein catabolism and prerenal uremia of thyrotoxicosis [9]. Most studies have shown relatively lower pretreatment urea concentrations in hyperthyroid cats [16–20] when compared with posttreatment values, however. This is presumably related to the elevated glomerular filtration rate (GFR) associated with hyperthyroidism, resulting from increased cardiac output and renal afferent arteriolar vasodilation [13,16–18]. In hyperthyroid cats without azotemia, the serum creatinine concentration is significantly lower compared with age-matched healthy animals [12] and significant increases have been documented after treatment [13]. These low values may be related to reduced muscle mass rather than to any effect of thyrotoxicosis on tubular secretion of creatinine, because this is not considered to occur in cats. Together with the effects of hyperthyroidism on urea concentrations, this has significant implications when assessing renal function before deciding on the best option for treatment.

Several other clinicopathologic abnormalities have been described in hyperthyroid cats. Hypokalemia has been reported in up to 17% of hyperthyroid cats, [21] but although the etiology remains unclear, it is rarely clinically significant [22]. In a study of 15 hyperthyroid and 40 healthy cats, there was no significant difference in circulating ionized or total magnesium concentrations between the two groups [23]. This contrasts to other species, in which hyperthyroidism increases magnesium excretion and lowers circulating concentrations. There was a negative correlation between ionized magnesium concentrations and logarithmically transformed total T_4 concentrations in the hyperthyroid group, however, suggesting some correlation with lowered magnesium concentration and the severity of the hyperthyroid state.

Blood glucose concentrations may be elevated in hyperthyroid cats, presumably reflecting a stress response [3]. Hyperthyroidism is also associated with glucose intolerance characterized by delayed clearance of administered glucose from the plasma despite increased secretion of insulin [24]. Two separate studies have examined the effect of hyperthyroidism on circulating fructosamine concentration [25,26]. In both studies, the serum fructosamine concentration was significantly lower in hyperthyroid cats compared with healthy cats, presumably as a result of increased protein turnover. Importantly, 17% to 50% of cases had values lower than the respective reference range, and caution is advised in interpreting the serum fructosamine concentration in hyperthyroid cats, particularly if they are concurrently diabetic. Almost 50% of hyperthyroid cats have detectable serum troponin I concentrations, with a marked reduction in this percentage after therapy, consistent with hyperthyroid-induced myocyte damage [27]. Abnormal coagulation parameters were detected in 3 of 21 cats before methimazole therapy [28]. All 3 cats had elevated proteins induced by vitamin K absence or antagonism; 1 cat also had an elevated prothrombin time. This could be attributable to the reduced fat absorption seen in some hyperthyroid cats [3] or to concurrent small intestinal disease. A separate study reported serum folate and cobalamin concentrations lower than the reference range in 5 (38.5%) and 3 (23.1%) of 13 hyperthyroid cats, respectively [29]. The cause warrants further investigation but may be associated with malabsorption or increased metabolism.

Other biochemical parameters, such as cholesterol, sodium, chloride, bilirubin, albumin, and globulin, are rarely, if ever, affected by hyperthyroidism. Of all the possible biochemical abnormalities, elevated liver enzyme activities remain the change most commonly associated with hyperthyroidism. The other reported changes are variably associated with hyperthyroidism and provide little diagnostic information.

Urinalysis

Routine urinalysis in thyrotoxic cats seems to be noncontributory. Urine specific gravity values are extremely variable and ranged from 1.009 to 1.050 (mean = 1.031) in 57 hyperthyroid cats, with only two values (4%) less than 1.015 [3]. This was not significantly different when compared with values obtained from hyperthyroid cats 10 years later [2].

Proteinuria is common in hyperthyroid cats. In one study, the urinary protein/creatinine ratio (UPC) was elevated (>0.5) in 15 (34%) of 44 hyperthyroid cats that were nonazotemic and had no evidence of a urinary tract infection [30]. In the same study, 27 cats (61%) had a urinary albumin/creatinine ratio (UAC) greater than 30 mg/g, with 18% having a ratio greater than 82 mg/g, which are cutoff points representing established limits for albumin excretion. The severity of the proteinuria decreased in most cats after treatment. Neither an elevated UPC nor an elevated UAC was predictive of the development of renal failure, and their pathogenic significance remains unclear.

Urinary corticoid/creatinine ratios are significantly higher in untreated hyperthyroid cats, with 15 (47%) of 32 cats having concentrations greater than the upper limit of the reference range (42.0×10^{-6}) [31]. In these cats, values reached up to four times this upper limit and presumably reflect increased metabolic clearance of cortisol and activation of the hypothalamic-pituitary-adrenal axis by the disease. Therefore, elevated urinary corticoid/creatinine ratios should be interpreted with caution, and hyperthyroidism should be ruled out if hyperadrenocorticism is being considered.

DEFINITIVE DIAGNOSTIC TESTS
The diagnosis of hyperthyroidism is confirmed by the demonstration of increased thyroidal radioisotope uptake or circulating concentrations of the thyroid hormones.

Thyroidal Radioisotope Uptake
Uptake of radioactive iodine isotopes (^{131}I or ^{123}I) and technetium Tc 99m as pertechnetate (^{99m}TcO$_4^-$) is increased in hyperthyroid cats [3,32–35]. The radioactive iodine isotopes and pertechnetate are trapped and concentrated within the thyroid gland. Unlike ^{131}I and ^{123}I, however, pertechnetate is not organically bound to thyroglobulin or stored within the thyroid gland. The relatively long half-life, higher γ-energy, and β-emission of ^{131}I and the higher expense of ^{123}I make their routine use in feline thyroid scintigraphy uncommon. Because of availability, lower cost, and superior image quality, pertechnetate is preferred.

Percentage thyroid uptake of pertechnetate is routinely measured between 20 and 60 minutes after intravenous injection [32,33]. Values are significantly higher in hyperthyroid cats compared with healthy cats and correlate well with circulating thyroid hormone concentrations [36]. Calculation of the percentage uptake of pertechnetate is not routinely performed, however, because it requires accurate assessment of the injected dose together with correction for background radioactivity. Similar if not more diagnostically efficient results are obtained if the thyroid/salivary (T/S) ratio is calculated, and this provides the best correlation with serum total T_4 concentrations [36]. It is generally accepted that the T/S ratio in healthy cats is <1 [36], although values as high as 1.66 have been reported [37], indicating the need for validation in individual centers. For assessment of the T/S ratio, pertechnetate may be administered subcutaneously or intravenously [38].

It is clear that quantitative thyroid imaging is not required for the diagnosis of hyperthyroidism in most cats. Theoretically, however, it could provide important diagnostic information in some cats. Nonthyroidal illness likely exerts less effect on the results of scintigraphy than basal total T_4 concentration and could potentially exclude hyperthyroidism in those few euthyroid cats with an elevated free T_4 concentration. In addition, results of scintigraphy may be abnormal in cats with early hyperthyroidism and reference range circulating thyroid hormone concentrations. In a preliminary study of 6 occult hyperthyroid cats, the diagnostic value of pertechnetate scans was considered greater than that of thyroid hormone measurements [39]. In a further study of 23 cats with palpable thyroid nodules and reference range circulating total T_4 values,

16 were diagnosed as hyperthyroid on the basis of scintigraphy (T/S ratio >1), and these cats had, as a group, significantly higher serum free T_4 concentrations than those with a normal T/S ratio [40].

Thyroid scintigraphy is expensive, requiring access to sophisticated equipment, and is not without limitations as a diagnostic tool. One study demonstrated positive scintigraphy results in 14 cats in which there was a clinical suspicion of hyperthyroidism but reference range serum total T_4 concentrations [41]. Three of these cats exhibited >60% T_4 stimulation after administration of thyrotropin-releasing hormone (TRH), however, and, subsequently, no histopathologic evidence of thyroid disease was found. Therefore, the specificity of thyroid scintigraphy warrants further investigation.

Methimazole administration may also affect scintigraphy findings. Methimazole and other related drugs inhibit the thyroid peroxidase enzyme, reducing organification of iodine and inhibiting coupling of iodotyrosines. Although methimazole exerts no direct effect on thyroidal iodide uptake, a reduction in T_4 and a consequent elevation in the thyroid-stimulating hormone (TSH) concentration are potentially associated with increased iodide uptake. One study of five healthy cats showed a significant increase in the percentage uptake of pertechnetate and the T/S ratio at 20 minutes after 3 weeks of methimazole therapy to maximal T_4 suppression, from a mean of 0.23% to 1.05% and 0.81 to 1.36, respectively [42]. A similar study in 19 hyperthyroid cats showed no significant change in either of these parameters after a minimum of 30 days of methimazole therapy [43]. At that time, all cats had total T_4 concentrations less than 51.5 nmol/L but circulating TSH concentrations remained suppressed, suggesting that the mechanism of increased trapping had not yet been activated. Two of the cats with unilateral disease seemed to have bilateral disease after treatment, possibly reflecting increased thyroidal radioisotope uptake, and in these cats, this diagnosis was supported by the greatest increase in TSH concentrations. Therefore, recent administration of methimazole must be considered during quantitative interpretation of thyroid scintigraphy.

Radioactive iodine is also affected by methimazole therapy, with mean 8-hour uptake values representing iodide trapping, increasing from a mean of 2.1% to 4.1% after 3 weeks of therapy [42]. Interestingly, the 24-hour uptake in this same group fell from a mean of 7.04% to 5.16%, presumably reflecting methimazole-induced reduction in organification and coupling within the thyroid gland. Withdrawal of methimazole was associated with markedly increased 8- and 24-hour uptake values peaking between 4 and 9 days after cessation of therapy and continuing out to 24 days after withdrawal. This supports a short-term rebound effect that may enhance the efficacy of radioactive iodine therapy but has implications when used as a diagnostic test in cats previously treated with methimazole.

Qualitative scintigraphic imaging, conversely, remains a useful procedure in hyperthyroid cats to determine unilateral or bilateral involvement, alterations in the position of thyroid lobes, the site of hyperfunctioning accessory or ectopic thyroid tissue, or distant metastases from a functioning thyroid carcinoma

[44]. Care must be taken in qualitative assessment of lobe involvement in cats previously treated with methimazole, however [43].

Circulating Thyroid Hormone Concentrations

The elevated circulating thyroid hormone concentration remains the biochemical hallmark of hyperthyroidism. Several reports have evaluated the efficacy of total T_4, total T_3, and free T_4 in confirming a diagnosis of hyperthyroidism. Measurement of TSH, although frequently used in people and long awaited in cats, has not been fully evaluated in the diagnosis of feline hyperthyroidism, because a species-specific assay is not yet available.

Basal total thyroid hormone concentration

The basal total T_4 concentration is greater than the reference range in most hyperthyroid cats [3,4,45]. Serum total T_3 values are often concurrently elevated [3,4,45]. Serum total T_3 values are within the reference range in a significant proportion of hyperthyroid cats; however, 4 (3%) of 131 cats [3], 11 (9%) of 122 cats [4], and, more recently, 59 (29%) of 202 cats [2] had a significantly higher percentage than previously described. In the largest study of 917 hyperthyroid cats thus far studied, the serum total T_3 concentration was within the reference range in 307 (33.5%) cases, representing 163 (79.5%) of 205 cats categorized as mildly hyperthyroid with a serum total T_4 concentration less than 65 nmol/L (Fig. 1) [45]. In most other cases, the total T_4 concentration is usually less than 100 nmol/L, and it is likely that the serum total T_3 concentration would increase into the thyrotoxic range if the disorder were allowed to progress untreated. Severe concurrent nonthyroidal illness may play a role in suppressing the T_3 concentration by inhibiting peripheral conversion of T_4 to T_3, as it does in people, although this seems to be a less common phenomenon in cats [4]. It is becoming increasingly recognized that the serum total T_4 concentration may also be within the middle to high end of the reference range (>30 nmol/L) in a significant percentage (up to and exceeding 10%) of hyperthyroid cats, presumably because of earlier diagnosis or sampling a group of mildly affected animals that would not have been tested previously (Fig. 2) [2,45].

Nonspecific fluctuation of thyroid hormones may account for the reference range total T_4 and T_3 values found in hyperthyroid cats. In one study of 14 mildly affected cats, serum total T_4 and total T_3 concentrations were measured hourly for 10 hours and daily for 15 days in 7 of the cats [46]. In both time frames, serum thyroid hormone concentrations fluctuated to a degree exceeding normal assay variation, with greater fluctuation occurring over the 15-day rather than the 10-hour sampling period. Provided that basal thyroid hormone concentrations are only mildly elevated, the degree of fluctuation can result in reference range values. Increased thyroidal production could result in an increased circulating concentration, but because the serum half-life of thyroid hormones is measured in hours, acute decreases presumably reflect fluctuations in binding proteins or other unclear hemodynamic changes. In cats with markedly elevated serum thyroid hormone concentrations, the degree of fluctuation is of little diagnostic significance [46,47].

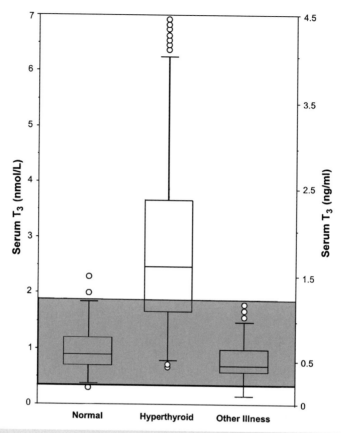

Fig. 1. Box plots of serum T₃ concentrations in 172 clinically normal cats, 917 cats with untreated hyperthyroidism, and 221 cats with nonthyroidal disease (other illness). The box represents the interquartile range (25th–75th percentile range or the middle half of the data). The horizontal bar in the box represents the median value. For each box plot, the T-bars represent the main body of data, which is equal to the range in most instances. Outlying data points are represented by open circles. The shaded area indicates the reference range for the serum T₃ concentration. (*From* Peterson ME, Melian C, Nichols R. Measurement of serum concentrations of free thyroxine, total thyroxine, and total triiodothyronine in cats with hyperthyroidism and cats with nonthyroidal disease. J Am Vet Med Assoc 2001;218:531; with permission).

The presence of concurrent nonthyroidal illness can also affect the circulating total T₄ concentration in hyperthyroid cats. In 494 cats with a variety of nonthyroidal illnesses, 63 had a palpable thyroid nodule and a significantly higher mean (±SD) serum total T₄ concentration of 21.7 (±10.4) nmol/L than the concentration of 12.7 (±8.1) nmol/L in the cats without a palpable thyroid nodule [48]. Subsequently, the serum total T₄ concentration increased into the thyrotoxic range in 4 of these cats, and adenomatous hyperplasia of the thyroid glands was found at necropsy in 2 other cats. In another study of 110 hyperthyroid cats, 39 had a concurrent nonthyroidal illness [49]. These cats

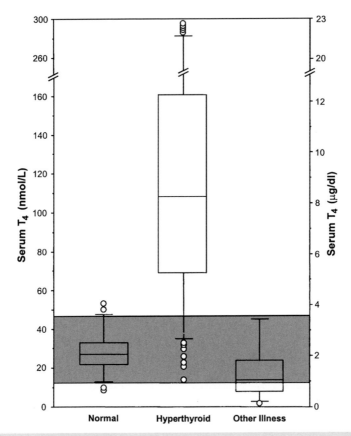

Fig. 2. Box plots of serum total T_4 concentrations from 172 clinically normal cats, 917 cats with untreated hyperthyroidism, and 221 cats with nonthyroidal disease (other illness). See Fig. 1 for key. (*From* Peterson ME, Melian C, Nichols R. Measurement of serum concentrations of free thyroxine, total thyroxine, and total triiodothyronine in cats with hyperthyroidism and cats with nonthyroidal disease. J Am Vet Med Assoc 2001;218:531; with permission.)

had a significantly lower serum total T_4 concentration than the hyperthyroid cats without a concurrent illness. In total, a reference range serum total T_4 concentration was found in 14 (13%) cats, but this only represented 3 (4%) of 71 cats without concurrent disease compared with 11 (28%) of 39 cats with such disorders. In a larger study of 917 hyperthyroid cats, a concurrent illness was identified in 17 (22%) of 80 cats with mild hyperthyroidism and a reference range serum total T_4 concentration [45]. In 12 of these cats, the serum total T_4 concentration was within the middle to high end of the reference range (>30 nmol/L), whereas values were within the middle to low end of the reference range in the remaining 5 cats, but these had the most severe concurrent illnesses. The mechanisms remain unclear but are more likely to involve changes in protein binding or metabolism rather than any effect on the hypothalamic-pituitary-thyroid axis [8,48]. Reference range values resulting from the suppressive effect of nonthyroidal disease are only expected in cats with early or mild hyperthyroidism, because the degree of suppression has little diagnostic significance in hyperthyroid cats with a markedly elevated serum total T_4 concentration [4,48,49]. Despite the possibility of encountering middle to high reference range values in mildly hyperthyroid cats with concurrent disease, they usually do not pose a diagnostic dilemma, because serum total T_4 concentrations also decline in euthyroid individuals with similar illnesses [45,48,50]. In euthyroid cats, the degree of suppression is correlated with the severity rather than with the type of illness and can be used as a prognostic indicator (Figs. 3 and 4) [45,48,50]. Low total T_4 values are only expected in

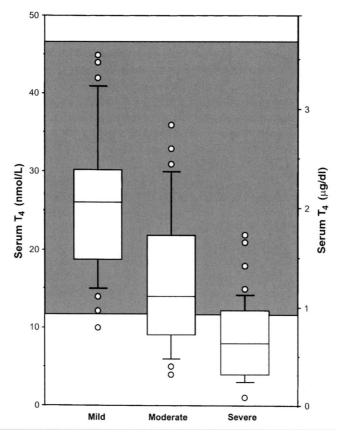

Fig. 3. Box plots of serum total T_4 concentrations from 221 cats with nonthyroidal disease, grouped according to severity of illness. Of the 221 cats, 65 had mild disease, 83 had moderate disease, and 73 had severe disease. See Fig. 1 for key. (*From* Peterson ME, Melian C, Nichols R. Measurement of serum concentrations of free thyroxine, total thyroxine, and total triiodothyronine in cats with hyperthyroidism and cats with nonthyroidal disease. J Am Vet Med Assoc 2001;218:533; with permission.)

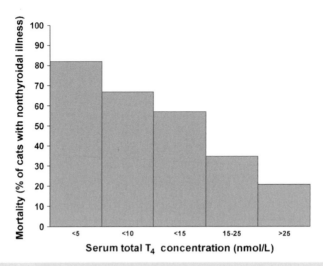

Fig. 4. Relation between mortality and serum total T$_4$ concentration in 98 cats with nonthyroidal illness. (*From* Mooney CT, Little CJ, Macrae AW. Effect of illness not associated with the thyroid gland on serum total and free thyroxine concentrations in cats. J Am Vet Med Assoc 1996;208:2005; with permission.)

hyperthyroid cats with the most severe concurrent disorders, and in these cases, other criteria, particularly detection of a palpable thyroid nodule, may indicate the need to investigate hyperthyroidism further [45].

Despite the number of drugs that are known to affect circulating thyroid hormone concentrations in people and dogs, there are few reports concerning such an effect in hyperthyroid cats. In eight hyperthyroid cats treated with an immunosuppressive dose of prednisolone administered intramuscularly, there was no significant decrease in the serum total T$_4$ concentration when assessed 24 hours later [51]. The effects of other drugs have not yet been evaluated.

Free thyroxine concentration
In human thyrotoxicosis, assessment of free T$_4$ is considered a better diagnostic test for hyperthyroidism because it is less affected by nonthyroidal factors than is total T$_4$ and provides a more accurate reflection of thyroid status. Notably, when the serum total T$_4$ concentration is increased, the concentration of free T$_4$ is disproportionately increased, and this may be related, in part, to relative saturation of binding proteins by T$_4$ and a subnormal concentration of the primary binding proteins. In addition, the serum free T$_4$ concentration remains elevated in hyperthyroid patients with nonthyroidal illnesses when the total T$_4$ concentration is suppressed into the reference range. Measurement of the free T$_4$ concentration has recently been evaluated in hyperthyroid cats and seems to be a useful diagnostic test, particularly in cats with a reference range serum total T$_4$ concentration (Fig. 5) [45]. The serum free T$_4$ concentration was elevated in 903 (98.5%) of 917 hyperthyroid cats, whereas the

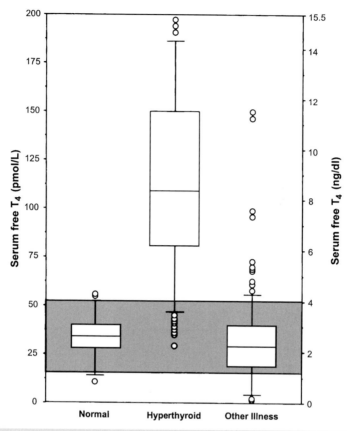

Fig. 5. Box plots of serum free T_4 concentrations in 172 clinically normal cats, 917 cats with untreated hyperthyroidism, and 221 cats with nonthyroidal disease (other illness). See Fig. 1 for key. (*From* Peterson ME, Melian C, Nichols R. Measurement of serum concentrations of free thyroxine, total thyroxine, and total triiodothyronine in cats with hyperthyroidism and cats with nonthyroidal disease. J Am Vet Med Assoc 2001;218:532; with permission.)

corresponding serum total T_4 concentration was elevated in 837 (91.3%) cases. In all cats with a markedly elevated serum total T_4 concentration, the free T_4 concentration was concurrently elevated, adding little diagnostic information to that already obtained. In 205 of these cats categorized as mildly hyperthyroid with or without a concurrent illness, however, the serum free and total T_4 concentrations were elevated in 191 (93.2%) and 125 (61%) cases, respectively (Fig. 6). The increased diagnostic sensitivity of free T_4 measurement is complicated by a loss of specificity, because 6% to 12% of sick euthyroid cats have elevated concentrations [45,50]. The specificity of free T_4 measurement may be substantially lower in certain disease states. In one study comparing free T_4 concentrations in cats with chronic renal failure and hyperthyroidism (n = 16) and hyperthyroidism alone (n = 16), free T_4 concentrations were

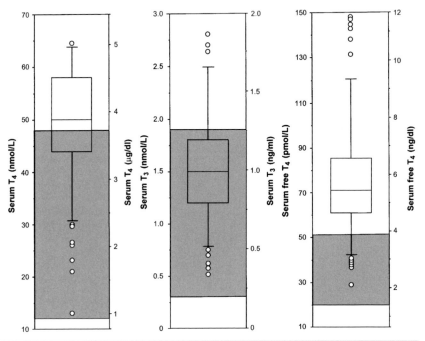

Fig. 6. Box plots of serum total T_4, T_3, and free T_4 concentrations in 205 cats with mild hyperthyroidism (defined as total T_4 concentration <66 nmol/L). See Fig. 1 for key. (*From* Peterson ME, Melian C, Nichols R. Measurement of serum concentrations of free thyroxine, total thyroxine, and total triiodothyronine in cats with hyperthyroidism and cats with nonthyroidal disease. J Am Vet Med Assoc 2001;218:533; with permission.)

falsely elevated in 31% of the euthyroid cats [52]. The serum free T_4 concentration should therefore be interpreted with caution if used as the sole diagnostic criterion for confirmation of hyperthyroidism. More reliable information is obtained when it is interpreted together with the serum total T_4 concentration. A middle to high reference range total T_4 concentration and an elevated free T_4 concentration are consistent with hyperthyroidism [45]. By contrast, a low total T_4 value and elevated free T_4 value are usually associated with nonthyroidal illness [45,50].

Feline thyroid-stimulating hormone

In human beings, measurement of the circulating TSH concentration is generally used as a first-line discriminatory test of thyroid function. Commercially available assays are second or third generation, with a functional sensitivity up to 30 times lower than the lower limit of the reference range. In addition, there is a log-linear negative feedback relation between free T_4 and TSH, such that marked changes in TSH concentration can be induced by relatively small changes in free T_4. To date, a feline-specific TSH assay has not been developed commercially, and most studies have focused on using assays designed for canine or human use.

One study has investigated the use of a TSH assay developed for use in dogs for diagnosing hyperthyroidism in cats [53]. The serum TSH concentration was measured in a group of 17 cats with chronic renal failure alone and in 17 cats with hyperthyroidism and renal failure. All the hyperthyroid cats had TSH concentrations at or lower than the lower limit of detection of the canine assay (0.03 ng/mL), whereas 15 of the cats with chronic renal failure had detectable TSH concentrations, with a median of 0.05 ng/mL. Thus, although canine TSH values are statistically lower in hyperthyroid cats compared with euthyroid cats, the assay, because of its relatively high sensitivity, is not helpful in confirming hyperthyroidism in individual cats. Its only value may be in eliminating hyperthyroidism in cats with readily detectable concentrations.

A separate study compared 12 euthyroid cats and 22 hyperthyroid cats using an assay developed for measuring human TSH concentration [54]. The median circulating TSH concentration of 0.14 mIU/L in euthyroid cats was higher than that of 0 mIU/L in hyperthyroid cats. The validity of measuring feline TSH using a human assay is currently unknown, however.

Recently, feline TSH has been expressed and purified in vitro, allowing future development to standardize and improve clinical assays for feline TSH. The development of such an assay would also be invaluable in studies of the pathogenesis of this disorder in cats [55,56].

Dynamic Thyroid Function Tests

Because of the possibility of finding reference range serum thyroid hormone concentrations in hyperthyroid cats, several additional diagnostic tests have been suggested to be useful in confirming a diagnosis (Table 1). In most cases, however, the serum total T_4 concentration increases into the thyrotoxic range if retested several weeks later, obviating the need for further diagnostic tests. Such tests may be required in some cats with clinical signs suggestive of hyperthyroidism, however, when a repeated serum total T_4 concentration remains equivocal and a serum free T_4 measurement is unavailable or unhelpful.

Thyroid-stimulating hormone response test

In an early study, it was suggested that the TSH response test, utilizing bovine TSH, was useful in confirming a diagnosis of hyperthyroidism [3]. In 11 hyperthyroid cats, the mean serum post-TSH total T_4 concentration of 144.1 nmol/L was not significantly different from the mean basal concentration of 127.4 nmol/L, suggesting that the thyroid glands in these cats secrete thyroid hormones independently of TSH control or are producing T_4 at a maximal rate with minimal reserve capacity. Nevertheless, in a larger study of 40 hyperthyroid cats, although the overall limited T_4 response to TSH stimulation was confirmed, it was shown that hyperthyroid cats with equivocal basal total T_4 concentrations exhibit a response indistinguishable from that in healthy cats [57]. The negative correlation between the relative increment and the baseline total T_4 suggests that the abnormal thyroid glands do retain the ability to

Table 1
Dynamic thyroid function tests in cats

	T_3 suppression	TSH response test		TRH response test
Drug	Liothyronine	Bovine TSH	Human TSH	TRH
Dose	15–25 μg every 8 hours for 7 doses	0.5 IU/kg	0.025–0.2 mg per cat	0.1 mg/kg
Route	Oral	Intravenous	Intravenous	Intravenous
Sampling times	0 and 2–4 hours after last dose	0 and 6 hours	1 and 6–8 hours	0 and 4 hours
Assay	Total T_4 (and total T_3 to check compliance/absorption)	Total T_4	Total T_4	Total T_4
Interpretation				
Euthyroidism	<20 nmol/L with >50% suppression	100% increase	100% increase	>60% increase
Hyperthyroidism	>20 nmol/L ± <35% suppression	Minimal/no increase	Not determined	<50% increase

Abbreviations: T_3, triiodothyronine; T_4, thyroxine; TRH, thyrotropin-releasing hormone; TSH, thyroid-stimulating hormone.

respond to TSH but are producing T_4 at maximal rates. Presumably, hyperthyroid cats with the lowest basal total T_4 concentrations have the greatest potential to respond to TSH, although it has been suggested that this response may be related to stimulation of normal thyroid tissue often found within hyperplastic glands [57]. Measurement of the serum total T_3 concentration adds little diagnostic information because of the more variable response found in healthy and hyperthyroid individuals.

Bovine TSH is no longer available as a pharmaceutic preparation. A recent study evaluating the use of recombinant human TSH (rhTSH) for this test in seven euthyroid cats suggested that this was a safe alternative capable of inducing similar T_4 stimulation [58]. Concurrent measurement of free T_4 was also evaluated but added little additional information. Given the expense of rhTSH, this test has limitations in the evaluation of hyperthyroidism in cats.

Thyrotropin-releasing hormone response test
There is a limited total T_4 response to TRH stimulation in hyperthyroid cats. In one study, there was a significant increase in the mean serum total T_4 concentration after TRH administration in 31 healthy cats, 35 mild to moderate hyperthyroid cats, and 15 cats with nonthyroidal illnesses [59]. The percentage increase in total T_4 was considerably less in the hyperthyroid cats compared

with healthy cats and those with other diseases, however. From the results of this study, it was suggested that a relative increase in total T_4 of less than 50% is consistent with mild hyperthyroidism, a value greater than 60% is suggestive of euthyroidism, and values between 50% and 60% remain equivocal. Discriminant analysis, taking into account the basal and absolute difference between basal and post-TRH total T_4 concentrations, can also be used to distinguish hyperthyroidism from euthyroidism. Similar to the TSH response test, measurement of the total T_3 concentration was considered unhelpful because of the greater variability in response within and between groups. A recent study evaluated the ability of the TRH response test to differentiate between hyperthyroid and severely sick euthyroid cats [60]. Of the 36 critically ill cats reported, 22 had clinical and histopathologic evidence of hyperthyroidism, whereas hyperthyroidism was not suspected in the remaining 14 animals. Of these 14 euthyroid cats, 6 had serum total T_4 increases less than 50% of baseline, 2 had increases between 50% and 60%, and 6 had increases greater than 60% after TRH administration. Although 18 of the hyperthyroid cats had a total T_4 increase less than 50% of baseline, 2 had increases between 50% and 60% and 2 had increases greater than 60%. The authors concluded that it was not possible to use this test to differentiate between hyperthyroid cats and those with severe nonthyroidal illness. Adverse reactions to TRH administration seem to be common and include vomiting, excessive salivation, tachypnea, and defecation. These reactions are transient, develop within a few minutes of TRH administration, and usually resolve by the end of the 4-hour test.

Triiodothyronine suppression test

The T_3 suppression test relies on the ability of administered liothyronine, through negative feedback, to decrease T_4 production by the thyroid gland. In hyperthyroidism, because excess circulating thyroid hormone concentrations have already suppressed TSH production and secretion, additional T_3 has minimal effect on T_4 production. Therefore, the serum total T_4 concentration remains significantly higher after liothyronine administration in hyperthyroid compared with euthyroid (healthy and sick) cats, and the percentage decrease is consequently significantly lower [61,62]. Although individual laboratories vary, as a general guideline, the postliothyronine serum total T_4 concentration tends to be greater than 20 nmol/L in hyperthyroid cats and less than 20 nmol/L in euthyroid cats. There is a greater overlap of results in hyperthyroid and euthyroid cats when the percentage change in total T_4 is calculated. Nevertheless, suppression of 50% or more is consistent with euthyroidism, whereas hyperthyroid cats rarely have values exceeding 35%. Discriminant analysis can also be applied to the results to identify those variables providing the best diagnostic sensitivity and specificity, but the overall performance of the test tends to be unaffected [62,63]. Although the T_3 suppression test is capable of diagnosing hyperthyroidism, some authors suggest that it is most useful in confirming euthyroidism and ruling out hyperthyroidism [61]. Unlike the TRH response test, it is not associated with any adverse reactions. It is a relatively prolonged test, however, and highly depends on good owner compliance in reliably administering liothyronine tablets and adequate gastrointestinal absorption, necessitating confirmation by before and after serum total T_3 measurement [61,63].

ADDITIONAL DIAGNOSTIC TESTS

Ultrasonography has been used to document the dimensions and volume of the thyroid glands in euthyroid and hyperthyroid cats [64]. Mean dimensions of 20.4 mm × 2.5 mm × 3.2 mm and 21.1 mm × 6.7 mm × 6.8 mm (length × width × height) and lobar volumes of 85 mm^3 and 578 mm^3 were recorded in euthyroid and hyperthyroid cats, respectively. Eight of the 16 hyperthyroid cats had unilateral disease, which may have affected results in these cases. Ultrasonography had 85.7% agreement with scintigraphy in defining normal and abnormal thyroid lobes. Thyroid ultrasonography is technically demanding and likely to be operator dependent, however.

A more recent study used helical CT to determine the dimensions and volume of thyroid tissue in clinically healthy cats [65]. The mean thyroid dimensions were 16.5 mm × 2.0 mm × 4.31 mm (length × width × height) as determined by transverse images, and the mean lobar volume measured 113.75 mm^3. The value of such imaging in the diagnosis of hyperthyroidism remains undocumented. The cost and availability of such technically demanding imaging techniques make their wide use unlikely, however.

SUMMARY

Hyperthyroidism remains a common endocrine disorder of cats. Although relatively easy to diagnose in classically presenting cats, the increased frequency of testing cats with early or mild disease has had significant implications for the diagnostic performance of many of the routine tests currently used. Further advances in the etiopathogenesis and earlier diagnosis are only likely with the advent of a species-specific feline TSH assay.

References

[1] Gordon JM, Ehrhart EJ, Sisson DD, et al. Juvenile hyperthyroidism in a cat. J Am Anim Hosp Assoc 2003;39:67–71.

[2] Broussard JD, Peterson ME, Fox PR. Changes in clinical and laboratory findings in cats with hyperthyroidism from 1983 to 1993. J Am Vet Med Assoc 1995;206:302–5.

[3] Peterson ME, Kintzer PP, Cavanagh PG, et al. Feline hyperthyroidism: pretreatment clinical and laboratory evaluation of 131 cases. J Am Vet Med Assoc 1983;183:103–10.

[4] Thoday KL, Mooney CT. Historical, clinical and laboratory features of 126 hyperthyroid cats. Vet Rec 1992;131:257–64.

[5] Christopher MM. Relation of endogenous Heinz bodies to disease and anemia in cats: 120 cases (1978–1987). J Am Vet Med Assoc 1989;194:1089–95.

[6] Sullivan P, Gompf R, Schmeitzel L, et al. Altered platelet indices in dogs with hypothyroidism and cats with hyperthyroidism. Am J Vet Res 1993;54:2004–9.

[7] Foster DJ, Thoday KL. Tissue sources of serum alkaline phosphatase in 34 hyperthyroid cats: a qualitative and quantitative study. Res Vet Sci 2000;68:89–94.

[8] Mooney C, Thoday KL, Doxey DL. Carbimazole therapy of feline hyperthyroidism. J Small Anim Pract 1992;33:228–35.

[9] Feldman EC, Nelson RW. Feline hyperthyroidism (thyrotoxicosis). In: Feldman EC, Nelson RW, editors. Canine and feline endocrinology and reproduction. St. Louis (MO): Saunders; 2004. p. 152–218.

[10] Archer FJ, Taylor SM. Alkaline phosphatase bone isoenzyme and osteocalcin in the serum of hyperthyroid cats. Can Vet J 1996;37:735–9.

[11] Horney BS, Farmer AJ, Honor DJ, et al. Agarose gel electrophoresis of alkaline phosphatase isoenzymes in the serum of hyperthyroid cats. Vet Clin Pathol 1994;23:98–102.

[12] Barber PJ, Elliott J. Study of calcium homeostasis in feline hyperthyroidism. J Small Anim Pract 1996;37:575–82.

[13] Slater LA, Jackson B, Stevens KB, et al. Evaluation of bone cell activity in four hyperthyroid cats before and after treatment with iodine-131 [abstract]. Presented at the Proceedings of the British Small Animal Veterinary Association. Birmingham (UK), April 1–4, 2004. p. 522.

[14] Declercq J, Bhatti S. Calcinosis involving multiple paws in a cat with chronic renal failure and in a cat with hyperthyroidism. Vet Dermatol 2005;16:74–8.

[15] Abboud B, Sleilaty G, Mansour E, et al. Prevalence and risk factors for primary hyperparathyroidism in hyperthyroid patients. Head Neck 2006;28:420–6.

[16] Adams WH, Daniel GB, Legendre AM. Investigation of the effects of hyperthyroidism on renal function in the cat. Can J Vet Res 1997;61:53–6.

[17] Adams WH, Daniel GB, Legendre AM, et al. Changes in renal function in cats following treatment of hyperthyroidism using ^{131}I. Vet Radiol Ultrasound 1997;38:231–8.

[18] Becker TJ, Graves TK, Kruger JM, et al. Effects of methimazole on renal function in cats with hyperthyroidism. J Am Anim Hosp Assoc 2000;36:215–23.

[19] DiBartola SP, Broome MR, Stein BS, et al. Effect of treatment of hyperthyroidism on renal function in cats. J Am Vet Med Assoc 1996;208:875–8.

[20] Graves TK, Olivier NB, Nachreiner RF, et al. Changes in renal function associated with treatment of hyperthyroidism in cats. Am J Vet Res 1994;55:1745–9.

[21] Milner RJ, Channell CD, Levy JK, et al. Survival times for cats with hyperthyroidism treated with iodine 131, methimazole, or both: 167 cases (1996–2003). J Am Vet Med Assoc 2006;228:559–63.

[22] Nemzek JA, Kruger JM, Walshaw R, et al. Acute onset of hypokalemia and muscular weakness in four hyperthyroid cats. J Am Vet Med Assoc 1994;205:65–8.

[23] Gilroy CV, Horney BS, Burton SA, et al. Evaluation of ionized and total serum magnesium concentrations in hyperthyroid cats. Can J Vet Res 2006;70:137–42.

[24] Hoenig M, Ferguson DC. Impairment of glucose tolerance in hyperthyroid cats. J Endocrinol 1989;121:249–51.

[25] Graham PA, Mooney CT, Murray M. Serum fructosamine concentrations in hyperthyroid cats. Res Vet Sci 1999;67:171–5.

[26] Reusch CE, Tomsa K. Serum fructosamine concentration in cats with overt hyperthyroidism. J Am Vet Med Assoc 1999;215:1297–300.

[27] Connolly DJ, Guitian J, Boswood A, et al. Serum troponin I levels in hyperthyroid cats before and after treatment with radioactive iodine. J Feline Med Surg 2005;7: 289–300.

[28] Randolph JF, DeMarco J, Center SA, et al. Prothrombin, activated partial thromboplastin, and proteins induced by vitamin K absence or antagonists clotting times in 20 hyperthyroid cats before and after methimazole treatment. J Vet Intern Med 2006;14:56–9.

[29] Steiner JM, Petersen MA, Ruaux CG, et al. Serum folate and cobalamin concentrations in cats with hyperthyroidism. [abstract]. J Vet Intern Med 2005;19:474.

[30] Syme HM, Elliott J. Prevalence and significance of proteinuria in cats with hyperthyroidism [abstract]. Presented at the Proceedings of the British Small Animal Veterinary Association. Birmingham (UK), April 3–6, 2003. p. 533.

[31] de Lange MS, Galac S, Trip MRJ, et al. High urinary corticoid/creatinine ratios in cats with hyperthyroidism. J Vet Intern Med 2004;18:152–5.

[32] Mooney CT, Thoday KL, Nicoll JJ, et al. Qualitative and quantitative thyroid imaging in feline hyperthyroidism using technetium-99m as pertechnetate. Vet Radiol Ultrasound 1992;33: 313–20.

[33] Nap AM, Pollak YW, van den Brom WE, et al. Quantitative aspects of thyroid scintigraphy with pertechnetate ($^{99m}TcO_4$-) in cats. J Vet Intern Med 1994;8:302–3.

[34] Peterson ME. Feline hyperthyroidism. Vet Clin North Am Small Anim Pract 1984;14: 809–26.

[35] Sjollema BE, Pollak YW, van den Brom WE, et al. Thyroidal radioiodine uptake in hyperthyroid cats. Vet Q 1989;11:165–70.

[36] Daniel GB, Sharp DS, Nieckarz JA, et al. Quantitative thyroid scintigraphy as a predictor of serum thyroxin concentration in normal and hyperthyroid cats. Vet Radiol Ultrasound 2002;43:374–82.

[37] Henrikson TD, Armbrust LJ, Hoskinson JJ, et al. Thyroid to salivary ratios determined by technetium-99m pertechnetate imaging in thirty-two euthyroid cats. Vet Radiol Ultrasound 2005;46:521–3.

[38] Page RB, Scrivani PV, Dykes NL, et al. Accuracy of increased thyroid activity during pertechnetate scintigraphy by subcutaneous injection for diagnosing hyperthyroidism in cats. Vet Radiol Ultrasound 2005;47:206–11.

[39] Smith TA, Bruyette DS, Hoskinson JJ, et al. Total thyroxine, free thyroxine, pertechnetate scan, and T3 suppression test results in cats with occult hyperthyroidism [abstract]. J Vet Intern Med 1996;10:185.

[40] Marsolais ME, Mott J, Berry CR. Diagnosis of feline hyperthyroidism using thyroid scintigraphy [abstract]. J Vet Intern Med 2003;17:393.

[41] Tomsa K, Hardeggar R, Glaus T, et al. ^{99m}Tc-pertechnetate scintigraphy in hyperthyroid cats with normal serum thyroxine concentrations [abstract]. J Vet Intern Med 2001;15:299.

[42] Nieckarz JA, Daniel GB. The effect of methimazole on thyroid uptake of pertechnetate and radioiodine in normal cats. Vet Radiol Ultrasound 2001;42:448–57.

[43] Fischetti AJ, Drost WT, DiBartola SP, et al. Effects of methimazole on thyroid gland uptake of ^{99m}TC-pertechnetate in 19 hyperthyroid cats. Vet Radiol Ultrasound 2005;46:267–72.

[44] Peterson ME, Becker DV. Radionuclide thyroid imaging in 135 cats with hyperthyroidism. Vet Radiol Ultrasound 1984;25:23–7.

[45] Peterson ME, Melian C, Nichols R. Measurement of serum concentrations of free thyroxine, total thyroxine, and total triiodothyronine in cats with hyperthyroidism and cats with nonthyroidal disease. J Am Vet Med Assoc 2001;218:529–36.

[46] Peterson ME, Graves TK, Cavanagh I. Serum thyroid hormone concentrations fluctuate in cats with hyperthyroidism. J Vet Intern Med 1987;1:142–6.

[47] Broome MR, Feldman EC, Turrel JM. Serial determination of thyroxine concentrations in hyperthyroid cats. J Am Vet Med Assoc 1988;192:49–51.

[48] Peterson ME, Gamble DA. Effect of nonthyroidal illness on serum thyroxine concentrations in cats: 494 cases. J Am Vet Med Assoc 1988;197:1203–8.

[49] McLoughlin MA, DiBartola SP, Birchard SJ, et al. Influence of systemic nonthyroidal illness on serum concentration of thyroxine in hyperthyroid cats. J Am Anim Hosp Assoc 1993;29:227–34.

[50] Mooney CT, Little CJ, Macrae AW. Effect of illness not associated with the thyroid gland on serum total and free thyroxine concentrations in cats. J Am Vet Med Assoc 1996;208:2004–8.

[51] Peterson ME, Ferguson DC. Effect of glucorticoids on thyroid function in normal cats and cats with hyperthyroidism [abstract]. J Vet Intern Med 1989;3:123.

[52] Syme HM, Elliott J, Dixon RM. Evaluation of free thyroxine measurement for the diagnosis of hyperthyroidism in cats with chronic renal failure [abstract]. J Vet Intern Med 2002;16:633.

[53] Moore KL, Syme H, Groves E, et al. Use of endogenous thyroid stimulating hormone measurement to diagnose hyperthyroidism in cats with chronic renal failure [abstract]. Presented at the Proceedings of the British Small Animal Veterinary Association. Birmingham (UK), April 1–4, 2004. p. 521.

[54] Otero T, Archer J, Billings H, et al. Serum TSH in hyperthyroid cats pre- and post-therapy [abstract]. Presented at the Proceedings of European Congress of Veterinary Internal Medicine–Companion Animals/European Society of Veterinary Internal Medicine. Munich (Germany), September 19–23, 2002. p. 173.

[55] Rayalam S, Eizenstat LD, Hoenig M, et al. Cloning and sequencing of feline thyrotropin (fTSH): heterodimeric and yoked constructs. Domest Anim Endocrinol 2006;30:203–17.

[56] Rayalam S, Eizenstat LD, Davis RR, et al. Expression and purification of feline thyrotropin (fTSH): Immunological detection and bioactivity of heterodimeric and yoked glycoproteins. Domest Anim Endocrinol 2006;30:185–202.

[57] Mooney CT, Thoday KL, Doxey DL. Serum thyroxine and triiodothyronine responses of hyperthyroid cats to thyrotropin. Am J Vet Res 1996;57:987–91.

[58] Stegeman JR, Graham PA, Hauptman JG. Use of recombinant human thyroid-stimulating hormone for thyrotropin-stimulation testing of euthyroid cats. Am J Vet Res 2003;64:149–52.

[59] Peterson ME, Broussard JD, Gamble DA. Use of the thyrotropin releasing hormone stimulation test to diagnose mild hyperthyroidism in cats. J Vet Intern Med 1994;8:279–86.

[60] Tomsa K, Glaus TM, Kacl GM, et al. Thyrotropin-releasing hormone stimulation test to assess thyroid function in severely sick cats. J Vet Intern Med 2001;15:89–93.

[61] Peterson ME, Graves TK, Gamble DA. Triiodothyronine (T3) suppression test. An aid in the diagnosis of mild hyperthyroidism in cats. J Vet Intern Med 1990;4:233–8.

[62] Refsal KR, Nachreiner RF, Stein BE, et al. Use of the triiodothyronine suppression test for diagnosis of hyperthyroidism in ill cats that have serum concentration of iodothyronines within normal range. J Am Vet Med Assoc 1991;199:1594–601.

[63] Peterson ME, Randolph JF, Mooney CT. Endocrine diseases. In: Sherding RG, editor. 2nd edition, The cat. Diseases and clinical management, vol. 2. New York: Churchill Livingstone; 1984. p. 1403–506.

[64] Wisner ER, Theon AP, Nyland TG, et al. Ultrasonographic examination of the thyroid gland of hyperthyroid cats: comparison to $^{99m}TcO_4$- scintigraphy. Vet Radiol Ultrasound 1994;35:53–8.

[65] Drost WT, Mattoon JS, Weisbrode SE. Use of helical computed tomography for measurement of thyroid glands in clinically normal cats. Am J Vet Res 2006;67:467–71.

Vet Clin Small Anim 37 (2007) 693–708

VETERINARY CLINICS
SMALL ANIMAL PRACTICE

Calcium Homeostasis in Thyroid Disease in Dogs and Cats

Patricia A. Schenck, DVM, PhD

Diagnostic Center for Population and Animal Health, Department of Pathobiology and Diagnostic Investigation, Endocrine Diagnostic Section, Michigan State University, 4125 Beaumont Road, Lansing, MI 48910, USA

H yperthyroidism is the most common endocrine disorder of cats, and hypothyroidism is the most common endocrine disorder of dogs (Fig. 1). Relations between thyroid disorders and calcium metabolism, particularly the effects on bone, have been the subject of many studies in human medicine. Little is known regarding the effects of hyperthyroidism, hypothyroidism, or treatment of these disorders on calcium metabolism in the dog or cat, however, especially any potential effects on bone.

REVIEW OF CALCIUM METABOLISM

Regulation of serum calcium concentration requires the integrated actions of parathyroid hormone (PTH), vitamin D metabolites, and calcitonin. PTH and calcitriol (1,25-dihydroxyvitamin D_3) are the main regulators of calcium homeostasis [1], and the intestine, kidney, and bone are the major target organs involved. The interactions of calcium regulatory hormones allow conservation of calcium by renal tubular reabsorption, increased intestinal absorption of calcium, and internal redistribution of calcium from bone. Normally, more than 98% of the filtered calcium is reabsorbed in the renal tubules. The intestine and kidneys are the major regulators of calcium balance in health, but bone provides a major supply of calcium and phosphorus when intestinal absorption and renal reabsorption inadequately maintain normal serum calcium concentration. Approximately 99% of body calcium resides in the skeleton and is stored as hydroxyapatite. Bone calcium mobilization is important in the acute regulation of calcium. Less than 1% of skeletal calcium is readily available and arises from the extracellular fluid (ECF) in bone that is present between osteoblasts and osteocytes and bone matrix. Calcium and phosphorus can be mobilized from this ECF compartment, but these stores are rapidly depleted. The osteoblast is critical in limiting the distribution of calcium and phosphate between bone and ECF, and for prolonged release of calcium from bone, there must be activation of osteoclastic bone resorption.

E-mail address: schenck5@msu.edu

0195-5616/07/$ – see front matter
doi:10.1016/j.cvsm.2007.03.007

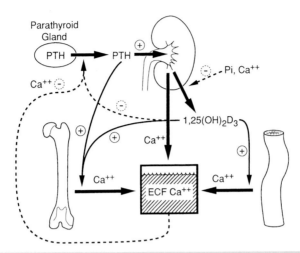

Fig. 1. Regulation of extracellular fluid (ECF) calcium concentration by the effects of parathyroid hormone (PTH) and calcitriol (1,25-dihydroxyvitamin D_3) on the gut, kidney, bone, and parathyroid gland. The principal effect of PTH is to increase ECF calcium concentration by mobilizing calcium from bone, increase tubular calcium reabsorption, and, acting indirectly on the gut, increase calcitriol synthesis. The principal effect of calcitriol is to increase intestinal absorption of calcium, but it also exerts negative regulatory control of PTH synthesis and further calcitriol synthesis. (*Modified from* Habner JF, Rosenblatt M, Pott JT. Parathyroid hormone: biochemical aspects of biosynthesis, secretion, action, and metabolism. Physiol Rev 1984;64:100; with permission.)

Parathyroid Hormone

PTH is synthesized by the chief cells of the parathyroid glands. After secretion, PTH has a short half-life (3–5 minutes) in serum; thus, a steady rate of secretion is necessary to maintain serum PTH concentrations. The most important biologic effects of PTH on calcium are to (1) increase blood extracellular ionized calcium (iCa) concentration; (2) increase tubular reabsorption of calcium, resulting in decreased calcium loss in the urine; (3) increase bone resorption and the numbers of osteoclasts on bone surfaces; and (4) accelerate the formation of calcitriol by the kidney by activating the 1α–hydroxylase in mitochondria of renal epithelial cells in the proximal convoluted tubules.

In bone, the important action of PTH is to mobilize calcium. The immediate effect is to increase the activity of existing bone cells by means of an interaction of PTH with osteoblast receptors. The long-term actions on bone occur by means of increasing osteoclast numbers. PTH can also serve as an anabolic agent in bone and stimulate osteoblastic bone formation [2,3].

Vitamin D Metabolites

Dogs and cats inefficiently photosynthesize vitamin D in their skin; consequently, they depend on vitamin D in their diet [4]. Vitamin D ingested in the diet is absorbed intact from the intestine. Vitamin D–binding protein

Bone turnover is increased in hyperthyroidism. Markers of bone formation, such as bone-specific alkaline phosphatase (BALP) [46,49,51–53], osteocalcin [47,49,51,54], and collagen type C-terminal propeptide (PICP) [49], are increased. Markers of bone resorption, such as urinary hydroxyproline [38,39,47], collagen telopeptide (ICTP) [49], and urinary deoxypyridinoline (DPD) [48,49,54], are also usually increased in hyperthyroidism, indicating a higher rate of bone turnover. There is a significant correlation between thyroid hormones and serum osteocalcin [39,47] and also a significant correlation between thyroid hormones and urinary DPD [51]. With the decrease in PTH and calcitriol, the increase in bone turnover is most likely attributable to the direct actions of thyroid hormones on bone, and the lack of negative effect of TSH by means of the TSH receptor.

Bone mineral density is decreased in hyperthyroidism [49,54–61]. In hyperthyroidism, the decrease in bone mineral density is significant in the femoral neck [58,61], tibia [60], and radius [59], with no difference in bone mineral density noted in the lumbar spine compared with that in euthyroid patients [58]. There is an increased risk of fracture at the time of diagnosis of hyperthyroidism [55], and the risk of hip fracture increases with age at the time of diagnosis of hyperthyroidism [56].

An interesting association has been noted in human patients with thyroid disorders. The prevalence of primary hyperparathyroidism is significantly increased in euthyroid goiter and in thyroid carcinoma as a result of unknown mechanisms [62].

Feline hyperthyroidism has a similar clinical, histologic, and pathologic resemblance to toxic nodular goiter in human beings [63]. Toxic nodular goiter is characterized by thyroid cells that grow and produce thyroid hormones in an autonomous fashion, independent of TSH. A few studies have begun to elucidate the effects of hyperthyroidism on calcium metabolism in cats. In one study, 30 hyperthyroid cats were compared with 38 euthyroid cats. The iCa concentration was significantly lower in hyperthyroid cats as compared with euthyroid cats, but the mean iCa concentration was still within the reference range. There was no significant difference in tCa concentration between groups. Secondary hyperparathyroidism with increased PTH concentration was found in 77% of the hyperthyroid cats. There was no significant difference in calcitriol concentration, but hyperthyroid cats tended to have a higher concentration, which is similar to the concentration of calcitriol noted in human patients with toxic nodular goiter [64]. Serum phosphorus concentration was increased and creatinine concentration was decreased in hyperthyroid cats, as has been seen in hyperthyroid human patients [39].

In a separate study of 29 hyperthyroid cats, 8 had elevated PTH concentrations (P.A. Schenck, DVM, PhD, unpublished data, 2006). Seven of these cats had secondary hyperparathyroidism characterized by a modest elevation in PTH concentration and normocalcemia; 1 cat had elevations of PTH and iCa. Three other cats had mild to moderate ionized hypercalcemia with normal concentration of PTH. There was a significant negative correlation between concentrations of total T_4 and serum iCa and between free T_4 by equilibrium dialysis and serum iCa.

Markers of increased bone turnover have been noted in several feline studies. Nine of 10 hyperthyroid cats in one study exhibited elevated BALP [65]. ALP was also characterized in 34 hyperthyroid cats to assess the occurrence of the bone isoenzyme. BALP was found in 88% of hyperthyroid cats, suggesting osteoblast activation [66]. In 36 hyperthyroid cats, BALP was increased in all cats and osteocalcin was elevated in 44% [67]. Increased serum phosphorus was observed in 35%, 50% had a decrease in serum iCa, and all had normal tCa concentrations.

Calcium Homeostasis After Treatment for Hyperthyroidism

In general, the goals of hyperthyroid treatment in regard to calcium metabolism are to return the serum calcium, PTH, calcitriol, phosphorus, and bone marker turnover concentrations to the normal state as seen in euthyroid patients. When hyperthyroid patients are treated with thyroidectomy, radioiodine therapy, or methimazole, a decrease in serum calcium [68–70] and phosphorus [70–72] concentrations from pretreatment levels has been observed, and levels are similar to those seen in euthyroidism. Concentration of PTH typically increases back to euthyroid levels or is mildly elevated after treatment [70,73], although some studies have shown no significant difference in serum calcium, phosphorus, or PTH concentrations with treatment [74]. With therapy for hyperthyroidism, PTH concentration increases as TSH concentration increases [73]. Calcitriol concentration has increased with treatment in some studies [64,70], but in other studies, there has been no significant change in calcitriol from pretreatment values [75]. There has been no change in 25-hydroxyvitamin D concentration noted after treatment [70]. Urinary excretion of calcium decreases [69,70], but urinary phosphorus excretion increases [70]. Even though calcitriol concentration typically increases with treatment for hyperthyroidism, 75% of treated patients showed a decrease in intestinal calcium absorption, most likely as a direct effect of the decreased thyroid hormones [76].

Concentration of serum and urine markers of bone turnover may decrease but may still remain at a higher level than expected. There is a decrease in BALP [69,70,77], osteocalcin [70,71], urinary hydroxyproline [69], and urinary N-telopeptides of type I collagen (NT_x) [70,78]; however, even after attaining euthyroidism, markers of bone turnover remain increased, indicating a higher rate of bone formation and resorption [71,79]. In one study of 13 hyperthyroid patients treated with methimazole, markers of bone turnover did not normalize after 1 year of therapy even though the euthyroid state had been attained, indicating an ongoing high rate of bone turnover [70]. Patients who attained a euthyroid state but still had suppressed TSH concentrations showed a higher level of bone turnover markers [80]. After 9 months of treatment for hyperthyroidism, bone mass was still less than expected [81], and bone mineral density of the lumbar spine, total skeleton, and legs continued to increase over a 2-year period after treatment of hyperthyroidism, indicating a long period of bone turnover [82].

Certainly, if thyroidectomy is the therapy for hyperthyroidism, calcium metabolism can be disturbed because of disruption of the parathyroid glands during surgery. If the parathyroid glands are removed or blood supply is disrupted to the parathyroid glands, there can be a decrease in PTH secretion with resulting hypocalcemia. In 101 hyperthyroid cats treated with partial thyroidectomy using a modified intracapsular dissection technique, 6% exhibited transient postoperative hypocalcemia [83]. In another study of hyperthyroid cats treated with thyroidectomy, hypocalcemia was noted in 33% in which a modified intracapsular technique was used, in 22% in which the intracapsular technique was used, and in 23% in which a modified extracapsular technique was used [84]. Hypocalcemia was present in 12% of human patients after subtotal thyroidectomy and in 22% after total thyroidectomy [68]. In another study, 37% of hyperthyroid human patients treated with a thyroidectomy required supplemental calcium and vitamin D in the postoperative period; 50% required supplementation for only 1 month [85].

At this time, there has been limited study of calcium metabolism in cats after treatment for hyperthyroidism. In 16 cats treated with methimazole, all exhibited a return to the euthyroid state (P.A. Schenck, DVM, PhD, unpublished data, 2006). There was no significant difference in serum iCa concentration compared with pretreatment values; however, several cats that had shown mild hypercalcemia before treatment became normocalcemic after methimazole treatment. PTH concentration decreased into the reference range in 8 cats that had an increased concentration of PTH before treatment, and 1 cat developed secondary hyperparathyroidism after treatment, most likely as a result of underlying renal disease.

HYPOTHYROIDISM

Calcium Homeostasis During Hypothyroidism

Less is known regarding bone remodeling in the presence of hypothyroidism, because clinically significant changes have not been evident. In adult-onset hypothyroidism, concentrations of tCa and phosphorus are typically within normal limits [48,58,86–88]. Concentrations of tCa and iCa may be significantly lower in hypothyroid patients but may still be within normal limits [89]. In congenital hypothyroidism, however, up to 23% of children exhibit hypercalcemia [90–92]. Concentration of PTH may be elevated, and calcitriol concentration is typically elevated [41,90,93]. Total thyroidectomy resulted in decreased calcium absorption, which may account for an elevation in PTH [76]. Even though serum tCa is usually normal, hypothyroid patients recover from hypocalcemia more slowly than do euthyroid patients. This blunted response has been attributed to decreased renal and bone sensitivity to PTH [94].

The prevalence of neuromuscular symptoms and musculoskeletal problems is higher in hypothyroid patients and is positively correlated with TSH concentration [89]. Carpal tunnel syndrome was present in 30% of hypothyroid patients [95], and the incidence of neuromuscular symptoms showed an inverse correlation with iCa concentration [89].

Some studies have shown a decrease in concentration of serum 25-hydroxyvitamin D [96], whereas others have shown no significant difference in 25-hydroxyvitamin D in hypothyroid patients compared with euthyroid patients [86]. A slight increase in vitamin D binding protein has been noted in hypothyroidism [41]. Fractional renal excretion of calcium increases in hypothyroidism, indicating less reabsorption of calcium by the renal tubules [30]. In adult-onset hypothyroidism, there is lower urinary hydroxyproline [86] and decreased osteocalcin concentrations [86,90], suggesting decreased osteoclastic bone resorption and sluggish osteoblastic bone formation and a general decrease in bone remodeling. Hyperosteoidosis with an increase in the thickness of osteoid has been noted in hypothyroidism and is a consequence of decreased basal osseous activity attributable to a decrease in thyroid hormone concentrations [87]. Calcitonin concentration also decreases in hypothyroidism [97]. In children with congenital hypothyroidism, there was no relation between VDR genotypes and bone mineral density or osteocalcin; however, VDR genotypes were related to a marker of bone resorption (urinary DPD) [98].

Calcium Homeostasis After Treatment for Hypothyroidism

The effects of T_4 therapy on calcium metabolism depend on the dose of T_4 used and the level of suppression of TSH. In studies in which a suppressive dose of T_4 was used, patients showed a significant decrease in bone mineral density, with an increase in BALP, osteocalcin, and urinary hydroxyproline [69,99] and with an inverse correlation between the length of T_4 supplementation and bone mineral density [99]. TSH-suppressive doses of T_4 also increased osteocalcin concentration in young rats, indicating an increase in bone turnover [100]. In addition, women with low TSH levels have an increased risk for hip and vertebral fracture as compared with those with normal TSH concentrations [101]. If TSH is administered to hypothyroid patients using TSH-suppressive doses of T_4, reversible inhibition of bone resorption is evident [102]. Carnitine supplementation may have a beneficial effect in the treatment of hyperthyroidism or in those receiving TSH-suppressive doses of T_4. Carnitine is an antagonist of thyroid hormone action and inhibits thyroid hormone entry into the nucleus of hepatocytes, neurons, and fibroblasts. In patients with low bone mineral density who are receiving T_4 supplementation, the addition of a carnitine supplement showed a beneficial effect on bone mineralization, with an increase in bone mineral density [103].

Other studies that have examined replacement T_4 doses have failed to show a negative effect on bone mineral density [79,104–107]. Serum thyroid hormone concentration and duration of T_4 replacement did not correlate with bone mineral density in the femoral neck, lumbar spine, or total hip [106]. With a mildly suppressive dose of T_4 and mild inhibition of TSH, there was no difference in bone mineral density or bone turnover markers in hypothyroid patients before or after treatment [104].

One study has evaluated the effects of female hormone replacement therapy alone or in combination with T_4 therapy in hypothyroid postmenopausal women [108]. Hypothyroid patients receiving no therapy showed a decrease in bone mineral density over time, as do healthy controls. Those hypothyroid patients receiving female hormone replacement therapy alone showed an increase in bone mineral density. The group that received female hormone replacement therapy in combination with T_4 therapy exhibited greater bone mineral density loss than the hypothyroid group receiving no therapy, however. Thus, the addition of T_4 prevented the beneficial effects of female hormone replacement on bone mineral density, most likely because of suppression of TSH concentration.

Dietary calcium may be important in hypothyroid patients being treated with T_4. Several studies have shown that increased calcium intake can decrease the absorption of T_4, resulting in lower serum thyroid hormone concentrations and higher TSH concentration [109–111]. T_4 binding to calcium occurs at an acidic pH, which decreases the bioavailability of T_4 [110]. If T_4 was given 4 hours before a calcium supplement, there were no apparent differences in serum thyroid hormone concentrations or TSH [112].

Unfortunately, calcium homeostasis has not been clinically assessed in hypothyroid pets before or after therapy.

SUMMARY

The impact of hyperthyroidism and hypothyroidism on calcium metabolism and bone density has been extensively studied in human patients. Hyperthyroidism in people is typically associated with hypercalcemia and an increase in bone turnover. With treatment for hyperthyroidism, increased bone turnover may persist for a time, even when therapy is apparently adequate. Hypothyroidism is not characterized by significant changes in calcium homeostasis; however, treatment of hypothyroidism may cause an increase in bone turnover with a loss in bone mineral density. Conflicting findings may be related to the differences in the pathogenesis of thyroid disorders. Little is known regarding the effects of thyroid disorders on calcium metabolism in cats and dogs. To date, no clinical signs of decreased bone mineral density or osteoporosis have been reported in hyperthyroid cats, even though there is evidence of increased bone turnover. With better diagnostic tools, better treatments, and increased longevity of pets, the clinical impact of thyroid disorders on calcium metabolism and bone may be uncovered.

References

[1] Schenck PA, Chew DJ, Nagode LA, et al. Disorders of calcium: hypercalcemia and hypocalcemia. In: DiBartola SP, editor. Fluid therapy in small animal practice. 3rd edition. St. Louis (MO): Elsevier; 2005. p. 122–94.

[2] Swarthout JT, D'Alonzo RC, Selvamurugan N, et al. Parathyroid hormone-dependent signaling pathways regulating genes in bone cells. Gene 2002;282(1–2):1–17.

[3] Frolik CA, Black EC, Cain RL, et al. Anabolic and catabolic bone effects of human parathyroid hormone (1–34) are predicted by duration of hormone exposure. Bone 2003;33(3): 372–9.

[4] How KL, Hazewinkel HA, Mol JA. Dietary vitamin D dependence of cat and dog due to inadequate cutaneous synthesis of vitamin D. Gen Comp Endocrinol 1994;96(1):12–8.

[5] Gascon-Barre M. The vitamin D 25-hydroxylase. In: Feldman D, editor. Vitamin D. New York: Academic Press; 1997. p. 41–56.

[6] DeLuca HF, Krisinger J, Darwish H. The vitamin D system: 1990. Kidney Int Suppl 1990;29: S2–8.

[7] Breslau NA. Normal and abnormal regulation of 1,25-(OH)2D synthesis. Am J Med Sci 1988;296(6):417–25.

[8] Zelikovic I, Chesney RW. Vitamin D and mineral metabolism: the role of the kidney in health and disease. World Rev Nutr Diet 1989;59:156–216.

[9] Bronner F. Mechanisms of intestinal calcium absorption. J Cell Biochem 2003;88(2): 387–93.

[10] Kumar R. Vitamin D and the kidney. In: Feldman D, editor. Vitamin D. New York: Academic Press; 1997. p. 275–92.

[11] Reichel H, Koeffler HP, Norman AW. The role of the vitamin D endocrine system in health and disease. N Engl J Med 1989;320(15):980–91.

[12] Aubin JE, Heersche JN. Vitamin D and osteoblasts. In: Feldman D, editor. Vitamin D. New York: Academic Press; 1997. p. 313–28.

[13] St. Arnaud R, Glorieux FH. Vitamin D and bone development. In: Feldman D, editor. Vitamin D. San Diego (CA): Academic Press; 1997. p. 293–303.

[14] Suda T, Takahashi N. Vitamin D and osteoclastogenesis. In: Feldman D, editor. Vitamin D. San Diego (CA): Academic Press; 1997. p. 329–40.

[15] Brown EM. Extracellular Ca2+ sensing, regulation of parathyroid cell function, and role of Ca2+ and other ions as extracellular (first) messengers. Physiol Rev 1991;71(2):371–411.

[16] Rosol TJ, Capen CC. Tumors of the parathyroid gland and circulating parathyroid hormone-related protein associated with persistent hypercalcemia. Toxicol Pathol 1989;17(2):346–56.

[17] Okada H, Merryman JI, Rosol TJ, et al. Effects of humoral hypercalcemia of malignancy and gallium nitrate on thyroid C cells in nude mice: immunohistochemical and ultrastructural investigations. Vet Pathol 1994;31(3):349–57.

[18] Galliford TM, Murphy E, Williams AJ, et al. Effects of thyroid status on bone metabolism: a primary role for thyroid stimulating hormone or thyroid hormone? Minerva Endocrinol 2005;30(4):237–46.

[19] Abu EO, Bord S, Horner A, et al. The expression of thyroid hormone receptors in human bone. Bone 1997;21(2):137–42.

[20] Abu EO, Horner A, Teti A, et al. The localization of thyroid hormone receptor mRNAs in human bone. Thyroid 2000;10(4):287–93.

[21] Gruber R, Czerwenka K, Wolf F, et al. Expression of the vitamin D receptor, of estrogen and thyroid hormone receptor alpha- and beta-isoforms, and of the androgen receptor in cultures of native mouse bone marrow and of stromal/osteoblastic cells. Bone 1999;24(5): 465–73.

[22] Robson H, Siebler T, Stevens DA, et al. Thyroid hormone acts directly on growth plate chondrocytes to promote hypertrophic differentiation and inhibit clonal expansion and cell proliferation. Endocrinology 2000;141(10):3887–97.

[23] Mundy GR, Shapiro JL, Bandelin JG, et al. Direct stimulation of bone resorption by thyroid hormones. J Clin Invest 1976;58(3):529–34.

[24] Britto JM, Fenton AJ, Holloway WR, et al. Osteoblasts mediate thyroid hormone stimulation of osteoclastic bone resorption. Endocrinology 1994;134(1):169–76.

[25] Kanatani M, Sugimoto T, Sowa H, et al. Thyroid hormone stimulates osteoclast differentiation by a mechanism independent of RANKL-RANK interaction. J Cell Physiol 2004;201(1):17–25.

[26] Davies T, Marians R, Latif R. The TSH receptor reveals itself. J Clin Invest 2002;110(2): 161–4.

[27] Abe E, Marians RC, Yu W, et al. TSH is a negative regulator of skeletal remodeling. Cell 2003;115(2):151–62.

[28] Sun L, Davies TF, Blair HC, et al. TSH and bone loss. Ann N Y Acad Sci 2006;1068: 309–18.

[29] Morimura T, Tsunekawa K, Kasahara T, et al. Expression of type 2 iodothyronine deiodinase in human osteoblast is stimulated by thyrotropin. Endocrinology 2005;146(4): 2077–84.

[30] Kumar V, Prasad R. Molecular basis of renal handling of calcium in response to thyroid hormone status of rat. Biochim Biophys Acta 2002;1586(3):331–43.

[31] Kano K. Rapid changes in serum vitamin D metabolites in response to TRH. Horm Metab Res 1984;16(10):553–4.

[32] Kumar V, Prasad R. Thyroid hormones stimulate calcium transport systems in rat intestine. Biochim Biophys Acta 2003;1639(3):185–94.

[33] Cross HS, Polzleitner D, Peterlik M. Intestinal phosphate and calcium absorption: joint regulation by thyroid hormones and 1,25-dihydroxyvitamin D3. Acta Endocrinol (Copenh) 1986;113(1):96–103.

[34] Obermayer-Pietsch BM, Fruhauf GE, Chararas K, et al. Association of the vitamin D receptor genotype BB with low bone density in hyperthyroidism. J Bone Miner Res 2000;15(10): 1950–5.

[35] Kohri K, Kodama M, Umekawa T, et al. Calcium oxalate crystal formation in patients with hyperparathyroidism and hyperthyroidism and related metabolic disturbances. Bone Miner 1990;8(1):59–67.

[36] Ford HC, Crooke MJ, Murphy CE. Disturbances of calcium and magnesium metabolism occur in most hyperthyroid patients. Clin Biochem 1989;22(5):373–6.

[37] Burman KD, Monchik JM, Earll JM, et al. Ionized and total serum calcium and parathyroid hormone in hyperthyroidism. Ann Intern Med 1976;84(6):668–71.

[38] Wang X, Wu H, Chao C. Effect of propranolol on calcium, phosphorus, and magnesium metabolic disorders in Graves' disease. Metabolism 1992;41(5):552–5.

[39] Popelier M, Jollivet B, Fouquet B, et al. [Phosphorus-calcium metabolism in hyperthyroidism]. Presse Med 1990;19(15):705–8.

[40] Auwerx J, Bouillon R. Mineral and bone metabolism in thyroid disease: a review. Q J Med 1986;60(232):737–52.

[41] Bouillon R, Muls E, De Moor P. Influence of thyroid function on the serum concentration of 1,25-dihydroxyvitamin D3. J Clin Endocrinol Metab 1980;51(4):793–7.

[42] Jastrup B, Mosekilde L, Melsen F, et al. Serum levels of vitamin D metabolites and bone remodelling in hyperthyroidism. Metabolism 1982;31(2):126–32.

[43] Haldimann B, Kaptein EM, Singer FR, et al. Intestinal calcium absorption in patients with hyperthyroidism. J Clin Endocrinol Metab 1980;51(5):995–7.

[44] Karsenty G, Bouchard P, Ulmann A, et al. Elevated metabolic clearance rate of 1 alpha,25-dihydroxyvitamin D3 in hyperthyroidism. Acta Endocrinol (Copenh) 1985;110(1):70–4.

[45] Kashio Y, Iwasaki J, Chihara K, et al. Pituitary 1,25-dihydroxyvitamin D3 receptors in hyperthyroid- and hypothyroid-rats. Biochem Biophys Res Commun 1985;131(1):122–8.

[46] Cleeve HJ, Brown IR. Plasma 25-hydroxyvitamin D and alkaline phosphatase isoenzymes in hyperthyroidism. Ann Clin Biochem 1978;15(6):320–3.

[47] Roiter I, Legovini P, Da Rin G, et al. [Serum osteocalcin in hyperthyroidism]. Ann Ital Med Int 1990;5(2):95–9.

[48] Kisakol G, Kaya A, Gonen S, et al. Bone and calcium metabolism in subclinical autoimmune hyperthyroidism and hypothyroidism. Endocr J 2003;50(6):657–61.

[49] Isaia GC, Roggia C, Gola D, et al. Bone turnover in hyperthyroidism before and after thyrostatic management. J Endocrinol Invest 2000;23(11):727–31.

[50] Peerenboom H, Keck E, Kruskemper HL, et al. The defect of intestinal calcium transport in hyperthyroidism and its response to therapy. J Clin Endocrinol Metab 1984;59(5): 936–40.

[51] Akalin A, Colak O, Alatas O, et al. Bone remodelling markers and serum cytokines in patients with hyperthyroidism. Clin Endocrinol (Oxf) 2002;57(1):125–9.

[52] Simsek G, Karter Y, Aydin S, et al. Osteoporotic cytokines and bone metabolism on rats with induced hyperthyroidism; changes as a result of reversal to euthyroidism. Chin J Physiol 2003;46(4):181–6.

[53] Jodar Gimeno E, Munoz-Torres M, Escobar-Jimenez F, et al. Identification of metabolic bone disease in patients with endogenous hyperthyroidism: role of biological markers of bone turnover. Calcif Tissue Int 1997;61(5):370–6.

[54] Lakatos P, Foldes J, Horvath C, et al. Serum interleukin-6 and bone metabolism in patients with thyroid function disorders. J Clin Endocrinol Metab 1997;82(1):78–81.

[55] Vestergaard P, Mosekilde L. Fractures in patients with hyperthyroidism and hypothyroidism: a nationwide follow-up study in 16,249 patients. Thyroid 2002;12(5):411–9.

[56] Vestergaard P, Mosekilde L. Hyperthyroidism, bone mineral, and fracture risk—a meta-analysis. Thyroid 2003;13(6):585–93.

[57] Karga H, Papapetrou PD, Korakovouni A, et al. Bone mineral density in hyperthyroidism. Clin Endocrinol (Oxf) 2004;61(4):466–72.

[58] Lee WY, Oh KW, Rhee EJ, et al. Relationship between subclinical thyroid dysfunction and femoral neck bone mineral density in women. Arch Med Res 2006;37(4):511–6.

[59] Lakatos P, Foldes J, Nagy Z, et al. Serum insulin-like growth factor-I, insulin-like growth factor binding proteins, and bone mineral content in hyperthyroidism. Thyroid 2000;10(5):417–23.

[60] Ben-Shlomo A, Hagag P, Evans S, et al. Early postmenopausal bone loss in hyperthyroidism. Maturitas 2001;39(1):19–27.

[61] Ugur-Altun B, Altun A, Arikan E, et al. Relationships existing between the serum cytokine levels and bone mineral density in women in the premenopausal period affected by Graves' disease with subclinical hyperthyroidism. Endocr Res 2003;29(4):389–98.

[62] Wagner B, Begic-Karup S, Raber W, et al. Prevalence of primary hyperparathyroidism in 13,387 patients with thyroid diseases, newly diagnosed by screening of serum calcium. Exp Clin Endocrinol Diabetes 1999;107(7):457–61.

[63] Gerber H, Peter H, Ferguson DC, et al. Etiopathology of feline toxic nodular goiter. Vet Clin North Am Small Anim Pract 1994;24(3):541–65.

[64] Czernobilsky H, Scharla S, Schmidt-Gayk H, et al. Enhanced suppression of 1,25(OH)2D3 and intact parathyroid hormone in Graves' disease as compared to toxic nodular goiter. Calcif Tissue Int 1988;42(1):5–12.

[65] Horney BS, Farmer AJ, Honor DJ, et al. Agarose gel electrophoresis of alkaline phosphatase isoenzymes in the serum of hyperthyroid cats. Vet Clin Pathol 1994;23(3):98–102.

[66] Foster DJ, Thoday KL. Tissue sources of serum alkaline phosphatase in 34 hyperthyroid cats: a qualitative and quantitative study. Res Vet Sci 2000;68(1):89–94.

[67] Archer FJ, Taylor SM. Alkaline phosphatase bone isoenzyme and osteocalcin in the serum of hyperthyroid cats. Can Vet J 1996;37(12):735–9.

[68] Demeester-Mirkine N, Hooghe L, Van Geertruyden J, et al. Hypocalcemia after thyroidectomy. Arch Surg 1992;127(7):854–8.

[69] Bijlsma JW, Duursma SA, Roelofs JM, et al. Thyroid function and bone turnover. Acta Endocrinol (Copenh) 1983;104(1):42–9.

[70] Pantazi H, Papapetrou PD. Changes in parameters of bone and mineral metabolism during therapy for hyperthyroidism. J Clin Endocrinol Metab 2000;85(3):1099–106.

[71] Barsal G, Taneli F, Atay A, et al. Serum osteocalcin levels in hyperthyroidism before and after antithyroid therapy. Tohoku J Exp Med 2004;203(3):183–8.

[72] Murakami T, Noguchi S, Murakami N, et al. [The mechanism of postoperative tetany in Graves' disease]. Nippon Naibunpi Gakkai Zasshi 1989;65(8):771–80.

[73] Ross DS, Nussbaum SR. Reciprocal changes in parathyroid hormone and thyroid function after radioiodine treatment of hyperthyroidism. J Clin Endocrinol Metab 1989;68(6):1216–9.

[74] Langdahl BL, Loft AG, Eriksen EF, et al. Bone mass, bone turnover, calcium homeostasis, and body composition in surgically and radioiodine-treated former hyperthyroid patients. Thyroid 1996;6(3):169–75.

[75] Langdahl BL, Loft AG, Eriksen EF, et al. Bone mass, bone turnover, body composition, and calcium homeostasis in former hyperthyroid patients treated by combined medical therapy. Thyroid 1996;6(3):161–8.

[76] Bone HG 3rd, Deftos LJ, Snyder WH, et al. Mineral metabolic effects of thyroidectomy and long-term outcomes in a family with MEN 2A. Henry Ford Hosp Med J 1992;40(3–4): 258–60.

[77] Olkawa M, Kushida K, Takahashi M, et al. Bone turnover and cortical bone mineral density in the distal radius in patients with hyperthyroidism being treated with antithyroid drugs for various periods of time. Clin Endocrinol (Oxf) 1999;50(2):171–6.

[78] Mora S, Weber G, Marenzi K, et al. Longitudinal changes of bone density and bone resorption in hyperthyroid girls during treatment. J Bone Miner Res 1999;14(11):1971–7.

[79] Sabuncu T, Aksoy N, Arikan E, et al. Early changes in parameters of bone and mineral metabolism during therapy for hyper- and hypothyroidism. Endocr Res 2001;27(1–2): 203–13.

[80] Kumeda Y, Inaba M, Tahara H, et al. Persistent increase in bone turnover in Graves' patients with subclinical hyperthyroidism. J Clin Endocrinol Metab 2000;85(11):4157–61.

[81] Jodar E, Munoz-Torres M, Escobar-Jimenez F, et al. Antiresorptive therapy in hyperthyroid patients: longitudinal changes in bone and mineral metabolism. J Clin Endocrinol Metab 1997;82(6):1989–94.

[82] Acotto CG, Niepomniszcze H, Vega E, et al. Ultrasound parameters and markers of bone turnover in hyperthyroidism: a longitudinal study. J Clin Densitom 2004;7(2):201–8.

[83] Naan EC, Kirpensteijn J, Kooistra HS, et al. Results of thyroidectomy in 101 cats with hyperthyroidism. Vet Surg 2006;35(3):287–93.

[84] Welches CD, Scavelli TD, Matthiesen DT, et al. Occurrence of problems after three techniques of bilateral thyroidectomy in cats. Vet Surg 1989;18(5):392–6.

[85] Razack MS, Lore JM Jr, Lippes HA, et al. Total thyroidectomy for Graves' disease. Head Neck 1997;19(5):378–83.

[86] Foscolo G, Roiter I, De Menis E, et al. [Bone metabolism in primary hypothyroidism in the adult]. Minerva Endocrinol 1991;16(1):7–10.

[87] Duquesnoy B, Hardouin P, Wemeau JL, et al. [Bone effects of hypothyroidism in adults. Apropos of 20 cases]. Rev Rhum Mal Osteoartic 1985;52(10):555–61.

[88] Simsek G, Andican G, Karakoc Y, et al. Calcium, magnesium, and zinc status in experimental hypothyroidism. Biol Trace Elem Res 1997;60(3):205–13.

[89] Monzani F, Caraccio N, Del Guerra P, et al. Neuromuscular symptoms and dysfunction in subclinical hypothyroid patients: beneficial effect of L-T4 replacement therapy. Clin Endocrinol (Oxf) 1999;51(2):237–42.

[90] Verrotti A, Greco R, Altobelli E, et al. Bone metabolism in children with congenital hypothyroidism—a longitudinal study. J Pediatr Endocrinol Metab 1998;11(6):699–705.

[91] Leger J, Tau C, Garabedian M, et al. [Prophylaxis of vitamin D deficiency in hypothyroidism in the newborn infant]. Arch Fr Pediatr 1989;46(8):567–71.

[92] Tau C, Garabedian M, Farriaux JP, et al. Hypercalcemia in infants with congenital hypothyroidism and its relation to vitamin D and thyroid hormones. J Pediatr 1986;109(5): 808–14.

[93] Zaloga GP, Eil C, O'Brian JT. Reversible hypocalciuric hypercalcemia associated with hypothyroidism. Am J Med 1984;77(6):1101–4.

[94] Bouillon R, De Moor P. Parathyroid function in patients with hyper- or hypothyroidism. J Clin Endocrinol Metab 1974;38(6):999–1004.

[95] Cakir M, Samanci N, Balci N, et al. Musculoskeletal manifestations in patients with thyroid disease. Clin Endocrinol (Oxf) 2003;59(2):162–7.

[96] Arlet P, Latorzeff S, Bayard F, et al. [Bone and calcium metabolism in adult hypothyroidism (author's transl)]. Sem Hop 1979;55(33–34):1488–92.

[97] Poppe K, Verbruggen LA, Velkeniers B, et al. Calcitonin reserve in different stages of atrophic autoimmune thyroiditis. Thyroid 1999;9(12):1211–4.

[98] Leger J, Tourrel C, Ruiz JC, et al. Vitamin D receptor genotype and bone mineral density in Caucasian children with congenital hypothyroidism. J Pediatr Endocrinol Metab 2000;13(6):599–603.

[99] Affinito P, Sorrentino C, Farace MJ, et al. Effects of thyroxine therapy on bone metabolism in postmenopausal women with hypothyroidism. Acta Obstet Gynecol Scand 1996; 75(9):843–8.

[100] Ross DS, Graichen R. Increased rat femur osteocalcin mRNA concentrations following in vivo administration of thyroid hormone. J Endocrinol Invest 1991;14(9):763–6.

[101] Bauer DC, Ettinger B, Nevitt MC, et al. Risk for fracture in women with low serum levels of thyroid-stimulating hormone. Ann Intern Med 2001;134(7):561–8.

[102] Mazziotti G, Sorvillo F, Piscopo M, et al. Recombinant human TSH modulates in vivo C-telopeptides of type-1 collagen and bone alkaline phosphatase, but not osteoprotegerin production in postmenopausal women monitored for differentiated thyroid carcinoma. J Bone Miner Res 2005;20(3):480–6.

[103] Benvenga S, Ruggeri RM, Russo A, et al. Usefulness of L-carnitine, a naturally occurring peripheral antagonist of thyroid hormone action, in iatrogenic hyperthyroidism: a randomized, double-blind, placebo-controlled clinical trial. J Clin Endocrinol Metab 2001;86(8): 3579–94.

[104] Appetecchia M. Effects on bone mineral density by treatment of benign nodular goiter with mildly suppressive doses of L-thyroxine in a cohort women study. Horm Res 2005;64(6): 293–8.

[105] Nuzzo V, Lupoli G, Esposito Del Puente A, et al. Bone mineral density in premenopausal women receiving levothyroxine suppressive therapy. Gynecol Endocrinol 1998;12(5): 333–7.

[106] Hanna FW, Pettit RJ, Ammari F, et al. Effect of replacement doses of thyroxine on bone mineral density. Clin Endocrinol (Oxf) 1998;48(2):229–34.

[107] Salerno M, Lettiero T, Esposito-del Puente A, et al. Effect of long-term L-thyroxine treatment on bone mineral density in young adults with congenital hypothyroidism. Eur J Endocrinol 2004;151(6):689–94.

[108] Pines A, Dotan I, Tabori U, et al. L-thyroxine prevents the bone-conserving effect of HRT in postmenopausal women with subclinical hypothyroidism. Gynecol Endocrinol 1999;13(3):196–201.

[109] Csako G, McGriff NJ, Rotman-Pikielny P, et al. Exaggerated levothyroxine malabsorption due to calcium carbonate supplementation in gastrointestinal disorders. Ann Pharmacother 2001;35(12):1578–83.

[110] Singh N, Singh PN, Hershman JM. Effect of calcium carbonate on the absorption of levothyroxine. Jama 2000;283(21):2822–5.

[111] Singh N, Weisler SL, Hershman JM. The acute effect of calcium carbonate on the intestinal absorption of levothyroxine. Thyroid 2001;11(10):967–71.

[112] Chopra IJ, Baber K. Treatment of primary hypothyroidism during pregnancy: is there an increase in thyroxine dose requirement in pregnancy? Metabolism 2003;52(1):122–8.

Vet Clin Small Anim 37 (2007) 709–722

VETERINARY CLINICS
SMALL ANIMAL PRACTICE

ELSEVIER
SAUNDERS

Clinical Signs and Concurrent Diseases of Hypothyroidism in Dogs and Cats

J. Catharine Scott-Moncrieff, MA, MS, Vet MB, MRCVS

Department of Veterinary Clinical Sciences, School of Veterinary Medicine, Purdue University, VCS/LYNN, 625 Harrison Street, West Lafayette, IN 47907–2026, USA

Thyroid hormones influence the function of almost every organ in the body; therefore, canine hypothyroidism may present with a wide range of clinical signs. The most common clinical signs are those of a decreased metabolic rate and dermatologic manifestations; however, many other clinical signs have been reported, including reproductive, neurologic, and cardiovascular abnormalities.

There are several factors that make it hard to determine the true relation between hypothyroidism and many of the less common clinical associations attributed to the disease. One factor is the challenge of confirming a diagnosis of hypothyroidism in dogs. Diagnosis of hypothyroidism is hampered by the lack of specificity of the thyroxine (T_4) assay as well as the lack of sensitivity of the thyrotropin assay. In many cases, it is difficult to make a definitive diagnosis and a therapeutic trial is necessary. Many nonthyroidal factors, such as breed, age, concurrent or previous drug therapy, and presence of concurrent disease, not only influence baseline thyroid hormone concentrations but may influence the results of a therapeutic trial. Another complicating factor is that the predictive value of a diagnostic test depends on the prevalence of the disease in the population. A diagnosis of hypothyroidism is sometimes viewed as an easy answer for medical concerns like obesity, dermatologic abnormalities, and behavioral problems; this leads to testing of many dogs in which hypothyroidism is not likely. The prevalence of disease in the tested population is therefore low, which decreases the predictive value of a positive test result. Another factor that makes it hard to determine a causal relation between reported clinical signs and hypothyroidism is that hypothyroidism and the other associated disorders are common in certain breeds. A common breed predisposition or common pathogenesis (eg, immune-mediated disease) can account for other diseases occurring together with hypothyroidism. The presence of two diseases occurring concurrently should not be interpreted to mean that there is necessarily a causal relation between them. Criteria for diagnosis of hypothyroidism

E-mail address: scottmon@purdue.edu

0195-5616/07/$ – see front matter
doi:10.1016/j.cvsm.2007.03.003

have become more stringent over the years, and early veterinary reports of hypothyroidism and its associated clinical signs likely included some cases that were not truly hypothyroid. All these factors mean that the clinician needs to be critical in evaluating the associations between hypothyroidism and other disorders in the literature, particularly in relation to the less common and well-established clinical signs.

CAUSES OF CANINE HYPOTHYROIDISM

Hypothyroidism may result from dysfunction of any part of the hypothalamic-pituitary-thyroid axis and may be acquired (most common) or congenital. Most cases of acquired canine hypothyroidism are attributable to primary hypothyroidism and are caused by lymphocytic thyroiditis or idiopathic thyroid atrophy. More rarely, primary hypothyroidism may be caused by bilateral thyroid neoplasia or invasion of the thyroid by metastatic neoplasia. Secondary hypothyroidism (deficiency of thyrotropin) has been rarely described in dogs. Causes of acquired secondary hypothyroidism include pituitary malformations and pituitary neoplasia. Tertiary hypothyroidism (deficiency of thyrotropin-releasing hormone [TRH]) has yet to be documented in the dog.

Reported causes of congenital primary hypothyroidism include iodine deficiency, thyroid dysgenesis, and dyshormonogenesis [1]. Congenital hypothyroidism with goiter attributable to thyroid peroxidase deficiency was reported as an autosomal recessive trait in Toy Fox Terriers [2]. Secondary congenital hypothyroidism attributable to apparent isolated thyrotropin or TRH deficiency was reported in a family of young Giant Schnauzers and in a young Boxer [3,4]. Congenital secondary hypothyroidism is also a feature of panhypopituitarism.

Iatrogenic causes of hypothyroidism include ^{131}I treatment, administration of antithyroid drugs, and surgical thyroidectomy; however, because of the presence of accessory thyroid tissue, permanent hypothyroidism after thyroidectomy is rare.

Because most clinical consequences of hypothyroidism result from the effects of decreased production of the thyroid hormones T_4 and triiodothyronine (T_3) on all organs of the body, clinical signs of hypothyroidism are usually similar independent of the underlying cause of thyroid dysfunction. In some forms of hypothyroidism, however, (congenital hypothyroidism, secondary hypothyroidism, and hypothyroidism attributable to thyroid neoplasia), additional clinical signs, such as a goiter, growth retardation, other signs of pituitary dysfunction, or clinical signs caused by the presence of a cervical mass, may be recognized. Although thyroiditis may cause thyroid pain in human beings, this is not frequently recognized in dogs with thyroiditis.

EPIDEMIOLOGY OF CANINE HYPOTHYROIDISM

There have been two large retrospective studies of canine hypothyroidism published in the past 15 years [5,6]. Other older studies of canine hypothyroidism did not use the same stringent criteria for confirmation of the diagnosis; thus, their results need to be evaluated more critically. The prevalence of canine

Cricopharyngeal achalasia was reported as an unusual manifestation of polyneuropathy in a young dog with hypothyroidism and suspected polyneuropathy [21]. Clinical signs of hind limb weakness and dysphagia resolved with thyroid hormone supplementation.

Myopathy has also been rarely described in hypothyroid dogs. In one study, two hypothyroid dogs with no clinical signs of muscle disease had histopathologic evidence of myopathy with type II fiber atrophy [22]. In a more recent report, a dog with hypothyroidism and clinical signs of myopathy, had type I fiber predominance with nemaline rods present in the type I fibers [23]. Gait abnormalities and exercise intolerance in the affected dog resolved 2 weeks after L-thyroxine supplementation. Unilateral lameness has also been reported in hypothyroid dogs and may be a manifestation of generalized neuromyopathy. Affected dogs had unilateral forelimb lameness, pain on manipulation of the glenohumeral joint, and atrophy of the supraspinatus muscle [24]. Only one of the four affected dogs had other more classic signs of hypothyroidism. Electromyography revealed evidence of widespread denervation, with fibrillation potentials and positive sharp waves recorded in multiple muscles. Thyroid tests were supportive of hypothyroidism, and all clinical signs resolved with L-thyroxine supplementation. In two dogs, clinical signs recurred after withdrawal of treatment and resolved again with reinitiation of treatment.

Dysfunction of multiple cranial nerves (facial, trigeminal, and vestibulocochlear) with or without abnormal gait and postural reactions have been reported in hypothyroid dogs [20,25]. In many cases, the neurologic signs are multifocal and progressive over time. Other clinical signs of hypothyroidism are often absent. Peripheral and central vestibular dysfunction has been reported. Some hypothyroid dogs with vestibular deficits have abnormal brain stem auditory-evoked responses and electromyographic abnormalities of the appendicular muscles. In a report of 10 dogs with hypothyroid-associated progressive central vestibular dysfunction, lesions were localized to the myelencephalic region in 5 dogs and to the vestibulocerebellum in 5 dogs. Two dogs had paroxysmal clinical signs, whereas in the remainder, the signs were persistent and progressive. Lesions consistent with an infarct were identified by imaging studies in 3 dogs, and brain stem auditory evoked responses were abnormal in 3 of 4 dogs tested. Clinical signs in all affected dogs resolved with T_4 supplementation [18].

Megaesophagus has been reported to occur in association with hypothyroidism; however, treatment of hypothyroidism does not consistently result in resolution of clinical signs and a causal relation cannot be confirmed [20]. In one report of four hypothyroid dogs with megaesophagus, thyroid hormone supplementation resulted in mild improvement in three dogs and resolution of clinical signs in one dog, but radiographic evaluation revealed persistence of megaesophagus in all dogs after 2 months of treatment [20]. In another report of four hypothyroid dogs with megaesophagus, only one dog had improvement with thyroxine supplementation and the improvement persisted despite cessation of L-thyroxine treatment for 1 year [5]. A retrospective study of dogs with acquired megaesophagus did not identify hypothyroidism as a risk factor [26]. In the same study, myasthenia gravis was a risk factor for acquired megaesophagus, and myasthenia gravis has been reported in association with hypothyroidism [27]. Concurrent hypothyroidism may exacerbate clinical signs of myasthenia gravis, such as muscle weakness and megaesophagus.

Laryngeal paralysis has also been reported to occur in association with hypothyroidism. In one retrospective study of 140 dogs treated surgically for laryngeal paralysis, 30 (21%) were considered to be hypothyroid based on results of thyrotropin stimulation tests or a complete thyroid hormone profile [28]. In a study of 66 hypothyroid dogs, laryngeal paralysis was diagnosed in 5 dogs but laryngeal function did not improve in 2 dogs treated with L-thyroxine supplementation alone [5]. In a report of another 5 dogs with hypothyroidism and laryngeal paralysis, dogs with laryngeal paralysis had electrodiagnostic evidence of more diffuse polyneuropathy [20]. Only 1 of these dogs was treated with L-thyroxine supplementation alone, and this dog improved clinically, although laryngeal function was not re-evaluated. Most dogs with laryngeal paralysis are treated surgically, and there are few reports of improvements in laryngeal function after supplementation with L-thyroxine alone. There is currently little evidence to establish a causal relation between hypothyroidism and laryngeal paralysis.

Rarely, cerebral dysfunction may occur in hypothyroidism as a result of myxedema coma, atherosclerosis, or the presence of a pituitary tumor causing secondary hypothyroidism. In myxedema coma, profound mental dullness or stupor may be accompanied by severe weakness, altered mentation, hypothermia, bradycardia, hypoventilation, hypotension, and inappetence [29,30]. Deposition of glycosaminoglycans may result in a nonpitting edema of the skin, face, and jowls. The most common clinicopathologic changes in affected dogs include anemia, hyperlipidemia, hypoglycemia, hyponatremia, hypoxia, and hypercarbia. Treatment with intravenous L-thyroxine is recommended in myxedema coma. In a report of 7 hypothyroid dogs with thyroid crisis treated with intravenous administration of L-thyroxine, concurrent disease, such as infection, was a common precipitating factor [31]. Seizures, disorientation, and circling may occur in hypothyroid dogs because of cerebral atherosclerosis or severe hyperlipidemia; however, there is little evidence to suggest that hypothyroidism is a common cause of seizure disorders in dogs [32,33]. In a study of 113 dogs with seizure disorders, only 3 dogs with hypothyroidism were identified [34]. Idiopathic epilepsy may cause changes in the thyroid profile consistent with the euthyroid sick syndrome; thus, an inaccurate diagnosis of hypothyroidism is commonly made in dogs with seizure disorders [34]. Once anticonvulsant therapy is initiated in dogs with idiopathic epilepsy, the effect of drug therapy on thyroid hormone concentration can make it even more difficult to assess thyroid function accurately.

Early reports suggested an association between hypothyroidism and cervical spondylomyelopathy. This observed association is likely the result of a similar breed predisposition (Doberman Pinscher) for both disorders [35].

Behavioral abnormalities that have been attributed to canine hypothyroidism include aggression and cognitive dysfunction. Myxedema coma and atherosclerosis can clearly cause cognitive dysfunction in some individuals; however, these manifestations of hypothyroidism are rare. In one report of a dog with polyneuropathy and aggressive behavior, the polyneuropathy and aggression resolved with L-thyroxine supplementation [19]. Resolution of acquired aggression toward the owners in a Russian Wolfhound was reported after diagnosis and treatment of hypothyroidism, and there are a small number of other anecdotal reports in the literature of an association between aggression and hypothyroidism [36]. Documentation of a causal relation between common behavioral problems and hypothyroidism requires further prospective studies.

Cardiovascular Abnormalities

Abnormalities of the cardiovascular system, such as sinus bradycardia, weak apex beat, low QRS voltages, and inverted T waves, occur in hypothyroid dogs [35]. Reduced left ventricular pump function has also been documented [37]. Hypothyroidism alone rarely causes clinically significant myocardial failure in dogs; however, dilated cardiomyopathy and hypothyroidism may occur concurrently. In two groups of Doberman Pinschers with and without cardiomyopathy, there was no difference in the prevalence of hypothyroidism between the two groups [38]. Hypothyroidism may exacerbate clinical signs in dogs with underlying cardiac disease, however. A recent case report documented dramatic long-term improvement in cardiac function after treatment with L-thyroxine in two Great Danes with concurrent dilated cardiomyopathy and hypothyroidism [39]. Pericardial disease has also been associated with hypothyroidism. A cholesterol-based pericardial effusion that resolved after L-thyroxine supplementation and aortic thromboembolism was reported in a 9-year-old mixed-breed dog with hypothyroidism [40].

Hypothyroidism has been reported to be a risk factor for atherosclerosis in dogs [41]. Atherosclerosis probably occurs because of hypercholesterolemia and is a rare complication of canine hypothyroidism, but it can potentially lead to other manifestations of cardiovascular disease, such as impaired left ventricular function and atrial fibrillation. One study suggested that hypothyroidism is more common in dogs with atrial fibrillation than in normal dogs [42]. Further studies are necessary to support this association.

Ophthalmologic Abnormalities

Ocular changes reported in canine hypothyroidism include corneal lipidosis, corneal ulceration, uveitis, lipid effusion into the aqueous humor, secondary glaucoma, lipemia retinalis, and retinal detachment [43,44]. These changes likely occur because of hyperlipidemia and seem to be rare occurrences in hypothyroid dogs. Dogs with experimentally induced hypothyroidism did not develop ocular changes during 6 months of observation; however, it was not reported whether any of the hypothyroid dogs became hyperlipidemic [45]. Keratoconjunctivitis sicca in dogs has also been reported to be associated with hypothyroidism; however, there is currently no evidence to support this association [35].

Secondary Hypothyroidism

In secondary hypothyroidism, clinical signs are usually similar to those of primary hypothyroidism; however, in dogs with combined anterior pituitary hormone deficiency, signs related to deficiency of other pituitary hormones (eg, growth hormone) typically predominate [46]. In dogs with secondary hypothyroidism attributable to pituitary neoplasia, clinical signs depend on the hormonal function of the tumor as well as the extent of invasion or compression of surrounding structures. Clinical signs of hyperadrenocorticism, diabetes insipidus, or hypothalamic dysfunction are usually more obvious than those of hypothyroidism [46].

Congenital Hypothyroidism

Congenital hypothyroidism results in mental retardation and stunted disproportionate growth because of epiphyseal dysgenesis and delayed skeletal maturation [47]. Affected dogs are mentally dull and have large broad heads, short thick necks, short limbs, macroglossia, hypothermia, delayed dental eruption, ataxia, and abdominal distention [1–4,47]. Dermatologic findings are similar to those seen in the adult hypothyroid dog. Other clinical signs may include gait abnormalities, stenotic ear canals, sealed eyelids, and constipation. Affected puppies are often the largest in the litter at birth but start to lag behind their littermates within 3 to 8 weeks. Severely affected puppies often die without a diagnosis in the first few weeks of life. A vertebral physeal fracture causing tetraparesis has been reported in a dog with congenital hypothyroidism [48].

Congenital hypothyroidism with goiter, attributable to thyroid peroxidase deficiency, has been recognized in Toy Fox Terriers and Rat Terriers [2]. The defect is an autosomal recessive trait, and a nonsense mutation in the thyroid peroxidase gene of affected dogs has been identified. A DNA test that can detect carriers of the defect is available to screen breeding animals through the Laboratory of Comparative Medical Genetics at Michigan State University.

CLINICOPATHOLOGIC CHANGES

A mild nonregenerative anemia occurs in 30% to 40% of hypothyroid dogs [5,6]. Fasting hypercholesterolemia occurs in 75% of hypothyroid dogs, whereas hypertriglyceridemia occurs in up to 88% [5,6]. Less common abnormalities include mild increases in alkaline phosphatase, alanine aminotransferase, and creatine kinase. Mild hypercalcemia has been reported in congenital hypothyroidism. Serum fructosamine was reported to be mildly increased in 9 of 11 untreated hypothyroid dogs, despite a normal blood glucose level [49]. The increased fructosamine is hypothesized to be attributable to decreased protein synthesis, and the change is reversed by L-thyroxine supplementation. Increased growth hormone and insulin-like growth factor (IGF)-1 concentrations have also been reported in experimentally induced canine hypothyroidism [50].

HEMOSTASIS

Decreased plasma von Willebrand factor antigen (vWf/Ag) concentration has been reported in hypothyroid dogs; however, studies have failed to demonstrate a relation between vWf/Ag or factor VIII activity and thyroid hormone status [51–54]. Canine hypothyroidism does not cause a clinical bleeding disorder, and platelet function and bleeding times are normal. Concentrations of vWf/Ag do not consistently increase during L-thyroxine treatment of hypothyroid dogs or euthyroid dogs with von Willebrand disease [53,54]. The reported association between von Willebrand disease and hypothyroidism is likely the result of a similar breed predisposition (Doberman Pinscher) for both disorders.

POLYENDOCRINOPATHIES

Canine hypothyroidism may occur in association with other immune-mediated endocrine disorders, such as hypoadrenocorticism and diabetes mellitus [55–57]. Insulin resistance has been reported in diabetic dogs with hypothyroidism [57]. Increased fructosamine concentrations in hypothyroid dogs suggest that fructosamine concentrations may not be a good indicator of glycemic control in dogs with concurrent diabetes mellitus and hypothyroidism. In dogs with concurrent hypothyroidism and hypoadrenocorticism, hypothyroidism may mask the classic electrolyte changes of hypoadrenocorticism. Concurrent hypothyroidism may also be a cause of poor clinical response to treatment in dogs with hypoadrenocorticism [55].

FELINE HYPOTHYROIDISM

Naturally occurring hypothyroidism is rare in cats, and the most common cause of low serum T_4 in cats is nonthyroidal illness. Iatrogenic hypothyroidism most commonly occurs after treatment for hyperthyroidism. Causes of spontaneous feline hypothyroidism include congenital hypothyroidism in domestic shorthair cats and Abyssinian cats [58–60], and lymphocytic thyroiditis was reported in a 5-year-old cat and in young kittens [61,62]. Clinical signs of hypothyroidism in cats are similar to those reported for dogs, with lethargy and obesity being the most common manifestations [63]. In contrast to dogs, however, a reduced appetite despite weight gain is common. Other reported clinical signs in cats include puffy facial features associated with myxedema, symmetric truncal or tail head alopecia, hypothermia, and bradycardia.

SUMMARY

The most common clinical signs of hypothyroidism are those of a decreased metabolic rate and dermatologic manifestations. There is strong evidence for a causal relation between hypothyroidism and a variety of neurologic abnormalities; however, the association between hypothyroidism and other manifestations, such as reproductive dysfunction, clinical heart disease, and behavioral abnormalities, is less compelling. Further studies are necessary to determine the full spectrum of disorders caused by hypothyroidism.

References

[1] Chastain CB, McNeel SV, Graham CL, et al. Congenital hypothyroidism in a dog due to an iodide organification defect. Am J Vet Res 1983;44:1257–65.

[2] Fyffe JC, Kampschmidt K, Dang V, et al. Congenital hypothyroidism with goiter in toy fox terriers. J Vet Intern Med 2003;17:50–7.

[3] Greco DS, Feldman EC, Peterson ME, et al. Congenital hypothyroid dwarfism in a family of giant schnauzers. J Vet Intern Med 1991;5:57–65.

[4] Mooney CT, Anderson TJ. Congenital hypothyroidism in a boxer dog. J Small Anim Pract 1993;34:31–4.

[5] Panciera DL. Hypothyroidism in dogs: 66 cases (1987–1992). J Am Vet Med Assoc 1994;204:761–7.

[6] Dixon RM, Reid SWJ, Mooney CT. Epidemiological, clinical, haematological and biochemical characteristics of canine hypothyroidism. Vet Rec 1999;145:481–7.

[7] Greco DS, Rosychuk AW, Ogilvie GK, et al. The effect of levothyroxine treatment on resting energy expenditure of hypothyroid dogs. J Vet Intern Med 1998;12:7–10.

[8] Credille KM, Slater MR, Moriello KA, et al. The effects of thyroid hormones on the skin of beagle dogs. J Vet Intern Med 2001;15:539–46.

[9] Campbell KL, Davis CA. Effects of thyroid hormones on serum and cutaneous fatty acid concentrations in dogs. Am J Vet Res 1990;51:752–6.

[10] Doliger S, Delverdier M, Moré J, et al. Histochemical study of cutaneous mucins in hypothyroid dogs. Vet Pathol 1995;32:628–34.

[11] Miller WH, Buerger RG. Cutaneous mucinous vesiculation in a dog with hypothyroidism. J Am Vet Med Assoc 1990;196:757–9.

[12] Beale KM, Bloomberg MS, Van Gilder J, et al. Correlation of racing and reproductive performance in greyhounds with response to thyroid function testing. J Am Anim Hosp Assoc 1992;28:263–9.

[13] Buckrell BC, Johnson WH. Anestrus and spontaneous galactorrhea in a hypothyroid bitch. Can Vet J 1986;27:204–5.

[14] Chastain CB, Schmidt B. Galactorrhea associated with hypothyroidism in intact bitches. J Am Anim Hosp Assoc 1980;16:851–4.

[15] Cortese L, Oliva G, Verstegen J, et al. Hyperprolactinemia and galactorrhea associated with primary hypothyroidism in a bitch. J Small Anim Pract 1997;38:572–5.

[16] Johnson C, Olivier NB, Nachreiner R, et al. Effect of ^{131}I-induced hypothyroidism on indices of reproductive function in adult male dogs. J Vet Intern Med 1999;13:104–10.

[17] Fritz TE, Lombard LS, Tyler SA, et al. Pathology and familial incidence of orchitis and its relation to thyroiditis in a closed beagle colony. Exp Mol Pathol 1976;24:142–58.

[18] Higgins MA, Rossmeisl JH, Panciera DL. Hypothyroid associated central vestibular disease in 10 dogs: 1999–2005. J Vet Intern Med, 2006;20:1363–9.

[19] Indrieri RJ, Whalen LR, Cardinet GH, et al. Neuromuscular abnormalities associated with hypothyroidism and lymphocytic thyroiditis in three dogs. J Am Vet Med Assoc 1987;190:544–8.

[20] Jaggy A, Oliver JE, Ferguson DC, et al. Neurological manifestations of hypothyroidism: a retrospective study of 29 dogs. J Vet Intern Med 1994;8:328–36.

[21] Bruchim Y, Kushnir A, Shamir MH. L-thyroxine responsive cricopharyngeal achalasia associated with hypothyroidism in a dog. J Small Anim Pract 2005;46:553–4.

[22] Braund KG, Dillon AR, August JR, et al. Hypothyroid myopathy in two dogs. Vet Pathol 1981;18:589–98.

[23] Delauche AJ, Cudodn PA, Podell M, et al. Nemaline rods in canine myopathies: 4 case reports and literature review. J Vet Intern Med 1998;12:424–30.

[24] Budsberg SC, Moore GE, Klappenbach K. Thyroxine-responsive unilateral forelimb lameness and generalized neuromuscular disease in four hypothyroid dogs. J Am Vet Med Assoc 1993;202:1859–60.

[25] Bichsel P, Jacobs G, Oliver JE. Neurologic manifestations associated with hypothyroidism in four dogs. J Am Vet Med Assoc 1988;192:1745–7.

[26] Gaynor AR, Shofer FS, Washabau RJ. Risk factors for acquired megaesophagus in dogs. J Am Vet Med Assoc 1997;211:1406–12.

[27] Dewey CW, Shelton GD, Bailey CS, et al. Neuromuscular dysfunction in five dogs with acquired myasthenia gravis and presumptive hypothyroidism. Prog Vet Neurol 1996;6: 117–23.

[28] MacPhail CM, Monnet E. Outcome of and postoperative complications in dogs undergoing surgical treatment of laryngeal paralysis: 140 cases (1985–1998). J Am Vet Med Assoc 2001;218:1949–56.

[29] Kelly MJ, Hill JR. Canine myxedema stupor and coma. The Compendium on Continuing Education 1984;6:1049–55.

[30] Henik RA, Dixon RM. Intravenous administration of levothyroxine for treatment of suspected myxedema coma complicated by severe hypothermia in a dog. J Am Vet Med Assoc 2000;216:713–7.

[31] Pullen WH, Hess RS. Hypothyroid dogs treated with intravenous levothyroxine. J Vet Intern Med 2006;20:32–7.

[32] Zeiss CJ, Waddle G. Hypothyroidism and atherosclerosis in dogs. The Compendium on Continuing Education 1995;17:1117–22.

[33] Liu S-K, Tilley LP, Tappe JP, et al. Clinical and pathologic findings in dogs with atherosclerosis: 21 cases (1970–1983). J Am Vet Med Assoc 1986;189:227–32.

[34] von Klopmann T, Boettcher IC, Rotermund A, et al. Euthyroid sick syndrome in dogs with idiopathic epilepsy before treatment with anticonvulsant drugs. J Vet Intern Med 2006; 20:516–22.

[35] Panciera DL. Conditions associated with canine hypothyroidism. Vet Clin North Am Small Anim Pract 2001;31:935–50.

[36] Beaver BV, Haug LI. Canine behaviors associated with hypothyroidism. J Am Anim Hosp Assoc 2003;39:431–4.

[37] Panciera DL. An echocardiographic and electrocardiographic study of cardiovascular function in hypothyroid dogs. J Am Vet Med Assoc 1994;205:996–1000.

[38] Calvert CA, Jacobs GJ, Medleau L, et al. Thyroid stimulating hormone stimulation tests in cardiomyopathic Doberman pinschers: a retrospective study. J Vet Intern Med 1998;12:343–8.

[39] Phillips DE, Harkin KR. Hypothyroidism and myocardial failure in two Great Danes. J Am Anim Hosp Assoc 2003;39:133–7.

[40] MacGregor JM, Rozanski EA, McCarthy RJ, et al. Cholesterol-based pericardial effusion and aortic thromboembolism in a 9 year old mixed breed dog with hypothyroidism. J Vet Intern Med 2004;18:354–8.

[41] Hess RS, Kass PH, Van Winkle TJ. Association between diabetes mellitus, hypothyroidism or hyperadrenocorticism, and atherosclerosis in dogs. J Vet Intern Med 2003;17: 489–94.

[42] Gerritsen RJ, van der Brom WE, Stokhof AA. Relationship between atrial fibrillation and primary hypothyroidism in the dog. Vet Q 1996;18:49–51.

[43] Kern TJ, Riis RC. Ocular manifestations of secondary hyperlipidemia associated with hypothyroidism and uveitis in a dog. J Am Anim Hosp Assoc 1980;16:907–14.

[44] Crispin SM, Barnett KC. Arcus lipoids corneae secondary to hypothyroidism in the Alsatian. J Small Anim Pract 1978;19:127–42.

[45] Miller PE, Panciera DL. Effects of experimentally induced hypothyroidism on the eye and ocular adnexa in dogs. Am J Vet Res 1994;55:692–7.

[46] Feldman EC, Nelson RW. Hypothyroidism. In: Feldman EC, Nelson RW, editors. Canine and feline endocrinology and reproduction. Philadelphia: WB Saunders; 2004.

[47] Saunders HM, Jezyk PK. The radiographic appearance of canine congenital hypothyroidism: skeletal changes with delayed treatment. Veterinary Radiology 1991;32:171–7.

[48] Lieb AS, Grooters AM, Tyler JW, et al. Tetraparesis due to vertebral physeal fracture in an adult dog with congenital hypothyroidism. J Small Anim Pract 1997;38:364–7.

[49] Reusch CE, Gerber B, Boretti FS. Serum fructosamine concentrations in dogs with hypothyroidism. Vet Res Commun 2002;26:531–6.

[50] Lee WM, Diaz-Espineira M, Mol JA, et al. Primary hypothyroidism in dogs is associated with elevated GH release. J Endocrinol 2001;168:59–66.

[51] Avgeris S, Lothrop CD, McDonald TP. Plasma von Willebrand factor concentration and thyroid function in dogs. J Am Vet Med Assoc 1990;196:921–4.

[52] Panciera DL, Johnson GS. Plasma von Willebrand factor antigen concentration in dogs with hypothyroidism. J Am Vet Med Assoc 1994;205:1550–3.

[53] Panciera DL, Johnson GS. Plasma von Willebrand factor antigen concentration and buccal mucosal bleeding time in dogs with experimental hypothyroidism. J Vet Intern Med 1996;10:60–4.

[54] Heseltine JC, Panciera DL, Troy GC, et al. Effect of levothyroxine administration on hemostatic analytes in Doberman Pinschers with von Willebrand disease. J Vet Intern Med 2005;19:523–7.

[55] Melendez LD, et al. Concurrent hypoadrenocorticism and hypothyroidism in 10 dogs [abstract]. J Vet Intern Med 1996;10:182.

[56] Hargis AM, Stephens LC, Benjamin SA, et al. Relationship of hypothyroidism to diabetes mellitus, renal amyloidosis, and thrombosis in purebred beagles. Am J Vet Res 1981;42:1077–81.

[57] Ford SL, Nelson RW, Feldman EC, et al. Insulin resistance in three dogs with hypothyroidism and diabetes mellitus. J Am Vet Med Assoc 1993;202:1478–80.

[58] Tanase H, Kudo K, Horikoshi H, et al. Inherited primary hypothyroidism with thyrotrophin resistance in Japanese cats. J Endocrinol 1991;129:245–51.

[59] Arnold U, Opitz M, Grosser I, et al. Goitrous hypothyroidism and dwarfism in a kitten. J Am Anim Hosp Assoc 1984;20:753–8.

[60] Jones BR, Gruffydd-Jones TJ, Sparkes AH, et al. Preliminary studies on congenital hypothyroidism in a family of Abyssinian cats. Vet Rec 1992;131:145–8.

[61] Rand JS, Levine J, Best SJ, et al. Spontaneous adult-onset hypothyroidism in a cat. J Vet Intern Med 1993;7:272–6.

[62] Schumm-Draeger PM, Lamger E, Caspar G, et al. Spontaneous Hashimoto-like thyroiditis in cats. Verh Dtsch Ges Pathol 1996;80:297–301 [in German].

[63] Greco DS. Diagnosis of congenital and adult onset hypothyroidism in cats. Clin Tech Small Anim Pract 2006;21:40–3.

Cardiovascular and Renal Manifestations of Hyperthyroidism

Harriet M. Syme, BSc, BVetMed, PhD, MRCVS

Department of Veterinary Clinical Sciences, Royal Veterinary College, University of London,
Hawkshead Lane, North Mymms, Hatfield, Hertfordshire AL9 7TA, UK

In the simplest terms, hyperthyroidism is the clinical syndrome that results from an excess of thyroid hormones. This review considers the effects of hyperthyroidism on the cardiovascular and renal systems by reviewing the available literature on the clinical manifestations of this syndrome in the cat and also considering experimental studies and experience in other species, including human beings.

MECHANISMS OF THYROID HORMONE ACTION IN TARGET TISSUES

To understand the alterations in organ function that occur as a result of hyperthyroidism, it is necessary to review the mechanisms by which thyroid hormones act within the cell. Although thyroxine (T_4) is the major product secreted by the follicular cells of the thyroid gland, it is the metabolite triiodothyronine (T_3) that is responsible for the main hormonal activity. The biologic activity of thyroid hormone is controlled by the intracellular T_3 concentration. This, in turn, depends on the concentrations of the circulating thyroid hormones T_3 and T_4, factors controlling the entry of these hormones into cells, and the activity of deiodinase enzymes within the cell that can convert the prohormone T_4 into T_3 or convert the hormones into inactive metabolites (Fig. 1).

Although it was originally presumed that thyroid hormones simply passed through the cell membrane because of their lipophilic structure, it is now known that most thyroid hormone passes through the cell membrane by means of specific transporters, several of which have been characterized [1]. In general, the transporters responsible for thyroid hormone uptake into the cell are organic anion transporters and amino acid transporters. Expression of some of these transporters is tissue specific, resulting in one mechanism for control of intracellular thyroid hormone availability.

E-mail address: hsyme@rvc.ac.uk

0195-5616/07/$ – see front matter
doi:10.1016/j.cvsm.2007.05.011

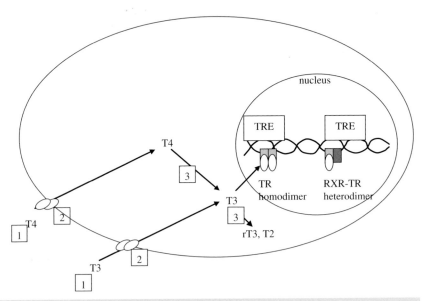

Fig. 1. Mechanisms for control of thyroid hormone activity within target tissue. (1) Concentration of circulating T_4 and T_3 is controlled by the thyroid gland and the peripheral actions of 5'-deiodinase type 1. (2) Entry of thyroid hormones into cells is controlled by specific membrane transporters. (3) Conversion of the prohormone T_4 into T_3 and of T_3 into inactive metabolites is, in turn, controlled by 5'-deiodinase enzymes (types 2 and 3). TR, thyroid receptor; TRE, thyroid hormone response element; RXR, retinoid X receptor.

Once thyroid hormone has entered the target cell, it may exert its biologic effects (T_3), be converted from an inactive precursor (T_4) into active hormone (T_3), or be metabolized (T_4 or T_3) into inactive hormones (rT_3 or T_2). All these conversions are controlled by iodothyronine deiodinase enzymes, a family of selenoproteins that catalyze the removal of specific iodine moieties from thyroid hormones. Deiodinases seem to be of critical importance in development, ensuring that there is regulated and coordinated exposure of specific tissues to thyroid hormones at different times. Expression of different deiodinase enzymes is, at least in part, responsible for the variable sensitivity of different tissues to thyroid hormones, because the intracellular production of T_3 is low in some tissues. There are recognized species differences in the tissue distribution and substrate selectivity of the deiodinase enzymes [2].

The classic mechanism of thyroid hormone action once in the cell is by means of interaction with nuclear receptors that bind to regulatory regions of genes, and thus act to up- or downregulate their expression. Thyroid hormone (T_3) regulates nuclear gene expression by binding to the thyroid hormone receptors, TRα and TRβ, each of which, in turn, has several different isoforms. At the target gene promoter, TR interacts with a distinct DNA sequence, termed the *thyroid hormone response element* (TRE), as a homodimer or, more often, as a heterodimer with retinoid X receptor (RXR) [3]. Target genes may be positively or negatively regulated by T_3, although negative regulation seems to be more common, at least in the liver [4]. At negatively regulated TREs, unliganded TRs mediate constitutive gene expression and T_3 binding induces active repression of gene transcription. Conversely, at positively regulated TREs, unliganded TRs mediate basal transcriptional repression and T_3 binding stimulates the active induction of gene transcription. Numerous families of coactivator and corepressor proteins exist, and binding or displacement of these proteins serves to amplify the effect of ligand-induced transcriptional repression or activation.

Classic genomic effects of steroid hormone binding have a considerable latency with response times in hours to days. Several thyroid hormone–mediated actions are known to occur within a few minutes, however, and are therefore incompatible with the classic genomic model of action. Nongenomic actions of thyroid hormones have been described at the plasma membrane, in the cytoplasm, and in cellular organelles, particularly the mitochondrion [5]. Nongenomic effects include the modulation of ion flux into and within the cell and the activation of numerous second-messenger systems. These effects are not, however, totally independent of the genomic actions of thyroid hormone, because activation of signaling pathways by nongenomic mechanisms may result in phosphorylation of TRs, augmenting their transcriptional activity and stability.

PHYSIOLOGIC EFFECTS OF THYROID HORMONE ON THE CARDIOVASCULAR SYSTEM

Thyroid hormones have profound effects on the cardiovascular system. Many of the clinical manifestations of hyperthyroidism are attributable to the ability of thyroid hormones to alter cardiovascular hemodynamics [6]. This has resulted in considerable study of the pathophysiologic effects of thyroid hormones on the cardiovascular system in human beings and animal models and at the cellular and molecular level.

Heart Rate

Thyroid hormone has a consistent positive chronotropic effect, and resting sinus tachycardia is the most common cardiovascular sign of hyperthyroidism in people. Circadian rhythm is preserved and may even be exaggerated [7]. Analysis of heart rate variability in hyperthyroid human patients supports a relative decrease in parasympathetic tone [8]. Beta-blockade reduces the tachycardia but does not completely abrogate it, supporting the notion also demonstrated by cell culture experiments that thyroid hormone is directly able to increase the rate of sinus node firing [9]. A direct effect is also supported by the positive chronotropic effect of thyroid hormone in isolated denervated hearts [10].

Autonomic Effects

The effects of sympathomimetic agents and thyroid hormones (such as increases in heart rate and contractility) are similar, and treatment of patients with beta-blockers ameliorates many of the clinical signs of hyperthyroidism. This has resulted in the hypothesis that some of the effects of thyroid hormone are mediated by increased activity of the sympathoadrenal system, but this theory has been difficult to substantiate. Because plasma and urine catecholamine concentrations are not elevated in thyrotoxicosis [11], it has been proposed that the sensitivity of the sympathoadrenal system is increased, but investigations in this area have yielded contradictory results [12,13]. Baroreceptor function, although blunted in hypothyroidism, seems to be similar in hyperthyroid and euthyroid rats [14]. Perhaps the most convincing evidence for adrenergic hyperresponsiveness in the hyperthyroid state comes from recent studies using transgenic mice [15]. In these mice, the human type 2 iodothyronine deiodinase (D2) gene is expressed in the myocardium, resulting in mild chronic thyrotoxicosis that is limited to cardiac tissue; circulating thyroid hormone concentrations are normal. Cardiomyocytes from these D2 transgenic mice exhibit an increase in β-adrenergic responsiveness.

Systemic Vascular Resistance and Blood Pressure

Thyrotoxicosis may be associated with as much as a 50% decline in systemic vascular resistance (SVR) [3]. T_3 causes this decrease in SVR by dilating the resistance arterioles of the peripheral circulation. This effect is greater than can be accounted for by thyroid hormone–induced increases in tissue metabolism and consequent release of locally acting vasodilators. Indeed, a direct relaxant effect of T_3 on vascular smooth muscle cells has been demonstrated in isolated skeletal muscle arteries [16] and in cell culture [17]. The rapidity with which the relaxation occurs in these studies favors a nongenomic mechanism. Endothelial denudation attenuates but does not abolish the T_3-mediated effect on arteriolar tone [16]. Altered secretion of atrial natriuretic peptide and adrenergic tone may also contribute to the T_3-induced changes in vascular resistance [18].

Administration of T_3 to healthy euthyroid human volunteers results in a reduction in SVR and increase in cardiac output (CO) within minutes, also supporting a nongenomic mechanism of thyroid hormone action in this setting. Supraphysiologic doses of T_3 were used in those experiments, however, so the physiologic relevance of the effects is not clearly established [19].

In the clinical setting, hyperthyroidism causes only a minor reduction in mean arterial blood pressure, because decreases in diastolic pressure attributable to peripheral vasodilation are offset by increases in systolic pressure caused by increases in stroke volume [20]. The increase in heart rate that occurs in hyperthyroidism may also contribute to the observed increases in systolic arterial pressure as the result of a reduction in the dynamic compliance of the arterial tree. This is because when the heart rate is elevated, the reflected pressure wave from the peripheral arterial tree may summate with the forward pressure wave from a subsequent cardiac contraction, increasing systolic pressure [21].

Cardiac Output

One of the predominant cardiovascular effects in hyperthyroidism is the increase in CO that occurs. This has been studied extensively in human patients and in animal models; however, the relative contribution of alterations in peripheral hemodynamics and myocardial contractility is still the subject of some debate [21]. Although these mechanisms of action are not mutually exclusive, whether the vascular or myocardial mechanism predominates may be of clinical significance, because modulation of loading status is thought to be a more energetically favorable method for increasing cardiac performance than increases in contractility. The importance of SVR to the increase in CO that occurs in hyperthyroidism was demonstrated by an experiment in which arterial vasoconstrictors were administered to human volunteers, resulting in a decrease in CO of 34% in those with hyperthyroidism but with no net effect in euthyroid subjects [22].

As a result of the decrease in SVR that occurs with hyperthyroidism, effective arterial filling volume falls, causing stimulation of the renin-angiotensin-aldosterone system (RAAS) [23]. Activation of the RAAS, in turn, stimulates renal sodium reabsorption, leading to an increase in plasma volume. In addition, thyroid hormone stimulates erythropoietin secretion [24]. The increase in blood volume that results from these actions increases cardiac preload, and this is one mechanism by which CO is increased in hyperthyroidism. The increase in cardiac preload that occurs in thyrotoxicosis may trigger secretion of atrial natriuretic peptide, although a stimulatory effect on ANP gene transcription by T_3 is also reported [25].

Within the cardiac myocyte, thyroid hormones regulate numerous genes that are intimately related to contractile function. One of the key events controlling systolic contraction and diastolic relaxation is the rate at which the free calcium concentration in the cytosol appears and disappears, limiting the availability of calcium to troponin C of the thin filament of the myofibrils. The increase in systolic contractile activity in the hyperthyroid heart is largely attributable to the increase in calcium release from the ryanodine channels in the sarcoplasmic reticulum [3,26]. Hyperthyroidism also results in a reduction in diastolic relaxation time. Numerous ion pumps play a role in the decline in cytosolic calcium concentration that controls this, but the sarcoplasmic reticulum Ca^{++} ATPase makes the greatest contribution. Expression of the gene coding for this pump (SERCA2) is markedly increased by T_3 [27]. The activity of the sarcoplasmic reticulum Ca^{++} ATPase is also regulated by phospholamban, and this, in turn, is also influenced by thyroid hormones. Numerous other plasma membrane transporters (including Na^+/K^+ ATPase, Na^+/Ca^{++} exchanger, and voltage-gated potassium channels) are also regulated at the translational and posttranslational levels by thyroid hormones [28]. These and other proteins modulated by thyroid hormones have been the subject of a recent review [3].

Hyperthyroidism can also alter the expression of genes encoding structural proteins within the cardiac myocyte. A typical example of T_3-induced alterations in cardiac contractile proteins is the altered myosin heavy chain isoform (from MHCβ to MHCα) that occurs in the hearts of hyperthyroid rats, resulting in accelerated cardiac contraction [29]. In human beings and other species, however, including the cat, in which MHCβ is the dominant isoform expressed in adult life, it is not clear whether an alteration in myosin isoform occurs to any significant extent in the hyperthyroid state [30,31]. Thyroid hormones also cause a marked change in numerous other contractile proteins, including cardiac actin, at least in rodents [32].

Although these and numerous other cellular mechanisms may contribute to an intrinsic increase in cardiac contractility in hyperthyroidism, there are studies suggesting that the consequences may be relatively trivial compared with those induced by hemodynamic alterations, predominantly driven by the decrease in SVR. In one study of human beings subjected to cardiac catheterization, left ventricular function in patients with hyperthyroidism was compared with that of volunteers who were atrially paced at identical heart rates. The authors concluded that there was no significant increase in myocardial contractility in hyperthyroid human patients independent of changes in heart rate and cardiac preload [33]. Also, experiments with rodents that have a heterotopically transplanted heart (an additional heart that is perfused from the abdominal aorta) have shown that although hyperthyroidism causes the expected increases in heart rate and switching of MHC isoforms in the native heart and the heterotopic heart, cardiac hypertrophy only develops in the native hemodynamically loaded heart [10].

CARDIOVASCULAR MANIFESTATIONS OF HYPERTHYROIDISM IN CATS

Several derangements of the cardiovascular system have been reported in cats diagnosed with hyperthyroidism. As in human beings, one of the more consistently documented abnormalities is tachycardia. This is reportedly found in approximately half of all hyperthyroid cats at presentation, although it seems that its prevalence is decreasing, presumably because of earlier diagnosis of the disease [34–36].

Systolic murmurs and gallop rhythms are frequently documented in hyperthyroid cats [36,37]. Hyperkinetic femoral pulses and a prominent left apical precordial beat are also common physical examination findings [37]. Murmurs are most often grade I to grade III/VI, and their intensity often varies with heart rate. In older reports, the murmurs were generally attributed to mitral or tricuspid regurgitation [37,38]. More recently, the murmurs have often been documented with color-flow Doppler echocardiography as being caused by dynamic left or right ventricular outflow tract obstruction [39,40]. The gallop rhythm is attributed to rapid ventricular filling.

Respiratory abnormalities, particularly tachypnea and panting, are relatively common clinical findings and may be precipitated by the stress of visiting the veterinary clinic or the physical examination process itself [36]. It is important to recognize that not all hyperthyroid cats with tachypnea or dyspnea actually have overt congestive heart failure (CHF). Causes for the respiratory signs are likely multifactorial, including heat intolerance as well as a decreased ability to increase the already elevated CO in response to stress or exercise. Exertional dyspnea in hyperthyroid human patients is often related to weakness of the respiratory muscles rather than to cardiac abnormalities [3].

Electrocardiography

Various ECG changes have been described with feline hyperthyroidism. The most common finding is sinus tachycardia, although with earlier diagnosis of the disease, the frequency of this finding is decreasing [35]. Other arrhythmias are also documented, although at a relatively low frequency, including atrial and ventricular arrhythmias and intraventricular conduction defects. The sinus tachycardia usually resolves with treatment for hyperthyroidism, but resolution of the other arrhythmias is less consistent. Coincident disease may be responsible for at least some of the observed abnormalities in this geriatric population of cats and, at least in some instances, the arrhythmias may not be directly related to hyperthyroidism. In people, the prevalence of atrial fibrillation and atrial tachycardia is increased in patients with hyperthyroidism compared with age-matched controls and falls with antithyroid therapy, but the prevalence of ventricular arrhythmias and conduction disturbances is not different in the two populations and does not alter with therapy [41].

The amplitude and duration of the P-QRS-T complexes may be abnormal in hyperthyroid cats. An increase in R-wave amplitude (0.9 mV) was observed in 29% of cats examined by one group in 1979 to 1982 [38], but this abnormality was only found in 8% of cats at the same institution in 1992 to 1993 [35]. The correlation between increased R-wave amplitude and radiographic or echocardiographic evidence of left ventricular enlargement in hyperthyroid cats was found to be poor in one study [42].

Diagnostic Imaging

Thoracic radiographs may show evidence of left-sided cardiomegaly in cats with hyperthyroidism, and in a small proportion, there is evidence of CHF. Echocardiographic abnormalities classically associated with hyperthyroidism include left ventricular hypertrophy, left atrial and ventricular dilation, and increased fractional shortening [37]. It is important to realize, however, that alterations in ventricular wall thickness and chamber dimensions are typically subtle in hyperthyroid cats; indeed, most echocardiographic measurements are within the normal range [39,43–45]. Consistent with this observation, changes in chamber dimension and wall thickness associated with establishment of euthyroidism are usually small [39,43]. The variable that is most consistently decreased by treatment is the fractional shortening [39,44].

It is helpful to consider that from a pathophysiologic standpoint, the anticipated changes that occur with hyperthyroidism are those of volume loading of the left ventricle (eccentric hypertrophy) [46]. This occurs because of an increase in blood volume, together with a shift from the arterial compartment to the venous compartment, resulting in an increase in cardiac preload. Therefore increases in chamber dimension may occur, together with hypertrophy of the ventricular wall, but this is expected to be mild. If marked cardiac hypertrophy is evident, particularly if the ventricular lumen is diminished, the possibility of concurrent idiopathic hypertrophic cardiomyopathy and hyperthyroidism should be considered.

Congestive Heart Failure

The prevalence of CHF in cats with hyperthyroidism also seems to be declining. In cats diagnosed with hyperthyroidism at the Animal Medical Center in New York, CHF was present in 12% of cats in the early 1980s [38] but in only 2% in 1992 to 1993 [34]. Similarly, a study in the United Kingdom found that only 4 (3.1%) of 126 cats diagnosed with hyperthyroidism had CHF, and 2 of these 4 cats had concurrent intrinsic cardiac disease [36]. Taken together, these reports suggest that hyperthyroidism is an uncommon cause of cardiac failure in the absence of preexisting cardiac disease. The volume loading that occurs with hyperthyroidism may readily decompensate preexisting subclinical heart disease, however.

CHF occurs infrequently in hyperthyroid human patients. It may be precipitated by the development of atrial fibrillation, which is of particular hemodynamic significance with the short duration of diastole that occurs at high heart rates. Occasionally, CHF may develop as a result of "rate-related cardiomyopathy" [6]. Pulmonary hypertension and, occasionally, right heart failure have also been associated with thyrotoxicosis [47].

Circulating cardiac troponin I (cTnI) is a sensitive and specific marker for myocyte damage and is increased in cats with hypertrophic cardiomyopathy [48,49]. Troponin I has also been measured in hyperthyroid cats and was elevated infrequently, although none of the cats tested had CHF [39]. Cats with detectable cTnI in that study tended to have higher thyroid hormone concentrations.

Blood Pressure

Hyperthyroidism is frequently cited as an important cause of systemic hypertension in cats. Studies of cats presenting with hypertensive retinopathy or choroidopathy have included only a few cats with hyperthyroidism, however, suggesting that extreme elevation of blood pressure may be relatively infrequent with this condition [50–52] Similarly, ocular examinations performed in a large series of hyperthyroid cats did not identify changes consistent with hypertension [53].

Older studies measuring blood pressure of hyperthyroid cats indicated that hypertension was common [54,55]. The number of cats included in these studies was small, however, and, in the study by Kobayashi and colleagues [54], the cutpoint for diagnosing systemic hypertension was low. More recently, two studies of blood pressure measurement in hyperthyroid cats have been reported as scientific abstracts, although neither has been published in full [56,57]. In the first of these studies, cats were examined in a referral practice before radioactive iodine therapy [56]. When blood pressure was measured using a Doppler method by a single experienced operator in a quiet environment, only 19% of the cats were found to have systolic blood pressure measurements greater than 160 mm Hg. When blood pressure was measured in an uncontrolled manner, however, the prevalence of hypertension was much higher, suggesting that this population is particularly susceptible to the effects of "white-coat" hypertension. The second study was of 100 sequentially diagnosed hyperthyroid cats evaluated in first-opinion practice [57]. Of these cats, only 9 were hypertensive (5 of 9 had ocular lesions) at the time the hyperthyroidism was diagnosed. In addition, 3 cats were receiving amlodipine for previously diagnosed hypertension. These results indicate that hypertension is less common in cats with hyperthyroidism than has been previously supposed. This is in accordance with the observation from experimental studies, and from studies in human patients, that SVR is markedly reduced in hyperthyroidism, resulting in a reduction in diastolic blood pressure, and that although CO is elevated, increases in systolic blood pressure are typically modest.

Interestingly, a proportion of cats actually seem to develop hypertension after treatment for hyperthyroidism [57]. Initial indications are that this occurs in approximately 20% to 25% of cases. This finding needs to be substantiated by following the blood pressure of a larger number of cats during treatment for hyperthyroidism. It is unclear whether this change is associated with the decline in renal function that occurs as euthyroidism is achieved, although the development of hypertension with treatment has not been limited to cats that become azotemic with treatment. A study of the RAAS system did not show any marked differences between cats that developed hypertension and those that remained normotensive [58].

TREATMENT FOR THE CARDIOVASCULAR MANIFESTATIONS OF HYPERTHYROIDISM

Treatment considerations are primarily centered on control of the underlying hyperthyroid state rather than on directly addressing its cardiovascular consequences. Cardiovascular effects of hyperthyroidism may influence the choice of treatment modality (radioactive iodine, antithyroid drugs, or surgical thyroidectomy). In general, provided that antithyroidal drugs are well tolerated, it is sensible to stabilize the condition of hyperthyroid patients before general anesthesia, because a high occurrence of catecholamine-induced arrhythmias has been reported in this clinical setting. If treatment with thiourylenes (methimazole or carbimazole) results in unacceptable side effects, treatment with betablockers is usually successful in reversing many of the cardiovascular effects of hyperthyroidism in the short term.

RENAL MANIFESTATIONS OF HYPERTHYROIDISM

The alterations in renal function that occur in the cat coincident with changes in thyroid status are a source of great clinical concern to veterinarians. In contrast, changes in renal function are barely considered in human medicine, although similar changes do occur. This lack of clinical interest is probably attributable to the low incidence of chronic renal failure in the general human population, compounded by the fact that many people are only middle aged when they develop thyrotoxicosis. As a result of this lack of clinical interest, there has been relatively little basic research into the effect of thyroid hormones on renal function, and much of this has focused on the effects of hypothyroidism rather than hyperthyroidism.

PHYSIOLOGIC EFFECTS OF THYROID HORMONES ON THE RENAL SYSTEM
Renal Hypertrophy
Hyperthyroidism increases the kidney-to-body weight ratio in rats. The mechanism is not well understood, but the participation of the renin-angiotensin system (RAS) has been proposed [59,60]. As a result of renal hypertrophy, interpretation of experimental studies in which the glomerular filtration rate (GFR) has been measured is complicated, because in some studies, the GFR apparently decreases in hyperthyroidism, but this is attributable to normalization of results per gram of renal tissue.

Renal Hemodynamics and Glomerular Filtration Rate
Activation of the RAS has been implicated as a mechanism for the alteration in renal hemodynamics that occurs in the hyperthyroid state. Plasma renin activity (PRA) and plasma concentrations of angiotensin II and aldosterone are increased in experimental hyperthyroidism [61]. RAS activation has also been demonstrated in cats with naturally occurring hyperthyroidism [58]. Local tissue-specific regulation of angiotensin-converting enzyme (ACE) may also be important in the thyroid hormone–induced alterations in renal hemodynamics [60]. It has been suggested that RAS activation may be mediated, at least in part, by changes in β-adrenergic activity, because this is known to increase renin activity. An increase in β-adrenoceptor density within the renal cortex in hyperthyroidism has been reported [62]. Renal denervation does not prevent the T_4-induced increase in renin activity [63], however, and it has been shown that the renin gene has a TRE [64].

Increases in renal perfusion pressure usually result in increases in water and sodium excretion, a phenomenon referred to as the "pressure-diuresis-natriuresis response." This mechanism is thought to be a central component of the feedback mechanism responsible for controlling extracellular fluid volume and arterial pressure. In hyperthyroid rats, the pressure-diuresis-natriuresis mechanism is impaired, such that at any given renal perfusion pressure, less sodium is excreted than in control animals [65]. This may occur because of increased renal tubular reabsorption of sodium. This seems to explain how plasma volume can increase and sodium excretion can decrease in the hyperthyroid state in spite of increases in renal blood flow and GFR. Thyroid hormones also have been shown to enhance tubular reabsorption of other electrolytes, including phosphorus [66] and chloride [67].

Role of Thyroid Hormone in the Progression of Experimental Nephropathy
Thyroidectomy has been shown to reduce proteinuria and slow the progressive deterioration in renal function that occurs in rats with induced renal

insufficiency [68]. Amelioration of proteinuria by thyroidectomy has also been confirmed by other studies [69]. Reduction in proteinuria may occur as a result of changes in glomerular hemodynamics or alteration in proximal tubular protein reabsorption. Hemodynamic mechanisms may predominate in hypothyroidism, because a demonstrable decline in single-nephron glomerular filtration rate (SNGFR) and glomerular capillary pressure occurs in hypothyroid compared with euthyroid rats [69].

Conversely, hyperthyroid rats show increased renal protein excretion. In a study in which aminoguanidine (an inhibitor of inducible nitric oxide synthase [iNOS]) was administered to hyperthyroid rats, a marked increase in blood pressure was noted, but there was no corresponding increase in proteinuria, leading the authors of the study to conclude that the proteinuria occurring in hyperthyroidism does not have a hemodynamic cause [70]. Instead, the authors of the study proposed that the proteinuria occurring in hyperthyroidism may be attributable to a direct effect on the permeability of the glomerular barrier. An alternative explanation would be that the alterations in renal hemodynamics occurring in hyperthyroidism do not directly reflect those of the systemic circulation. The cause of proteinuria in hyperthyroidism should be considered unresolved.

RENAL MANIFESTATIONS OF HYPERTHYROIDISM IN CATS
Glomerular Filtration Rate
Several studies have been performed on cats and show that GFR decreases with treatment for hyperthyroidism. This has been demonstrated to occur with all treatment modalities (radioactive iodine, surgery, and medical treatment) [71–73] and should be considered to occur as a consequence of resolution of the hyperthyroid state rather than as a side effect of treatment. The decline in GFR is detectable 1 month after treatment for hyperthyroidism but then remains stable for at least 6 months [71]. It has also been shown that GFR and effective renal blood flow increase when normal cats are treated with exogenous thyroid hormone [74].

Urea and Creatinine
Urea and creatinine concentrations are inversely related to GFR; therefore, values typically increase after treatment of hyperthyroidism as GFR falls. Increases in creatinine concentration occur fairly consistently in hyperthyroid cats after treatment, although in many instances, these increases occur within the laboratory reference range. Creatinine concentration is also reflective of the patient's muscle mass; thus, in an emaciated hyperthyroid patient, the creatinine concentration may be low for several reasons before treatment.

Assessment of urea concentrations in hyperthyroid cats is more complicated. Urea concentrations tend to be decreased by hyperthyroidism because of the effects on GFR, but an increase in dietary protein intake and protein catabolism may tend to increase urea concentration. For this reason urea/creatinine ratios tend to be increased in hyperthyroid cats and to normalize with treatment

(Lucie Goodwin, unpublished data, 2005). Mild elevation of urea is common in untreated hyperthyroid cats and is poorly correlated with the development of significant azotemia after treatment. For these reasons, in the discussions that follow, only elevation of creatinine is considered as evidence of significant azotemia.

Urinalysis

Polyuria or polydipsia was observed in up to 74% of cats with hyperthyroidism in early reports of the condition [36]. The prevalence of these clinical signs is thought to be decreasing as a result of earlier diagnosis of hyperthyroidism [34]. Urine specific gravity does not seem to be strongly correlated with changes in GFR in cats with hyperthyroidism, because a consistent decrease in specific gravity does not occur with treatment [72,75,76]. Thus, it is important to recognize that some hyperthyroid cats are polyuric or polydipsic without having any evidence of renal disease and that this problem may resolve with treatment for hyperthyroidism. It has been suggested that psychogenic polydipsia, possibly caused by heat intolerance, may play a pathogenic role in some cats [77].

In one study, 12% of cats with hyperthyroidism were diagnosed with urinary tract infections, although, interestingly, none of the affected cats was showing any clinical signs of lower urinary tract disease [78]. Because only cats that remained nonazotemic after treatment for hyperthyroidism were included in that study, it is possible that the prevalence of infections might have been even higher had cats with renal compromise been included.

Mild proteinuria is frequently present in cats with hyperthyroidism. The proteinuria tends to resolve with treatment, even in cats that develop azotemia (Fig. 2) [79]. It is thought that the proteinuria is a reflection of the glomerular hypertension and hyperfiltration that is known to occur in the hyperthyroid state. Alternatively, changes in urinary protein excretion may reflect differences in tubular protein handling. Although, as discussed previously, a change in the structure of the glomerular barrier has been proposed as a cause for the proteinuria observed in hyperthyroid animals, the rapid decrease in protein excretion with treatment for hyperthyroidism seems to make this explanation less likely.

Prediction of Azotemia After Treatment

A significant proportion of cats that are treated for hyperthyroidism become azotemic, but objective data documenting exactly how common this is are lacking. Estimates vary, but in an unselected population of hyperthyroid cats seen in first-opinion clinics in central London, approximately a third become azotemic after treatment [80]. As discussed previously, this is considered to be attributable to the "unmasking" of chronic kidney disease (CKD) in patients with significantly increased GFR attributable to the hemodynamic effects of hyperthyroidism. Even cats that develop azotemia are likely to appear clinically improved after treatment for hyperthyroidism, leading to an underestimation of the proportion of cats that develop azotemia unless renal function is systematically retested in all cats that are treated.

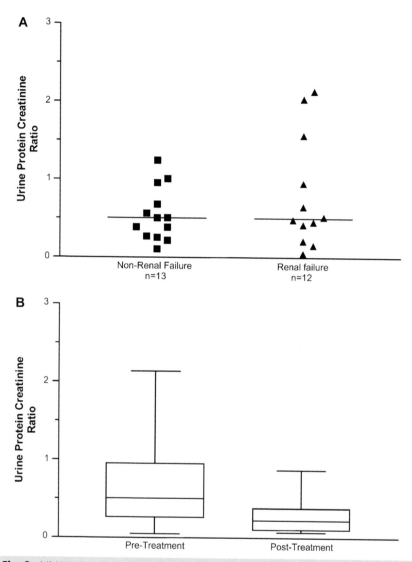

Fig. 2. (A) Urine protein creatinine ratios (UPCs) in untreated hyperthyroid cats. There was no difference in the UPCs of cats that developed azotemia (renal failure group) or remained non-azotemic (non-renal failure group) after treatment for hyperthyroidism. A reference range for UPC derived from normal geriatric cats in the same clinic had an upper limit of 0.43. More than half of the hyperthyroid cats in this study had a UPC ratio that exceeded this. (B) There was a significant ($P < .001$) decrease in UPC after treatment (n = 19) for hyperthyroidism.

Development of azotemia after treatment for hyperthyroidism can be predicted from pretreatment GFR measurements. In one study, a pretreatment GFR of <2.25 mL/kg/min had 100% sensitivity and 78% specificity for the development of posttreatment azotemia [76]. GFR measurements are not widely performed in general practice, however, so attempts have been made to predict the development of azotemia from data obtained from the history, physical examination, or routine biochemistry and urinalysis. It is suggested that azotemia is more likely to develop in older patients and in those with small or irregular kidneys [77,80]. Intuitively, higher creatinine concentrations (even when within the laboratory reference range), lower urine specific gravity, and extremely high pretreatment total T_4 concentrations increase the risk of a patient being azotemic after treatment for hyperthyroidism. No single parameter has been shown to be consistently useful in this prediction, however.

Interestingly, although many cats may be mildly azotemic after treatment for hyperthyroidism, it is not clear how clinically significant this finding is. A study comparing the survival of cats that developed azotemia with those that remained nonazotemic after treatment for hyperthyroidism in an unselected population of cats presented to first-opinion practice did not find any difference between the two groups [81]. Median survival time of the cats that developed azotemia was 595 (range: 62–2016) days compared with 584 (range: 29–2044) days for the cats that did not. These survival times are only slightly shorter than those of cats treated with radioactive iodine, of which it is estimated that 30% to 41% have significant renal problems at their time of death [82,83]. Cats that are treated with radioactive iodine are likely to be selected, to some extent, for a favorable response to treatment because of the cost, the requirement for a period of isolation, and the irreversible nature of the treatment.

A recent study reported that the activity of the tubular enzyme N-acetyl-β-D-glucosaminidase (NAG) was increased in hyperthyroid cats that went on to develop azotemia with treatment compared with hyperthyroid cats that remained nonazotemic [84]. The number of cats included in the study was small, but the result is worthy of further investigation.

Choice of Treatment Modality

It is generally recommended that hyperthyroidism in cats be initially treated medically for a sufficient period to determine whether significant azotemia is likely to develop with the return to euthyroidism. This approach is prudent and allows the owner of a patient to make an informed decision as to whether or not a more permanent form of treatment (radioactive iodine or surgery) should be undertaken. In light of the information given previously regarding survival times, the author does not discourage owners of cats that are mildly azotemic following medical treatment from treating these cats with radioactive iodine or surgical thyroidectomy, provided that the owners are well informed and the patient is acting clinically well.

Methimazole has antioxidant properties that confer a degree of protection against cisplatin- and gentamicin-induced renal injury in experimental models [85,86]. Because the decline in GFR with treatment for hyperthyroidism is related to hemodynamic changes rather than to nephrotoxicity, however, there is no reason to suppose that treatment with this drug confers an intrinsic benefit over the other treatment modalities other than its reversibility. Sometimes, cats that are nonazotemic after treatment with methimazole or carbimazole become azotemic when treated by thyroidectomy or with radioactive iodine. This is usually a result of better control of hyperthyroidism with these treatment methods.

In the author's opinion, it is rarely advisable to undertreat hyperthyroidism deliberately in an attempt to maintain renal parameters within the laboratory reference range, because glomerular hyperfiltration may ultimately be detrimental to renal function as discussed elsewhere in this article.

Treatment of Hyperthyroid Cats That Are Azotemic Before Therapy

Only a small number of hyperthyroid cats are azotemic (have elevated creatinine concentration) before treatment, but these patients can be challenging to diagnose and treat. A retrospective study of cats that had been diagnosed with azotemic CKD and were suspected, and eventually proven, to have concurrent hyperthyroidism found that only 43% had an elevated total T_4 concentration when it was first measured [87]. The diagnosis of hyperthyroidism in the remaining cats was eventually confirmed by repeated measurements of total T_4 or by a T_3 suppression test. The study also found a relatively high rate of false-positive test results using free T_4 measurements and recommended that this test not be used in isolation for the confirmation of hyperthyroidism, a finding that is in accordance with the work of other authors [88,89].

It is important to recognize that diagnosis of cats with concurrent CKD and hyperthyroidism is often not straightforward. Clinical suspicion that hyperthyroidism is present, or is developing, is facilitated by good clinical record keeping. Insidious weight loss in a patient that the owner believes is doing well otherwise and that is maintaining a reasonable appetite in spite of documented CKD should alert the clinician to the possibility of concurrent hyperthyroidism, as should unexplained increases in liver enzyme activities. It is worth noting that creatinine concentration may decrease quite significantly in a patient with renal failure that develops hyperthyroidism; this can be useful in alerting the clinician to the possibility that hyperthyroidism is developing, because there are few clinical conditions that actually cause GFR to increase over time.

When hyperthyroidism is diagnosed in a patient that is concurrently azotemic, medical treatment should be introduced gradually, starting with a low dose of methimazole or carbimazole. This should be increased gradually to the point at which optimum benefit seems to be achieved in terms of general demeanor and weight gain. This is almost inevitably accompanied by worsening azotemia. It is essential to treat the cat and not the numbers in this situation and to recognize that treating hyperthyroidism is likely to result in a decline in GFR (and therefore a worsening of the azotemia) in most patients but that, ultimately, the cat may be best served by controlling the hyperthyroidism. Because the total T_4 concentration is often not elevated before commencing treatment, it can be difficult to know what the therapeutic end point should be. Cats that are azotemic before commencing treatment for hyperthyroidism have short survival times compared with those that only develop azotemia after treatment; reviewing case records of cats treated at the first-opinion clinics of the Royal Veterinary College shows that the median survival time of 30 cats that were azotemic before commencing treatment was approximately 6 months (median survival = 213 days, range: 8–1617 days) (Jenny Wakeling, unpublished data, 2007). Many published studies have excluded cats that were azotemic before treatment; thus, few objective data are available in this regard.

Is Hyperthyroidism Damaging to the Feline Kidney?

As discussed previously, a significant number of hyperthyroid cats develop azotemia after treatment. What is not known is whether this proportion of middle-aged and elderly cats would be expected to have CKD or whether CKD is more common in hyperthyroid cats than in the population at large. There are few good estimates of the prevalence of CKD in the feline population. One study found that 15% of cats older than 15 years presented to North American veterinary schools had renal failure, although this figure may not be representative of the feline population as a whole [90]. As a result, it is impossible to reach firm conclusions regarding whether more hyperthyroid cats develop CKD than would be expected. Further epidemiologic studies are required in this area.

Glomerular hypertension has been demonstrated to cause progressive decline in renal function in the rat and has been proposed as a mechanism for intrinsic progression of CKD in the cat. Indirect evidence that glomerular hypertension occurs in hyperthyroid cats is provided by the observation that urinary protein excretion is increased in many cats at diagnosis, but this resolves rapidly with treatment [79]. Proteinuria has been associated with shortened survival times in cats with CKD or systemic hypertension [91] and also in older apparently healthy cats [92]. It is suggested that the proteinuria may be directly injurious to the kidney, because trafficking of protein through the tubulointerstitium in rats has been demonstrated to cause upregulation of various inflammatory mediators and profibrotic cytokines [93]. It is also possible that proteinuria is simply a marker for glomerular hypertension, with the damage being mediated by means of other mechanisms. Alternatively, proteinuria may be a reflection of a particular type of glomerular lesion that is intrinsically more rapidly progressive.

An additional mechanism that could contribute to renal injury in feline hyperthyroidism is hyperparathyroidism. Hyperthyroid cats have frequently been shown to have elevated parathyroid hormone (PTH) concentrations [94]. Hyperparathyroidism can result in calcification of soft tissues, including the kidney, and has been proposed as a mechanism for the intrinsic progression of CKD. Dietary phosphate restriction, which decreases PTH concentration, has been shown to prolong the survival of cats with CKD [95]. The role, if any, of hyperparathyroidism in the development of CKD in cats with hyperthyroidism is an interesting avenue for further study.

SUMMARY

CO is increased in the hyperthyroid state because of the combined effects of a decrease in SVR and an increase in resting heart rate, resulting in increases in left ventricular ejection fraction and increased blood volume. Cardiovascular manifestations of hyperthyroidism are common in the cat, although the occurrence of overt heart failure is low and seems to be decreasing as the disease is diagnosed earlier in its clinical course. Although CO is increased in hyperthyroidism, the concomitant decrease in SVR means that there is little overall change in systemic arterial pressure.

These hemodynamic alterations, together with activation of the RAS and direct tubular mechanisms, are responsible for marked increases in GFR that occur in the hyperthyroid state. Many cats become azotemic after treatment for hyperthyroidism as preexisting CKD is unmasked. What remains to be conclusively determined is whether the hyperthyroidism is intrinsically damaging to the feline kidney. If it is, this would have profound implications for the treatment of this common endocrine disease.

References

[1] Jansen J, Friesema EC, Milici C, et al. Thyroid hormone transporters in health and disease. Thyroid 2005;15:757–68.

[2] Foster DJ, Thoday KL, Beckett GJ. Thyroid hormone deiodination in the domestic cat. J Mol Endocrinol 2000;24:119–26.

[3] Kahaly GJ, Dillmann WH. Thyroid hormone action in the heart. Endocr Rev 2005;26: 704–28.

[4] Feng X, Jiang Y, Meltzer P, et al. Thyroid hormone regulation of hepatic genes in vivo detected by complementary DNA microarray. Mol Endocrinol 2000;14:947–55.

[5] Bassett JH, Harvey CB, Williams GR. Mechanisms of thyroid hormone receptor-specific nuclear and extra nuclear actions. Mol Cell Endocrinol 2003;213:1–11.

[6] Klein I, Ojamaa K. Thyroid hormone and the cardiovascular system. N Engl J Med 2001; 344:501–9.

[7] von Olshausen K, Bischoff S, Kahaly G, et al. Cardiac arrhythmias and heart rate in hyperthyroidism. Am J Cardiol 1989;63:930–3.

[8] Cacciatori V, Bellavere F, Pezzarossa, et al. Power spectral analysis of heart rate in hyperthyroidism. J Clin Endocrinol Metab 1996;81:2828–35.

[9] Sun ZQ, Ojamaa K, Nakamura TY, et al. Thyroid hormone increases pacemaker activity in rat neonatal atrial myocytes. J Mol Cell Cardiol 2001;33:811–24.

[10] Klein I, Hong C. Effects of thyroid hormone on cardiac size and myosin content of the heterotopically transplanted rat heart. J Clin Invest 1986;77:1694–8.

[11] Coulombe P, Dussault JH, Walker P. Catecholamine metabolism in thyroid disease. II. Norepinephrine secretion rate in hyperthyroidism and hypothyroidism. J Clin Endocrinol Metab 1977;44:1185–9.

[12] Hoit BD, Khoury SF, Shao Y, et al. Effects of thyroid hormone on cardiac beta-adrenergic responsiveness in conscious baboons. Circulation 1997;96:592–8.

[13] Hammond HK, White FC, Buxton IL, et al. Increased myocardial beta-receptors and adrenergic responses in hyperthyroid pigs. Am J Physiol 1987;252:H283–90.

[14] Foley CM, McAllister RM, Hasser EM. Thyroid status influences baroreflex function and autonomic contributions to arterial pressure and heart rate. Am J Physiol Heart Circ Physiol 2001;280:H2061–8.

[15] Carvalho-Bianco SD, Kim BW, Zhang, et al. Chronic cardiac-specific thyrotoxicosis increases myocardial beta-adrenergic responsiveness. Mol Endocrinol 2004;18:1840–9.

[16] Park KW, Dai HB, Ojamaa K, et al. The direct vasomotor effect of thyroid hormones on rat skeletal muscle resistance arteries. Anesth Analg 1997;85:734–8.

[17] Ojamaa K, Klemperer JD, Klein I. Acute effects of thyroid hormone on vascular smooth muscle. Thyroid 1996;6:505–12.

[18] Diekman MJ, Harms MP, Endert E, et al. Endocrine factors related to changes in total peripheral vascular resistance after treatment of thyrotoxic and hypothyroid patients. Eur J Endocrinol 2001;144:339–46.

[19] Schmidt BM, Martin N, Georgens AC, et al. Nongenomic cardiovascular effects of triiodothyronine in euthyroid male volunteers. J Clin Endocrinol Metab 2002;87:1681–6.

[20] Fazio S, Palmieri EA, Lombardi G, et al. Effects of thyroid hormone on the cardiovascular system. Recent Prog Horm Res 2004;59:31–50.

[21] Biondi B, Palmieri EA, Lombardi G, et al. Effects of thyroid hormone on cardiac function: the relative importance of heart rate, loading conditions, and myocardial contractility in the regulation of cardiac performance in human hyperthyroidism. J Clin Endocrinol Metab 2002;87:968–74.

[22] Theilen EO, Wilson WR. Hemodynamic effects of peripheral vasoconstriction in normal and thyrotoxic subjects. J Appl Physiol 1967;22:207–10.

[23] Resnick LM, Laragh JH. Plasma renin activity in syndromes of thyroid hormone excess and deficiency. Life Sci 1982;30:585–6.

[24] Caro J, Silver R, Erslev AJ, et al. Effects of thyroid hormones and glucose supplementation. J Lab Clin Med 1981;98:860–8.

[25] Mori Y, Nishikawa M, Matsubara H, et al. Stimulation of rat atrial natriuretic peptide (rANP) synthesis by triiodothyronine and thyroxine (T4): T4 as a prohormone in synthesizing rANP. Endocrinology 1990;126:466–71.

[26] Jiang M, Xu A, Tokmakejian S, et al. Thyroid hormone-induced overexpression of functional ryanodine receptors in the rabbit heart. Am J Physiol Heart Circ Physiol 2000;278: H1429–38.

[27] Rohrer D, Dillmann WH. Thyroid hormone markedly increases the mRNA coding for sarcoplasmic reticulum Ca2+-ATPase in the rat heart. J Biol Chem 1988;263:6941–4.

[28] Davis PJ, Davis FB. Nongenomic actions of thyroid hormone on the heart. Thyroid 2002;12: 459–66.

[29] Izumo S, Lompre AM, Matsuoka R, et al. Myosin heavy chain messenger RNA and protein isoform transitions during cardiac hypertrophy. Interaction between hemodynamic and thyroid hormone-induced signals. J Clin Invest 1987;79:970–7.

[30] Kinugawa K, Minobe WA, Wood WM, et al. Signaling pathways responsible for fetal gene induction in the failing human heart: evidence for altered thyroid hormone receptor gene expression. Circulation 2001;103:1089–94.

[31] Swynghedauw B. Developmental and functional adaptation of contractile proteins in cardiac and skeletal muscles. Physiol Rev 1986;66:710–71.

[32] Machackova J, Barta J, Dhalla NS. Molecular defects in cardiac myofibrillar proteins due to thyroid hormone imbalance and diabetes. Can J Physiol Pharmacol 2005;83:1071–91.

[33] Merillon JP, Passa P, Chastre J, et al. Left ventricular function and hyperthyroidism. Br Heart J 1981;46:137–43.

[34] Broussard JD, Peterson ME, Fox PR. Changes in clinical and laboratory findings in cats with hyperthyroidism from 1983 to 1993. J Am Vet Med Assoc 1995;206:302–5.

[35] Fox PR, Peterson ME, Broussard JD. Electrocardiographic and radiographic changes in cats with hyperthyroidism: comparison of populations evaluated during 1992–1993 vs. 1979–1982. J Am Anim Hosp Assoc 1999;35:27–31.

[36] Thoday KL, Mooney CT. Historical, clinical and laboratory features of 126 hyperthyroid cats. Vet Rec 1992;131:257–64.

[37] Fox PR, Broussard JD, Peterson ME. Hyperthyroidism and other high output states. In: Fox PR, Sisson D, Moise NS, editors. Textbook of canine and feline cardiology. Philadelphia: WB Saunders; 1999. p. 781–93.

[38] Peterson ME, Kintzer PP, Cavanagh PG, et al. Feline hyperthyroidism: pretreatment clinical and laboratory evaluation of 131 cases. J Am Vet Med Assoc 1983;183:103–10.

[39] Connolly DJ, Guitian J, Boswood A, et al. Serum troponin I levels in hyperthyroid cats before and after treatment with radioactive iodine. J Feline Med Surg 2005;7:289–300.

[40] Rishniw M, Thomas WP. Dynamic right ventricular outflow obstruction: a new cause of systolic murmurs in cats. J Vet Intern Med 2002;16:547–52.

[41] Osman F, Franklyn JA, Holder RL, et al. Cardiovascular manifestations of hyperthyroidism before and after antithyroid therapy: a matched case-control study. J Am Coll Cardiol 2007;49:71–81.

[42] Moise NS, Dietze AE, Mezza LE, et al. Echocardiography, electrocardiography, and radiography of cats with dilatation cardiomyopathy, hypertrophic cardiomyopathy, and hyperthyroidism. Am J Vet Res 1986;47:1476–86.

[43] Weichselbaum RC, Feeney DA, Jessen CR. Relationship between selected echocardiographic variables before and after radioiodine treatment in 91 hyperthyroid cats. Vet Radiol Ultrasound 2005;46:506–13.

[44] Bond BR, Fox PR, Peterson ME, et al. Echocardiographic findings in 103 cats with hyperthyroidism. J Am Vet Med Assoc 1988;192:1546–9.

[45] Moise NS, Dietze AE. Echocardiographic, electrocardiographic, and radiographic detection of cardiomegaly in hyperthyroid cats. Am J Vet Res 1986;47:1487–94.

[46] de Morais HA, Schwartz DS. Pathophysiology of heart failure. In: Ettinger SJ, Feldman EC, editors. Textbook of veterinary internal medicine. 6th edition. St. Louis: Elsevier Saunders; 2005. p. 915–21.

[47] Soroush-Yari A, Burstein S, Hoo GW, et al. Pulmonary hypertension in men with thyrotoxicosis. Respiration 2005;72:90–4.

[48] Herndon WE, Kittleson MD, Sanderson K, et al. Cardiac troponin I in feline hypertrophic cardiomyopathy. J Vet Intern Med 2002;16:558–64.

[49] Connolly DJ, Cannata J, Boswood A, et al. Cardiac troponin I in cats with hypertrophic cardiomyopathy. J Feline Med Surg 2003;5:209–16.

[50] Maggio F, DeFrancesco TC, Atkins CE, et al. Ocular lesions associated with systemic hypertension in cats: 69 cases (1985–1998). J Am Vet Med Assoc 2000;217:695–702.

[51] Littman MP. Spontaneous systemic hypertension in 24 cats. J Vet Intern Med 1994;8:79–86.

[52] Jepson RE, Syme HM, Elliott J. Feline hypertension: the associations between long term blood pressure control and survival. J Vet Intern Med 2005;19:938–938.

[53] van der Woerdt A, Peterson ME. Prevalence of ocular abnormalities in cats with hyperthyroidism. J Vet Intern Med 2000;14:202–3.

[54] Kobayashi DL, Peterson ME, Graves TK, et al. Hypertension in cats with chronic renal failure or hyperthyroidism. J Vet Intern Med 1990;4:58–62.

[55] Stiles J, Polzin DJ, Bistner SI. The prevalence of retinopathy in cats with systemic hypertension and chronic renal failure or hyperthyroidism. Journal of the American Animal Hospital Association 1994;30:564–72.

[56] Stepien RL, Rapoport GS, Henik RA, et al. Effect of measurement method on blood pressure findings in cats before and after therapy for hyperthyroidism. J Vet Intern Med 2003;17:754.

[57] Syme HM, Elliott J. The prevalence of hypertension in hyperthyroid cats at diagnosis and following treatment. J Vet Intern Med 2003;17:754–5.

[58] Jepson RE, Elliott J, Syme HM. The role of renin-angiotensin-aldosterone system (RAAS) in the development of systemic hypertension in cats treated for hyperthyroidism. J Vet Intern Med 2005;19:424–424.

[59] Kobori H, Ichihara A, Miyashita Y, et al. Mechanism of hyperthyroidism-induced renal hypertrophy in rats. J Endocrinol 1998;159:9–14.

[60] Carneiro-Ramos MS, Silva VB, Santos RA, et al. Tissue-specific modulation of angiotensin-converting enzyme (ACE) in hyperthyroidism. Peptides 2006;27:2942–9.

[61] Montiel M, Jimenez E, Navaez JA, et al. Aldosterone and plasma renin activity in hyperthyroid rats: effects of propranolol and propylthiouracil. J Endocrinol Invest 1984;7:559–62.

[62] Haro JM, Sabio JM, Vargas F. Renal beta-adrenoceptors in thyroxine-treated rats. J Endocrinol Invest 1992;15:605–8.

[63] Kobori H, Ichihara A, Suzuki H, et al. Thyroid hormone stimulates renin synthesis in rats without involving the sympathetic nervous system. Am J Physiol 1997;272:E227–32.

[64] Kobori H, Hayashi M, Saruta T. Thyroid hormone stimulates renin gene expression through the thyroid hormone response element. Hypertension 2001;37:99–104.

[65] Vargas F, Atucha NM, Sabio JM, et al. Pressure-diuresis-natriuresis response in hyperthyroid and hypothyroid rats. Clin Sci (Lond) 1994;87:323–8.

[66] Alcalde AI, Sarasa M, Raldua, et al. Role of thyroid hormone in regulation of renal phosphate transport in young and aged rats. Endocrinology 1999;140:1544–51.

[67] Santos OD, Grozovsky R, Goldenberg RC, et al. Thyroid hormone modulates ClC-2 chloride channel gene expression in rat renal proximal tubules. J Endocrinol 2003;178:503–11.

[68] Tomford RC, Karlinsky ML, Buddington B, et al. Effect of thyroparathyroidectomy and parathyroidectomy on renal function and the nephrotic syndrome in rat nephrotoxic serum nephritis. J Clin Invest 1981;68:655–64.

[69] Conger JD, Falk SA, Gillum DM. The protective mechanism of thyroidectomy in a rat model of chronic renal failure. Am J Kidney Dis 1989;13:217–25.

[70] Rodriguez-Gomez I, Wangensteen R, Moreno JM, et al. Effects of chronic inhibition of inducible nitric oxide synthase in hyperthyroid rats. Am J Physiol Endocrinol Metab 2005;288:E1252–7.

[71] Slater LA, Neiger R, Haller M, et al. Long-term changes in glomerular filtration rate in hyperthyroid cats following treatment with iodine-131. J Vet Intern Med 2003;17:742–742.

[72] DiBartola SP, Broome MR, Stein BS, et al. Effect of treatment of hyperthyroidism on renal function in cats. J Am Vet Med Assoc 1996;208:875–8.

[73] Graves TK, Olivier NB, Nachreiner RF, et al. Changes in renal function associated with treatment of hyperthyroidism in cats. Am J Vet Res 1994;55:1745–9.

[74] Adams WH, Daniel GB, Legendre AM. Investigation of the effects of hyperthyroidism on renal function in the cat. Can J Vet Res 1997;61:53–6.

[75] Becker TJ, Graves TK, Kruger JM, et al. Effects of methimazole on renal function in cats with hyperthyroidism. J Am Anim Hosp Assoc 2000;36:215–23.

[76] Adams WH, Daniel GB, Legendre AM, et al. Changes in renal function in cats following treatment of hyperthyroidism using 131I. Vet Radiol Ultrasound 1997;38:231–8.

[77] Feldman EC, Nelson RW. Feline hyperthyroidism (thyrotoxicosis). In: Canine and feline edocrinology and reproduction. 3rd edition. St. Louis: Elsevier Saunders; 2004. p. 118–66.

[78] Mayer-Ronne B, Goldstein RE, Erb HN. Urinary tract infections in cats with hyperthyroidism, diabetes mellitus, chronic renal failure and feline lower urinary tract disease. J Vet Intern Med 2006;18:777–8.

[79] Syme HM, Elliott J. Evaluation of proteinuria in hyperthyroid cats. J Vet Intern Med 2001;15:299.

[80] Elliott J. Chronic renal failure in hyperthyroid cats: diagnostic and therapeutic dilemmas. Proceedings of The North American Veterinary Conference: 2004;590–1.

[81] Wakeling J, Rob C, Elliott J, et al. Survival of hyperthyroid cats is not affected by post-treatment azotaemia. J Vet Intern Med 2006;20:1523–1523.

[82] Slater MR, Geller S, Rogers K. Long-term health and predictors of survival for hyperthyroid cats treated with iodine 131. J Vet Intern Med 2001;15:47–51.

[83] Peterson ME, Becker DV. Radioiodine treatment of 524 cats with hyperthyroidism. J Am Vet Med Assoc 1995;207:1422–8.

[84] Lapointe C, Belanger MC, Dunn M, et al. N-acetyl-β-D-glucosaminidase index as an early biomarker for chronic renal insufficiency in cats with hyperthyroidism. J Vet Intern Med 2006;20:740–1.

[85] Elfarra AA, Duescher RJ, Sausen PJ, et al. Methimazole protection of rats against gentamicin-induced nephrotoxicity. Can J Physiol Pharmacol 1994;72:1238–44.

[86] Braunlich H, Appenroth D, Fleck C. Protective effects of methimazole against cisplatin-induced nephrotoxicity in rats. J Appl Toxicol 1997;17:41–5.

[87] Wakeling J, Moore K, Elliott J, et al. Diagnosis of hyperthyroidism in cats with chronic renal failure, submitted for publication.

[88] Mooney CT, Little CJ, Macrae AW. Effect of illness not associated with the thyroid gland on serum total and free thyroxine concentrations in cats. J Am Vet Med Assoc 1996;208: 2004–8.

[89] Peterson ME, Melian C, Nichols R. Measurement of serum concentrations of free thyroxine, total thyroxine, and total triiodothyronine in cats with hyperthyroidism and cats with nonthyroidal disease. J Am Vet Med Assoc 2001;218:529–36.

[90] Lulich JP, O'Brien TD, Osborne CA, et al. Feline renal failure: questions, answers, questions. Compendium on Continuing Education for the Practicing Veterinarian 1992;14:127–52.

[91] Syme HM, Markwell PJ, Pfeiffer D, et al. Survival of cats with naturally occurring chronic renal failure is related to severity of proteinuria. J Vet Intern Med 2006;20:528–35.

[92] Walker D, Syme HM, Markwell PJ, et al. Predictors of survival in healthy, non-azotaemic cats. J Vet Intern Med 2004;18:417–417.

[93] Abbate M, Remuzzi G. Proteinuria as a mediator of tubulointerstitial injury. Kidney Blood Press Res 1999;22:37–46.

[94] Barber PJ, Elliott J. Study of calcium homeostasis in feline hyperthyroidism. J Small Anim Pract 1996;37:575–82.

[95] Elliott J, Rawlings JM, Markwell PJ, et al. Survival of cats with naturally occurring chronic renal failure: effect of dietary management. J Small Anim Pract 2000;41:235–42.

Vet Clin Small Anim 37 (2007) 745–754

VETERINARY CLINICS
SMALL ANIMAL PRACTICE

Feline Thyroid Storm

Cynthia R. Ward, VMD, PhD

Department of Small Animal Medicine, University of Georgia College of Veterinary Medicine,
501 DW Brooks Drive, Athens, GA 30602, USA

hyrotoxicosis is a term used to describe any condition in which there is an excessive amount of circulating thyroid hormone, whether from excess production and secretion from an overactive thyroid gland, leakage from a damaged thyroid gland, or an exogenous source. In most veterinary patients, thyrotoxicosis occurs from thyroid gland hyperfunction. Feline hyperthyroidism is a common endocrinopathy in middle-aged to older cats and is most often the cause of thyrotoxicosis seen by veterinarians. Although less common, active thyroid carcinomas in cats and dogs can also result in severe thyrotoxicosis. The clinical presentation of thyrotoxicosis in veterinary patients can vary tremendously from asymptomatic biochemical changes to life-threatening multisystemic disease. In human beings, one form of acute thyrotoxicosis is called thyroid storm and is a cause of significant mortality in human emergency rooms. Thyroid storm is uncommon, and the signs can go unrecognized, thus contributing to the high degree of mortality associated with this disease. In human beings, thyroid storm can occur at any age. It can be present in euthyroid patients as well as in treated and partially treated hyperthyroid patients.

Although thyroid storm is a rare but well-recognized syndrome in human medicine, it has not been described as a clinical entity in veterinary medicine. Most frequently, acute thyrotoxicosis is diagnosed in hyperthyroid cats, although dogs with functional carcinomas or after accidental oversupplementation with thyroid hormone are also presented. As with human medicine, early recognition of acute thyrotoxicosis and aggressive therapy can improve the clinical outcome of such patients.

PATHOGENESIS

Just what precipitates the actual thyroid storm syndrome in certain thyrotoxic patients is unknown [1]. Because multiple factors seem to be involved, the exact pathogenesis of the disease is even more clouded. Thyroid hormone causes a cellular effect by the free hormone diffusing into the cell and binding to response elements in the nucleus. The result is thyroid hormone–specific gene expression, resulting in altered cellular metabolism. Therefore, the

E-mail address: cward@vet.uga.edu

0195-5616/07/$ – see front matter
doi:10.1016/j.cvsm.2007.03.002

availability of free thyroid hormone would seem to be an important part of the pathogenesis of thyroid storm.

Initially, one might surmise that circulating thyroid hormones would be significantly higher in patients with thyroid storm than in other thyrotoxic patients. Early studies in thyrotoxic human patients attempted to show such a difference, and total and free thyroid hormone levels were compared between patients with thyroid storm and uncomplicated hyperthyroid patients. Some isolated case reports did show transient elevations in free hormone or changes in thyroxine (T_4)-binding globulin levels in patients with thyroid storm [2]. These biochemical parameter changes are consistent with the presence of nonthyroidal illness, however, and because nonthyroidal illness is a known precipitant of thyroid storm, they may not be diagnostic of thyroid storm itself [3,4]. Further studies have shown that there is no difference between serum total or free thyroid hormone levels in patients with thyroid storm and in more stable hyperthyroid patients in human medicine [5,6].

The rapidity and magnitude of change in the serum thyroid hormone level may be more important than the actual serum levels themselves. This would explain the occurrence of thyroid storm after radioactive iodine therapy and thyroidal surgery, both of which potentially damage the thyroid gland, causing rapid release of hormone [7]. Also supporting this theory is that thyroid storm has been reported to follow abrupt cessation of antithyroid medication or accidental thyroid hormone overdose, both resulting in the rapid rise of serum thyroid hormone levels [8,9]. Additionally, nonthyroidal illness is known to be a precipitating factor for thyroid storm in human medicine. Nonthyroidal illness has been shown to alter binding of thyroid hormones to their carriers. Changes in thyroid hormone–binding protein affinity could be responsible for a rapid increase of circulating free thyroid hormone available to activate cellular targets [10]. A sudden increase of inappropriately activated cells by thyroid hormone could certainly result in thyroid storm.

Activation of the sympathetic nervous system has been implicated in the onset of thyroid storm [11]. Evidence supporting this is that many of the clinical signs and physiologic symptoms seen in thyroid storm are similar to those seen during catecholamine excess. Additionally, medical adrenergic blockade can dramatically reduce clinical signs seen with thyroid storm. In human beings, it has been shown that serum and urine catecholamine levels are within normal limits during thyroid storm [12]. It is known that thyroid hormones can alter tissue sensitivity to catecholamines, however. This can occur at the cell surface receptor as well as at the intracellular signaling levels, and this increased sensitivity may result in the clinical signs seen during thyroid storm [13]. Beta-blockade does not completely prevent thyroid storm [14], however, although it may ameliorate some of the clinical signs. These findings lead to the conclusion that factors other than activation of the sympathetic nervous system are probably important in the development of clinical signs associated with thyroid storm.

There is some evidence that thyroid storm not only results from relative increases in circulating thyroid hormone but that cellular response to thyroid hormone may be enhanced. This effect has been implicated in the cause of thyroid storm resulting from infection, sepsis, hypoxemia, hypovolemia, and lactic or ketoacidosis [15]. Similar enhanced cellular responses may be present in thyrotoxic veterinary patients. In hyperthyroid cats, increased serum concentrations of cardiac troponin I, a marker of cardiac myocyte injury, have been demonstrated [16]. Successful treatment of the hyperthyroidism and reduction of the serum T_4 levels resulted in a decrease of the troponin. Additionally, thyroid hormone has been shown to increase Na^+ current and intracellular Ca^{++} in isolated feline atrial myocytes [17]. These data suggest that exposure to excess thyroid hormone may directly result in alteration of cellular response in the cat or at least in feline cardiac myocytes.

PRECIPITATING EVENTS

In most cases of thyroid storm in human beings, a precipitating event can be identified, although no known causes are found in up to 2% of cases [18]. The most common events are infection, thyroidal and nonthyroidal surgery, radioactive iodine therapy, administration of iodinated contrast dyes, administration of stable iodine, withdrawal of antithyroid medication, amiodarone therapy, ingestion of excessive amounts of exogenous thyroid hormone, vigorous palpation of the thyroid, severe emotional stress, and a variety of acute nonthyroidal illnesses. Common events that may precipitate thyroid storm in feline hyperthyroid patients include radioactive iodine therapy, thyroidal surgery [19], or vigorous thyroid palpation causing destruction of thyroid cells and release of thyroid hormone into the circulation (Box 1). Abrupt withdrawal

---

Box 1: Potential precipitating factors for feline thyroid storm

Associated with acute increase in circulating thyroid hormones

Abrupt withdrawal of methimazole or antithyroid medication

Iodine 131 therapy

Thyroidal surgery

Palpation of the thyroid

Administration of stable iodine compounds

Inappropriate ingestion of excessive thyroid hormone supplementation

Associated with nonthyroidal illness

Stress

Infection

Nonthyroidal surgery

Trauma

Thromboembolic disease

Vascular accidents

of antithyroid medication could result in an acute elevation of circulating thyroid hormone, as could the administration of stable iodine compounds, which result in an initial increase of thyroid hormone synthesis in the cells. Stress and nonthyroidal illness, especially infections, are most likely important for progression of the clinical course in hyperthyroid cats to thyroid storm. The presence of any of the other causes found as precipitating factors in human beings could also play a role in the precipitation of thyroid storm.

CLINICAL SIGNS

Thyroid storm is the acute exacerbation of clinical signs of thyrotoxicosis; however, the diagnosis of thyroid storm in human medicine is primarily a clinical one. In human beings, it is based on the prevalence of four major clinical signs. These include fever; central nervous system (CNS) effects ranging from mild agitation to seizures or coma; gastrointestinal-hepatic dysfunction ranging from vomiting or diarrhea and abdominal pain to unexplained jaundice; and cardiovascular effects, including sinus tachycardia, atrial fibrillation, and congestive heart failure. The combination of these clinical signs, along with identification of a precipitating event, allows for the diagnosis of thyroid storm [18]. In cats presenting with presumed thyroid storm, many of these clinical signs also occur (Box 2). Such cats often show mild to severe respiratory distress. Auscultation may reveal a cardiac murmur or arrhythmia, most often a gallop rhythm [20]. Crackles or dullness in the lung fields indicating pulmonary edema or pleural effusion, respectively, associated with congestive heart failure may also be auscultated [21]. Additional clinical signs that may be associated with thyroid storm in cats include mild to severe hypertension [22]. Retinopathies, including hemorrhage, edema, degeneration, or even retinal

---

Box 2: Clinical signs of feline thyroid storm

Tachypnea

Tachycardia

Hyperthermia

Respiratory distress

Cardiac murmur

Cardiac arrhythmia

Ausculatory crackles or dullness

Sudden blindness

Severe muscle weakness

Ventroflexion of the neck

Absent motor limb function

Neurologic abnormalities

Sudden death

detachment, may be found, especially in hypertensive thyrotoxic cats [23]. Tachypnea and hypothermia may be present, and absent limb motor function may be detected as a result of thromboembolic disease occurring from acute thyrotoxicosis [24]. Severe acute muscle weakness and ventroflexion of the neck may be seen in acutely thyrotoxic cats, often associated with hypokalemia [25]. Cats in thyroid storm may exhibit a myriad of neurologic abnormalities ranging from hyperexcitability to stupor [26]. Sudden death may also occur.

DIAGNOSIS

The diagnosis of thyroid storm is based on identification of the presence of thyrotoxicosis, appropriate clinical signs, and evidence of a precipitating event [18]. Thyrotoxicosis in hyperthyroid cats is demonstrated by an elevated total T_4 level or a total T_4 level in the high normal range combined with an elevated free T_4 level or with lack of suppression by triiodothyronine (T_3) [27]. In some cases, the total T_4 level may be in the normal range in a hyperthyroid cat, but in cases of thyroid storm, the total T_4 and free T_4 levels are expected to be higher than the reference range. The severity of clinical signs in hyperthyroid cats does not seem to correlate with the absolute level of circulating thyroid hormone. Therefore, as in people, the diagnosis of thyroid storm in cats probably cannot be based on absolute serum thyroid hormone levels. In human medicine, thyroid storm is diagnosed based on a point system assigned to each of the main clinical components: fever, CNS signs, gastrointestinal signs, and cardiovascular signs as well as the presence or absence of a precipitating event [18]. In hyperthyroid feline patients, thyroid storm may be diagnosed based on the presence of clinical signs of acute thyrotoxicosis, as described in the preceding paragraph. The owners should be questioned and the clinical case reviewed thoroughly to identify a precipitating event. If one can be found, it would further narrow the diagnosis to thyroid storm.

LABORATORY ABNORMALITIES

Laboratory abnormalities are those seen resulting from uncomplicated thyrotoxicosis [20,28]; there is no distinguishing laboratory value(s) for the diagnosis of feline thyroid storm. In the hyperthyroid cat, hematologic abnormalities may include mild erythrocytosis, macrocytosis, and Heinz body formation. In human patients with thyroid storm, leukocytosis with a left shift in the absence of active infection or inflammation has been identified [29]. In hyperthyroid cats, mature neutrophilia, lymphopenia, and eosinopenia are more commonly identified as stress responses. Biochemical abnormalities seen in people with thyroid storm include mild hyperglycemia and hypercalcemia. Elevated liver enzymes are seen as well, and hyperbilirubinemia may occur in severe cases. This finding carries a poor prognosis. In hyperthyroid cats, elevated liver enzymes, mild hyperglycemia, hyperbilirubinemia, and severe hypokalemia may be seen in acute thyrotoxicosis. A decreased sodium/potassium ratio may be seen in thyrotoxic cats that are presented in heart failure with pleural effusions [30]. Mild to severely elevated creatine kinase may be seen in cats presenting with thyroid storm. Radiographs may reveal an enlarged heart or evidence of congestive heart failure. Echocardiography may show hypertrophy of the left ventricular wall or left interventricular septum [31]. Myocardial contractility deficits also may be seen.

TREATMENT

Treatment of thyroid storm is aimed at controlling the four major problematic areas: (1) to reduce the production or secretion of thyroid hormones, (2) to counteract the peripheral effects of thyroid hormones, (3) to provide systemic support, and (4) to identify and eliminate the precipitating factor [32].

Reduction in the Production or Secretion of New Thyroid Hormones

The thioimidazole compound methimazole inhibits iodine incorporation into tyrosyl residues of thyroglobulin, and thus prevents the synthesis of active thyroid hormone. As a result, methimazole should be the first line of defense against thyroid storm. It does not prevent the secretion of already formed thyroid hormones, however. Methimazole may be given orally, transdermally, or even rectally in cats [33]. The dose should be toward the high end (5 mg administered twice daily) in cats that have normal renal function [34]. If there is suspected renal insufficiency or failure, the dose of methimazole should be reduced by half.

Methimazole blocks the formation of new active thyroid hormone, but other therapy must be instituted to prevent further secretion of formed hormone, which is stored in high concentrations in the thyroid gland. This can be done by treatment with stable iodine compounds, such as potassium iodine. In large doses, these compounds can also decrease the synthesis rate of thyroid hormone. They must be given 1 hour after methimazole administration, because a large load of iodine initially stimulates thyroid hormone production. Potassium iodate, a more stable form of potassium iodine, has been used successfully in cats and may be given at a dose of 25 mg every 8 hours [35]. Instead of potassium iodide, lipid-soluble radiographic contrast agents containing stable iodine, such as iopanoic acid, may be given. Such compounds have been used in hyperthyroid cats as an ancillary treatment for hyperthyroidism. Iopanoic acid or diatrizoate meglumine may be given at a dose of 100 mg by mouth twice daily [36]. Although iopanoic acid is available in a parenteral form, oral dosing is safer because it is a hyperosmolar agent. These compounds have the additional advantages of blocking peripheral conversion of T_4 to T_3, blocking T_3 binding to its receptor, and inhibiting thyroid hormone synthesis [37].

Inhibition of Peripheral Effects of Thyroid Hormone

The most rapid relief of signs caused by thyroid storm is by medications that block the β-adrenergic receptors, such as propranolol and atenolol. The nonselective beta-blocker propranolol, most commonly used as a sympatholytic in human medicine, is inherently difficult to use in cats because of its poor oral bioavailability and short half-life, requiring dosing every 8 hours. Its use has been largely superseded by that of atenolol because of its selectivity and the once-daily dosing regimen [38]. Propranolol has been shown to inhibit the peripheral conversion of T_4 to T_3, although this effect happens slowly [39]. Therefore, its use may be advantageous in severely thyrotoxic cats [35]. Additionally, it may be used intravenously. Propranolol should be used toward the high end of the dose range at 5 mg administered by mouth every 8 hours or 0.02 mg/kg administered intravenously over 1 minute to ensure β-adrenergic blockade. Alternatively, the selective β_1-adrenergic blocker atenolol may be used at a dose of 1 mg/kg administered every 12 to 24 hours. In acute situations, the short-acting β_1-adrenergic blocker esmolol may be used intravenously at a loading dose of 0.5 mg/kg administered intravenously over 1 minute, followed by a constant rate intravenous infusion of 10 to 200 μg/kg/min.

An extreme method to fight the peripheral actions of excess thyroid hormones is to reduce the systemic levels present. Peritoneal dialysis, plasmapheresis, and hemodialysis have been used in human medicine as well as cholestyramine, which inhibits enterohepatic circulation of thyroid hormones by binding to the gastrointestinal tract [40–42]. These methods are rarely used in human patients and probably have limited use in veterinary patients with thyroid storm.

Systemic Support

The third arm of treatment for thyroid storm involves reversing the effects of thyroid hormones on the body. Fever should be treated by the judicious use of ice packs and fans. Volume depletion is another common systemic effect of thyroid storm, and this should be treated aggressively with crystalloid fluid replacement. Because many cats have concurrent cardiomyopathy, they should be thoroughly evaluated for heart failure to ensure judicious fluid use. Colloid therapy is generally not indicated unless severe gastrointestinal disease or another syndrome resulting in low oncotic pressure is present. Serum potassium levels should be closely monitored, and potassium supplementation should be added as necessary, remembering that some patients with thyroid storm become acutely hypokalemic and demonstrate severe muscle weakness [25]. Dextrose supplementation of 5% to 10% should be considered as well as B vitamin supplementation to combat potential thiamine deficiency in hyperthyroid cats.

Cardiac disturbances are common with thyroid storm in people, and it is not uncommon for cats with thyroid storm to be presented with cardiac failure that must be managed. β-adrenergic blockade therapy, as described previously, may also be helpful to manage mild cardiac failure because of its effects in reducing the elevated heart rate caused by thyrotoxicosis; however, its use should be avoided in cats presenting with severe heart failure because it could cause lowering of the cardiac output to a dangerous level. Furosemide (1–4 mg/kg administered intravenously or intramuscularly as a bolus when needed, 0.5–2 mg/kg administered by mouth every day), angiotensin-converting enzyme (ACE) inhibitors (enalapril or benazepril at a dose of 0.5–2 mg/kg administered by mouth twice daily), isosorbide dinitrate (0.5–2 mg/kg administered by mouth every 8–12 hours), nitroglycerin (0.5–1.5 administered cutaneously every 8–12 hours), or hydralazine (0.5–1 mg/kg administered intravenously as a bolus as needed, 0.5–2 mg/kg administered by mouth every 12 hours) may be useful to manage feline heart failure but must be used with care in patients with renal compromise. In all cases, medications should be started at the lowest levels and titrated up to effect and blood pressure must be carefully monitored. Supraventricular arrhythmias are also common in human thyroid storm, with the most common disturbance being atrial fibrillation. In feline patients with thyroid storm, atrial fibrillation can also occur. β-adrenergic receptor blockade, as described previously, is a first-line defense in treating these arrhythmias. Thromboembolic disease may be a sequela in thyrotoxic feline patients, especially those with heart failure or atrial fibrillation [43]. Anticoagulation therapy should be considered to include low-dose aspirin (5 mg per cat every 72 hours), heparin (200–400 U/kg administered subcutaneously every hour until the partial thromboplastin time [PTT] is 1.5–2 times prolonged), and low-molecular-weight heparin (100 U/kg administered subcutaneously every 6 hours). Hypertension is often a complication of thyroid storm in cats. Blood pressure in these cats should be checked, and antihypertensive therapy should be instituted as appropriate to include beta-blockade, as discussed previously, or amlodipine (0.625–1.25 mg per cat every day). In acute cases of hypertension, nitroprusside may be used as a constant rate infusion at 0.5 to 5 µg/kg/min.

In human beings with thyroid storm, a relative adrenal insufficiency can be found because of increased cortisol clearance, leading some physicians to treat with glucocorticoids [42,44]. No such studies have been done in feline patients with thyroid storm, and the use of glucocorticoid therapy in these patients is controversial.

Eradication of the Precipitating Factor

In human thyroid storm, a precipitating factor is one of the criteria that define the disease. The presence of a precipitating factor should be thoroughly investigated in cats presenting with thyroid storm. A full workup, including a full hematologic examination, biochemical analysis, urinalysis, retroviral testing, blood pressure measurement, and imaging studies, should be performed on these cats. Abnormal findings should be further examined by specialized testing. If another abnormality is identified, it should be treated to prevent recurrence of thyroid storm.

OUTCOME

Although thyroid storm is an uncommon presentation in human emergency rooms, there is a significant rate of mortality in patients with this syndrome. Rapid recognition of the problem as well as aggressive treatment is necessary for a successful outcome. Thyroid storm is not as well defined a syndrome in feline medicine, although acute manifestations of thyrotoxicosis result in a syndrome that can be considered feline thyroid storm. Veterinary recognition of this syndrome may be lacking; thus, it is unknown what the true incidence and mortality from thyroid storm may be in cats. Nevertheless, it is certainly recognized that death may result from treated or untreated acute thyrotoxicosis. As in human patients, it is anticipated that early recognition and aggressive treatment of feline thyroid storm should improve the survival of veterinary patients.

References

[1] Dillmann WH. Thyroid storm. Curr Ther Endocrinol Metab 1997;6:81–5.

[2] Brooks MH, Waldstein SS. Free thyroxine concentrations in thyroid storm. Ann Intern Med 1980;93(5):694–7.

[3] Chopra IJ, Hershman JM, Pardridge WM, et al. Thyroid function in nonthyroidal illnesses. Ann Intern Med 1983;98(6):946–57.

[4] Colebunders R, Bourdoux P, Bekaert J, et al. Determination of free thyroid hormones and their binding proteins in a patient with severe hyperthyroidism (thyroid storm?) and thyroid encephalopathy. J Endocrinol Invest 1984;7(4):379–81.

[5] Jacobs HS, Mackie DB, Eastman CJ, et al. Total and free triiodothyronine and thyroxine levels in thyroid storm and recurrent hyperthyroidism. Lancet 1973;2(7823):236–8.

[6] Tietgens ST, Leinung MC. Thyroid storm. Med Clin North Am 1995;79(1):169–84.

[7] McDermott MT, Kidd GS, Dodson LE Jr, et al. Radioiodine-induced thyroid storm. Case report and literature review. Am J Med 1983;75(2):353–9.

[8] Mandel SH, Magnusson AR, Burton BT, et al. Massive levothyroxine ingestion. Conservative management. Clin Pediatr (Phila) 1989;28(8):374–6.

[9] Maussier ML, D'Errico G, Putignano P, et al. Thyrotoxicosis: clinical and laboratory assessment. Rays 1999;24(2):263–72.

[10] McIver B, Gorman CA. Euthyroid sick syndrome: an overview. Thyroid 1997;7(1):125–32.

[11] Silva JE. Catecholamines and the sympathoadrenal system in thyrotoxicosis. In: Braverman LE, Utiger RD, editors. Werner and Ingbar's the thyroid: a fundamental and clinical text. Philadelphia: Lippinkott, Williams and Wilkins; 2000. p. 642–51.

[12] Coulombe P, Dussault JH, Letarte J, et al. Catecholamines metabolism in thyroid diseases. I. Epinephrine secretion rate in hyperthyroidism and hypothyroidism. J Clin Endocrinol Metab 1976;42(1):125–31.

[13] Bilezikian JP, Loeb JN, Gammon DE. The influence of hyperthyroidism and hypothyroidism on the beta-adrenergic responsiveness of the turkey erythrocyte. J Clin Invest 1979;63(2): 184–92.

[14] Jamison MH, Done HJ. Post-operative thyrotoxic crisis in a patient prepared for thyroidectomy with propranolol. Br J Clin Pract 1979;33(3):82–3.

[15] Boelaert K, Franklyn JA. Thyroid hormone in health and disease. J Endocrinol 2005;187(1): 1–15.

[16] Connolly DJ, Guitian J, Boswood A, et al. Serum troponin I levels in hyperthyroid cats before and after treatment with radioactive iodine. J Feline Med Surg 2005;7(5):289–300.

[17] Wang YG, Dedkova EN, Fiening JP, et al. Acute exposure to thyroid hormone increases Na+ current and intracellular Ca2+ in cat atrial myocytes. J Physiol 2003;546(Pt 2): 491–9.

[18] Burch HB, Wartofsky L. Life-threatening thyrotoxicosis. Thyroid storm. Endocrinol Metab Clin North Am 1993;22(2):263–77.

[19] Naan EC, Kirpensteijn J, Kooistra HS, et al. Results of thyroidectomy in 101 cats with hyperthyroidism. Vet Surg 2006;35(3):287–93.

[20] Broussard JD, Peterson ME, Fox PR. Changes in clinical and laboratory findings in cats with hyperthyroidism from 1983 to 1993. J Am Vet Med Assoc 1995;206(3):302–5.

[21] Kienle RD, Bruyette D, Pion PD. Effects of thyroid hormone and thyroid dysfunction on the cardiovascular system. Vet Clin North Am Small Anim Pract 1994;24(3):495–507.

[22] Elliott J, Barber PJ, Syme HM, et al. Feline hypertension: clinical findings and response to antihypertensive treatment in 30 cases. J Small Anim Pract 2001;42(3):122–9.

[23] Maggio F, DeFrancesco TC, Atkins CE, et al. Ocular lesions associated with systemic hypertension in cats: 69 cases (1985–1998). J Am Vet Med Assoc 2000;217(5):695–702.

[24] Smith SA, Tobias AH, Jacob KA, et al. Arterial thromboembolism in cats: acute crisis in 127 cases (1992–2001) and long-term management with low-dose aspirin in 24 cases. J Vet Intern Med 2003;17(1):73–83.

[25] Nemzek JA, Kruger JM, Walshaw R, et al. Acute onset of hypokalemia and muscular weakness in four hyperthyroid cats. J Am Vet Med Assoc 1994;205(1):65–8.

[26] Joseph RJ, Peterson ME. Review and comparison of neuromuscular and central nervous system manifestations of hyperthyroidism in cats and humans. Progress in Veterinary Neurology 1992;3(4):114–8.

[27] Mooney CT. Hyperthyroidism. In: Ettinger SJ, Feldman EC, editors. 6th edition, Textbook of veterinary internal medicine, vol. 2. St. Louis (MO): Elsevier Saunders; 2005. p. 1544–60.

[28] Peterson ME, Kintzer PP, Cavanagh PG, et al. Feline hyperthyroidism: pretreatment clinical and laboratory evaluation of 131 cases. J Am Vet Med Assoc 1983;183(1):103–10.

[29] Pimentel L, Hansen KN. Thyroid disease in the emergency department: a clinical and laboratory review. J Emerg Med 2005;28(2):201–9.

[30] Bell R, Mellor DJ, Ramsey I, et al. Decreased sodium:potassium ratios in cats: 49 cases. Vet Clin Pathol 2005;34(2):110–4.

[31] Bond BR, Fox PR, Peterson ME, et al. Echocardiographic findings in 103 cats with hyperthyroidism. J Am Vet Med Assoc 1988;192(11):1546–9.

[32] Sarlis NJ, Gourgiotis L. Thyroid emergencies. Rev Endocr Metab Disord 2003;4(2): 129–36.

[33] Sartor LL, Trepanier LA, Kroll MM, et al. Efficacy and safety of transdermal methimazole in the treatment of cats with hyperthyroidism. J Vet Intern Med 2004;18(5):651–5.

[34] Trepanier LA, Hoffman SB, Kroll M, et al. Efficacy and safety of once versus twice daily administration of methimazole in cats with hyperthyroidism. J Am Vet Med Assoc 2003; 222(7):954–8.

[35] Foster DJ, Thoday KL. Use of propanolol and potassium iodate in the presurgical management of hyperthyroid cats. J Small Anim Pract 1999;40:307–15.

[36] Murray LAS, Peterson ME. Ipodate treatment of hyperthyroidism in cats. J Am Vet Med Assoc 1997;211(1):63–7.

[37] Fontanilla JC, Schneider AB, Sarne DH. The use of oral radiographic contrast agents in the management of hyperthyroidism. Thyroid 2001;11(6):561–7.

[38] Quinones M, Dyer DC, Ware WA, et al. Pharmacokinetics of atenolol in clinically normal cats. Am J Vet Res 1996;57(7):1050–3.

[39] Geffner DL, Hershman JM. Beta-adrenergic blockade for the treatment of hyperthyroidism. Am J Med 1992;93(1):61–8.

[40] Kokuho T, Kuji T, Yasuda G, et al. Thyroid storm-induced multiple organ failure relieved quickly by plasma exchange therapy. Ther Apher Dial 2004;8(4):347–9.

[41] Rosenberg R. Malabsorption of thyroid hormone with cholestyramine administration. Conn Med 1994;58(2):109.

[42] Migneco A, Ojetti V, Testa A, et al. Management of thyrotoxic crisis. Eur Rev Med Pharmacol Sci 2005;9:69–74.

[43] Smith SA, Tobias AH. Feline arterial thromboembolism: an update. Vet Clin North Am Small Anim Pract 2004;34(5):1245–71.

[44] Ringel MD. Management of hypothyroidism and hyperthyroidism in the intensive care unit. Crit Care Clin 2001;17(1):59–74.

Vet Clin Small Anim 37 (2007) 755–773

VETERINARY CLINICS
SMALL ANIMAL PRACTICE

Thyroid Tumors in Dogs and Cats

Lisa G. Barber, DVM

Department of Clinical Sciences, Cummings School of Veterinary Medicine, Tufts University, 200 Westboro Road, North Grafton, MA 01536, USA

T he prevalence and clinical significance of masses within the thyroid gland vary widely across species. Thyroid nodules are frequently encountered in human beings, particularly women, and most are benign [1,2]. Similarly, thyroid nodules are relatively common in older cats and are associated with clinical hyperthyroidism [3–5]. Most are functional adenomatous hyperplasia, but malignant tumors are occasionally recognized. In contrast, thyroid masses are rare in the dog. When they are seen, however, they are likely to be malignant [6,7]. For cats and dogs, a pet is often presented to the veterinarian for clinical signs related to the thyroid lesion. In cats, the signs are attributable to thyroid hormone excess. In dogs, the clinical signs more often arise from space-occupying effects of a cervical mass impinging on normal structures. In all three species, the risk of thyroid nodules increases with age [4,8,9].

Tumors of the thyroid gland in cats, dogs, and people usually arise from the epithelial cells that line the colloid follicles. In the normal state, these cells concentrate iodine and are involved in thyroid hormone production. The tumors that arise from these cells are adenomas or carcinomas of varying degrees of differentiation. In addition, tumors may arise from the parafollicular C cells, which are part of the amine precursor uptake decarboxylation (APUD) system. These cells produce calcitonin, and when neoplastic transformation occurs, they give rise to medullary thyroid carcinomas. Medullary thyroid carcinomas may be seen as part of the multiple endocrine neoplasia (MEN) syndromes. Medullary tumors are relatively rare, typically occurring in less than 10% of thyroid tumors in cats [7], dogs [7,8], and human beings [10], although recent evidence suggests that these tumors may be more common than previously recognized in the dog [11,12]. Lymphocytes and stromal cells within the thyroid may also give rise to lymphoma or sarcoma, respectively, but these tumor types are rare.

ETIOLOGY AND RISK FACTORS

The causes of thyroid neoplasia in domestic animals have not been studied extensively. In people, there is indisputable evidence that exposure of the neck to

E-mail address: lisa.barber@tufts.edu

0195-5616/07/$ – see front matter
doi:10.1016/j.cvsm.2007.03.008

external radiation is linked to the development of thyroid cancer. This relation has been demonstrated in children and adolescents who received radiation therapy for benign disorders, such as acne and ringworm, as well as in patients with Hodgkin's disease who received cervical irradiation [13,14]. Diagnostic testing using iodine 131 (^{131}I) presents negligible risk [15]. Ingestion of iodine radioisotopes from nuclear fallout poses a much greater threat. The most compelling evidence comes from Chernobyl, where the rate of thyroid cancer 10 years after the nuclear power reactor accident had increased 100-fold in some areas of Belarus among children who were younger than 15 years of age at the time of initial exposure [16]. Dogs have served as models in studies investigating the timing and dose of irradiation in the development of thyroid and other neoplasias [17], but these studies are not widely applicable to the pet population.

Other environmental factors, particularly dietary iodine intake, have been linked to the risk of thyroid cancer. Although some data have been conflicting, iodine-deficient diets or high intake of cruciferous vegetables that block iodine uptake may increase thyroid-stimulating hormone (TSH) levels, thereby promoting the development of thyroid neoplasia [1]. Additionally, in these areas, the proportion of follicular and anaplastic tumors is higher than average [18]. In contrast, areas where the incidence of papillary carcinoma is high correspond to diets with high iodine intake, such as Iceland and Norway [1]. The influence of iodine in the canine diet on the development of thyroid carcinoma is not known.

Hypothyroidism attributable to spontaneous lymphocytic thyroiditis was associated with tumor development in a colony of 276 beagle dogs that were allowed to live out their natural lives as part of a control group for another study [19]. Thyroid tumors were detected in approximately half (22 [54.5%] of 44 dogs) of hypothyroid dogs compared with approximately one quarter of asymptomatic dogs (53 [22.8%] of 232 dogs). Among dogs with thyroid masses, multiple tumors were also more common in hypothyroid dogs. Moreover, carcinomas were more common than benign tumors in hypothyroid dogs (34% versus 25%, respectively), whereas adenomas predominated in clinically euthyroid dogs (6.9% malignant versus 17.2% benign). Sibling pair analysis strongly supported a familial relationship in the occurrence of hypothyroidism, although independent risk for cancer was not evaluated.

In addition to a potential genetic component of canine thyroid carcinoma in this beagle colony, the study also supports the theory that chronic TSH exposure of thyroid follicular cells may act as a promoter of neoplastic growth, because none of these dogs received thyroxine supplementation. TSH has been shown to promote angiogenesis in thyroid cancer cell lines through the induction of vascular endothelial growth factor (VEGF) [20]. TSH binding in canine thyroid carcinomas did not differ significantly from that in normal canine thyroid tissue, which suggests that TSH may continue to act as a growth factor for canine thyroid tumors [21].

As with nearly all cancers, transformation of normal thymocytes to a malignant phenotype is believed to involve a series of genetic events. Somatic mutations in members of the RAS family of oncogenes (k-ras, n-ras, and h-ras) have been observed in human thyroid tumors, with k-ras mutation reported in 60% of radiation-induced thyroid tumors [22]. In addition, as might be expected, several chromosomal deletions have been detected in human follicular thyroid carcinomas, supporting the role of several tumor suppressor genes in the development of these neoplasms [18]. Interestingly, mutations in the p53 suppressor gene are uncommon in differentiated thyroid tumors but are frequently detected in anaplastic thyroid carcinomas [23]. The tumor suppressor gene p53 encodes for a protein that causes cell cycle arrest in the G1 phase, allowing for repair of damaged DNA or induction of apoptosis if the DNA damage is too great. In a single report in dogs, however, p53 mutation was detected in only 1 of 23 cases of thyroid carcinoma [24].

Aneuploidy is a common feature of canine thyroid carcinomas, occurring in more than half of primary tumors, with hypoploidy being most common [25]. The ploidy status of primary and recurrent tumors was similar, although there was some discordance between primary tumors and metastases. The authors speculated that the degree of aneuploidy may reflect differences in the average number of genetic events required to overcome the cell's innate protection mechanisms against malignant transformation. Risk factors for the development of malignant thyroid tumors in cats have not been described.

CANINE THYROID TUMORS

Thyroid tumors account for only 1% to 2% of reported neoplasia in dogs in most reports [6,26,27]. Yet, they are the most common form of endocrine neoplasia in this species. Benign adenomas and malignant carcinomas have been reported. In studies that review tissue specimens in pathology banks, the proportion of adenomas has been reported to be as high as 30% to 40%t [6,7,28]. Most adenomas are incidental findings at necropsy, however, because they tend to be small and freely moveable and do not produce clinical signs. Nevertheless, large size does not exclude benign disease, because adenomas reaching greater than 6 cm have been observed [6,7].

Most thyroid tumors detected in the clinic are carcinomas. The signalment of dogs with benign or malignant thyroid tumors is similar. Moreover, this holds true for follicular and parafollicular C-cell tumors. The median age at presentation is 9 to 10 years in almost all studies [6,7,11,12,26–40]. The reported age ranges in these studies are often around 5 to 18 years. The risk of thyroid cancer seems to increase with age, as evidenced by incremental increases in the incidence of these tumors from 1.1% per year in dogs aged 8 to 12 years to 4% per year in dogs aged 12 to 15 years. The cumulative risk was 67% in beagle dogs older than 17 years of age [9]. Unlike the case in human beings, no gender predilection has been observed in dogs [6,7,11,12,26–40]. An epidemiologic study noted that risk rises more steeply in older women, however [28]. Boxers, beagles, and Golden Retrievers have consistently been reported to be overrepresented [6,7,27–29]. Shetland Collies, Old English Sheepdogs, and Cairn Terriers were reported to be overrepresented in a case series in Scotland [34].

Nevertheless, a recent series of 237 dogs was composed mostly of mixed-breed dogs and retrievers, likely reflecting current breed popularity [41]. Similar findings were reported in another recent histopathologic study of 55 thyroid masses [31].

Biologic Behavior

Although most thyroid neoplasms arise in the thyroid gland located in the ventral neck, caudal to the larynx, tumors may also develop within vestigial thyroid tissue that may be present from the base of the tongue to the base of the heart [42–44]. The bilobed thyroid gland is not normally palpable in the dog; thus, any mass effect in this area warrants investigation. Benign thyroid adenomas are typically small, slow-growing, well-encapsulated nodules that have marginal clinical significance. In many cases, they may not be detectable on physical examination. In contrast, thyroid carcinomas tend to grow more quickly and have a proclivity for invasion of surrounding structures, including the trachea, larynx, jugular veins, and carotid sheath. The probability of a thyroid mass in a dog being malignant has been calculated to be 87.5% [26]. Tumors occur with equal frequency in the left and right lobes, and bilateral involvement may be seen in up to 40% of patients with carcinomas [6,7,29,33].

Metastasis has been reported in 16% to 38% of dogs at the time of diagnosis [11,27,29,31,34], whereas rates as high as 80% are reported at necropsy [6,7]. Size was significantly related to metastasis in one necropsy-based study in which all dogs with tumors that exceeded 100 cm^3 had documented distant metastasis. The metastatic rates were 74% and 14% for tumors from 21 to 100 cm^3 and 20 cm^3 or less, respectively [7]. The presence of metastasis has not been correlated to clinical signs [34]. The lungs are the most frequent site of metastasis, followed by the regional lymph nodes [6,7]. The developmental history of the thyroid also predicts the pattern of regional metastasis, with lymph node involvement typically seen in the retropharyngeal and mandibular nodes because of the rostral flow of lymphatic drainage. Nevertheless, the superficial cervical lymph nodes should not be overlooked during staging of thyroid tumors. Other sites of metastasis include the jugular vein, heart, kidney, adrenal gland, liver, brain, and other sites [6,7,27]. All dogs with metastasis had disease within the lungs or lymph nodes in one study [7]. Of dogs with spread to other sites, only 20% did not have recognized lung metastasis. In one study, bilateral thyroid neoplasia was 16 times more likely to metastasize than unilateral tumors [45].

Expected length of survival for dogs with untreated carcinomas is not well documented, because most reports describe outcomes for dogs that have received various interventions. One study evaluating surgical management of thyroid tumors included six dogs with inoperable tumors. The median survival in these dogs was 15 weeks, with a range of 2 to 38 weeks [46]. Similarly, seven untreated dogs in another study of radioiodide therapy had a reported median survival of 3 months [38]. A third study reported that all untreated dogs with metastatic disease were dead within 3 months [34]. An observational study of a colony of research beagle dogs that were monitored for spontaneous development of thyroid neoplasia did not report on survival times of dogs after the recognition of a thyroid tumor. The age at death was not statistically significantly different, however, whether dogs underwent surgery to remove the mass or not (14.7 versus 14.5 years, respectively). A likely difference in these dogs compared with companion animals is that they were monitored more closely for the presence of a cervical mass, which would presumably lead to diagnosis of the tumor while it was still small [19].

Diagnosis and Staging

An owner's discovery of a cervical mass is the most common presenting complaint in dogs diagnosed with thyroid tumors [6,11,29,33,34,38]. The time from the owner's recognition of the mass until diagnosis averaged 1 to 2 months in most studies, but a few studies reported delays of up to 1 to 2 years before a dog was presented for evaluation. These masses tend to be firm and nonpainful. They may be well circumscribed and freely moveable or diffusely infiltrative and fixed. The degree of mobility is often related to the size of the tumor. Incidental discovery of a cervical mass on routine physical examination is uncommon [6,29]. Although this may seem surprising in view of the large size of many thyroid tumors, it may relate to the lack of careful palpation as a routine part of physical examination for many veterinarians.

Clinical signs

Clinical signs related to a mass lesion are often the presenting complaint, including cough, dysphagia, and dysphonia [6,11,26,27]. Dyspnea may relate to upper airway disruption (eg, tracheal compression, laryngeal paralysis) or to lower airway compromise from pulmonary metastases. Rarely, obstruction of venous or lymphatic return may cause spectacular diffuse swelling of the head and neck [6]. Additionally, erosion of major blood vessels by the tumor may lead to rapid cervical swelling and, in extreme cases, cardiovascular collapse [47].

Thyroid hormone status

Most dogs do not exhibit signs of abnormal thyroid function. Thyroid function testing (eg, triiodothyronine [T_3], tetraiodothyronine [T_4], TSH measurements) are rarely reported in clinical studies, with most dogs described as clinically euthyroid. In two studies in which T_3 and T_4 levels were tested, 29% and 39% of dogs had low hormone levels [27,38] but only one dog with an adenoma showed clinical signs of hypothyroidism. It was not possible to determine whether the low thyroid levels preceded the thyroid tumors, indeed potentially predisposing the dogs to tumor development, or were a consequence of the neoplasm. In one of these two studies [27], thyroid hormone levels did not exceed the normal range in any of the dogs. In contrast, the other study [38] reported elevated T_4 levels in 31% of dogs, but only two exhibited clinical signs, such as polyuria, polydipsia, weight loss in the face of adequate food intake, heat intolerance, and restlessness. In another older study, 22% of dogs with thyroid tumors were clinically hyperthyroid [7]. Dogs in these studies exhibited abnormal iodine metabolism and had decreased radionuclide uptake within the contralateral thyroid lobe. Hyperthyroidism results from constitutive production of biologically active thyroid hormone by neoplastic cells.

Staging

Diagnosis of a thyroid tumor is best achieved through histologic examination of a biopsy sample, although cytology may be sufficient in some cases. Standard staging procedures for dogs with confirmed or suspected thyroid carcinomas include general health screening, including a physical examination, complete blood cell count, chemistry profile, urinalysis, thyroid hormone level with or without TSH stimulation testing, regional lymph node evaluation, and thoracic radiographs. Abdominal ultrasound should be considered in patients with pulmonary or lymph node metastasis but is of low yield in patients without evidence of disease at these sites. The World Health Organization (WHO) system is the standardized scheme for assigning disease stage (Box 1; Table 1) [48].

Evaluation of a cervical mass should include palpation to determine size and adherence to surrounding structures. Thorough evaluation may require sedation, because invasiveness of the tumor may be overestimated in the awake

---

Box 1: Clinical classification of canine thyroid tumors

T: primary tumor

T_0—no evidence of tumor (microscopic residual disease)

T_1—maximum tumor diameter less than 2 cm

T_2—maximum tumor diameter 2 to 5 cm

T_3—maximum tumor diameter greater than 5 cm

Substage a—tumor freely movable

Substage b—tumor fixed to surrounding structures

N: regional lymph nodes

N_0—no evidence of lymph node involvement

N_1—ipsilateral lymph node involvement

N_2—bilateral lymph node involvement

Substage a—lymph node freely movable

Substage b—lymph node fixed

M: distant metastasis

M_0—no evidence of distant metastasis

M_1—distant metastasis detected

From Owen LN, editor. TNM classification of tumours in domestic animals. Geneva, Switzerland: World Health Organization; 1980. p. 52; with permission.

Table 1
Clinical staging of canine thyroid tumors

Staging group	Primary tumor	Regional lymph nodes	Distant metastases
I	T_1 a, b	N_0	M_0
II	T_0	N_1	M_0
	T_1 a, b	N_1	M_0
	T_2 a, b	N_0 or N_1 a	M_0
III	T_3	Any N	M_0
	Any T	N_1 b or N_2 b	M_0
IV	Any T	Any N	M_1

From Owen LN, editor. TNM classification of tumours in domestic animals. Geneva, Switzerland: World Health Organization; 1980. p. 52; with permission.

dog. Plain radiographs of the neck often confirm a soft tissue mass and demonstrate deviation or compression of the trachea or larynx. Radiographs do not provide information on vascularity or invasion of neighboring structures. Ultrasound may provide greater detail with respect to these properties and is used routinely in some hospitals as a rapid, inexpensive, noninvasive method for evaluation of a thyroid mass before further diagnostics (Fig. 1). CT and particularly MRI may provide more sensitive information on the degree of invasiveness of a thyroid mass. Although MRI has the advantage of better soft tissue discrimination, CT scans may also include the thorax to investigate the presence of potential metastases to lungs and other intrathoracic structures.

Scintigraphy
Imaging the thyroid gland with technetium-99m (^{99}mtc)–pertechnetate is another diagnostic and staging procedure that has become routine in many

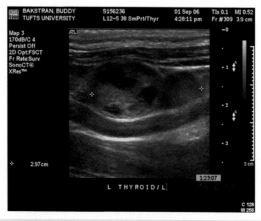

Fig. 1. Ultrasound image of a tumor in the left thyroid gland. Note the hypoechoic areas suggestive of hemorrhage.

veterinary hospitals (Fig. 2). Pertechnetate localizes in the iodine trapping mechanism within thyroid cells. The most common scintigraphic appearance in dogs with thyroid tumors is unilaterally increased uptake of radionuclide relative to the parotid salivary gland. The pattern of radionuclide uptake does not seem to correlate with the histologic type of tumor but has predicted the histologic degree of capsular invasion [32]. Tumors with extensive capsular invasion had poorly circumscribed heterogeneous uptake of pertechnetate by the tumor, whereas well-circumscribed homogeneous uptake was more common in tumors without capsular invasion. The intensity of uptake has also been reported to be consistently greater and more homogeneous in hyperthyroid dogs with thyroid tumors. Pertechnetate scans may be helpful in identifying ectopic thyroid tumors, particularly in locations that are difficult to biopsy.

Scintigraphy has also been used as a staging procedure to investigate pulmonary metastasis, to search for nodules not detectable by plain radiography, or to characterize nodules seen on plain films further. Although anecdotal reports of revealing occult metastases have fueled enthusiasm for such testing, others have

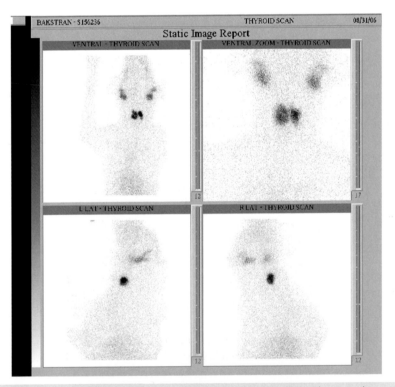

Fig. 2. Pertechnetate scan of a dog with bilateral thyroid tumors. This is the same dog as in Fig. 1. Note the large irregular areas of increased uptake in the neck. The uptake in the tumors is greater than in the parotid salivary glands.

found that scintigraphy has been less rewarding [27,32], adding little over standard radiography. Failure of scintigraphy to identify pulmonary lesions that were later histologically confirmed to be metastatic thyroid carcinoma has been speculatively attributed to loss of the cellular pertechnetate trapping mechanism stemming from loss of differentiation in some metastatic cells [32].

Biopsy and cytology
Scintigraphy has been used to make a presumptive diagnosis of thyroid neoplasia when biopsy or fine-needle aspirate cytology of the mass is not feasible or is declined by the pet owner. Nevertheless, biopsy remains the "gold standard" for diagnosis. For small freely moveable tumors, excisional biopsy has the advantage of being diagnostic and therapeutic. For large invasive tumors, however, incisional or needle core biopsies may be necessary. Because thyroid carcinomas tend to be highly vascular, some authors have suggested that ultrasound guidance may be helpful in minimizing the risk of significant hemorrhage [41]. Fine-needle aspirate cytology is often discounted as being unrewarding because of the low cellularity of samples secondary to hemodilution. Although this complication may be encountered, one study supports a high percentage of concordance of cytologic and histopathologic findings [49]. Among dogs with cervical masses, fine-needle aspirate cytology correctly identified the mass to be of thyroid origin in 10 of 11 samples. Convincing cytologic features of malignancy were present in 5 samples, and malignancy was suspected in another 5 samples. Aspirates from only one dog had insufficient cellularity.

A few simple steps have been helpful for the author in obtaining diagnostic fine-needle aspirate cytology samples from cervical masses. First, a 22-gauge or smaller needle is inserted into the tumor in one direction, followed by aspiration with a syringe no larger than 6 mL. This tends to result in less blood contamination than redirecting with a bare needle or using a larger syringe. Gentle digital pressure over the aspiration site for 1 to 2 minutes has been helpful in minimizing bruising, thereby allowing multiple aspirations if needed. In addition, preparation of the smear by a manual wedge method (as used for making blood smears) concentrates the larger epithelial cells toward the feathered edge.

Differential diagnoses
Although thyroid tumors are the primary differential diagnosis for a ventral cervical mass, other disorders must be considered, such as salivary mucocele, abscess, or granuloma secondary to wounds or foreign bodies (eg, ingestion of a stick); cervical lymph node metastasis from another cancer (eg, tonsillar squamous cell carcinoma); carotid body tumor; rhabdomyosarcoma; or fibrosarcoma. For masses within the cranial mediastinum and heart base, other differential diagnoses to consider include lymphoma, thymoma, chemodectoma, and hemangiosarcoma in addition to inflammatory processes.

Histopathologic findings
Most canine thyroid tumors are well to moderately differentiated [6,7,27,29,33]. The hallmark of malignancy in well-differentiated tumors that

distinguishes them from benign adenomas is the presence of capsular invasion. Vascular invasion is another feature of malignancy that may be seen [31]. Most canine thyroid tumors arise from the follicular epithelium and are classified as compact, follicular, or a mixture of the two patterns (compact-follicular). These forms account for approximately three quarters of canine thyroid neoplasias [6,7,26–29,33,38]. Papillary carcinoma, the most common thyroid cancer in human beings, has been reported only sporadically in dogs [7,38]. In people, this histologic type carries the most favorable prognosis [50]. In contrast, several studies have not found prognostic significance of histologic subtype among well-differentiated tumors in dogs [26,27,31,33]. In addition, microvessel density was not shown to predict metastasis or survival [31]. High histologic grade and anaplastic carcinomas, as might be expected, tend to be associated with the least favorable outcomes [46].

Thyroid tumors arising from the parafollicular C-cells often have a compact cellular pattern and may be difficult to distinguish from follicular tumors with a similar histologic appearance with routine light microscopy alone. Tumors derived from follicular elements routinely stain positively for thyroglobulin [51,52]. In contrast, C-cell tumors have demonstrated strong immunoreactivity to calcitonin and calcitonin gene–related peptide, more variable staining for synaptophysin, and consistent absence of staining for neurotensin [12,52,53]. The lack of immunohistochemical staining of tumor specimens in most studies of canine thyroid carcinoma suggests that the prevalence of medullary thyroid carcinomas may have been underestimated. This may have clinical relevance, because evidence suggests that medullary tumors may be more slowly growing; may be less invasive, and thereby more amenable to complete surgical resection; and may possess lower metastatic potential [11]. Lymphomas and sarcomas are rare in human beings and are exceedingly rare in dogs. Most sarcomas in the neck are believed to arise from structures other than the thyroid gland in dogs.

Treatment

Appropriate treatment strategies for canine thyroid carcinomas depend in large part on the size and invasiveness of the tumor as well as on the presence of metastasis.

Surgery

As with almost all solid tumors, surgery is the preferred modality for local control for thyroid tumors. In the case of adenomas, surgery is expected to be curative if complete excision is achieved. Local control of well-circumscribed carcinomas is often possible with surgery (Fig. 3). The surgical approach is usually through a ventral midline incision. Care must be taken in identifying the recurrent laryngeal nerve, jugular vein, and carotid artery. These structures may be sacrificed unilaterally with an acceptable clinical outcome. When bilateral tumors are present, however, it is typically recommended to spare one of the parathyroid glands, if possible, to preserve calcium homeostasis. In one retrospective study of 20 dogs with freely moveable tumors, the median overall

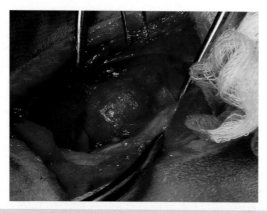

Fig. 3. Thyroid tumor as seen at surgery. This is the same dog as in Figs. 1 and 2. The tumor was well encapsulated, and complete excision was achieved.

survival was 20.5 months [33]. When animals were censored for death attributable to other causes, the median survival was estimated to be greater than 36 months by means of Kaplan-Meier product limit survival analysis. Many dogs are not good candidates for surgery, however, because of the invasiveness of many tumors at the time of diagnosis. The prior case series included only approximately one quarter of all dogs with thyroid carcinomas that were presented to the hospital, because the recommendation for surgery alone was based on the mobility of the mass and absence of metastatic disease.

Another study of 33 dogs reported that 80% of medullary thyroid carcinomas (which comprised approximately one third of tumors) were amenable to complete surgical excision compared with half of the thyroid adenocarcinomas [11]. One-year survival rates for completely resected medullary and follicular cell tumors were 33% and 55%, respectively. For nonresectable thyroid adenocarcinomas, the 1-year survival rate was 26% with surgery alone. Even with seemingly resectable tumors, treatment-related morbidity and mortality were considerable. Reported postoperative complications include laryngeal paralysis, megaesophagus, tracheostomy complications, upper airway distress, and hypocalcemia [29]. Such complications were responsible for five or seven tumor-related deaths in one study [33].

For fixed tumors, surgery often results in incomplete excision because of the lack of encapsulation and extensive local invasion. The tumors tend to be highly vascular, with the regional vessels described as large, tortuous, and often incompletely filled with tumor thrombi. Additionally, massive aneurysmal vascular dilations within the tumor have been the source of major hemorrhage [29]. Invasion into the larynx, trachea, and esophagus may preclude complete excision. In general, dogs with large invasive tumors, particularly if they are bilateral, should be considered poor surgical candidates, and other means of disease control should be considered.

External beam radiation therapy

Despite early anecdotal reports that canine thyroid tumors are relatively resistant to irradiation, recent studies have demonstrated that external beam radiation therapy is helpful in achieving local control of tumors that cannot be completely resected surgically [35,36,45]. The misconception may have stemmed from the slow decrement in tumor size after treatment, such that reported maximal response may not be achieved until 8 to 22 months after the completion of therapy [45]. In a prospective study of 25 dogs with measurable thyroid carcinomas, the mean progression-free interval was 45 months, with a median not achieved at the time of the report. The 1- and 3-year progression-free survival rates were 80% and 72%, respectively [45]. A smaller case series of 8 dogs reported a median survival time of 24.5 months, with none of the dogs exhibiting regrowth of the primary tumor [35]. In both studies, the dogs were treated with megavoltage [54] cobalt radiation therapy. The tumor dose was 46.8 to 48 Gy delivered over 12 fractions three times weekly. Acute side effects included alopecia; erythema; and acute mucositis involving the esophagus, trachea, or larynx, resulting in dysphagia, hoarseness, or cough in approximately half of the dogs. In most cases, these effects were self-limiting within 2 to 3 weeks. Late complications noted at greater than 1 year after treatment included skin fibrosis and permanent alopecia, chronic tracheitis, and dry cough in less than 20% of the patients. No late effects were noted in the second study. Despite these toxicities, the complication rate and severity compare favorably for dogs with large invasive tumors undergoing surgery.

A palliative protocol has also been assessed in which four weekly 9-Gy fractions of external beam radiation therapy were given to 13 dogs with large nonresectable tumors [36]. The mean size of the tumors was 6 cm in the largest diameter (range: 3.5–9 cm). Radiation therapy was successful in halting the growth of all the tumors, with one tumor regressing to undetectable levels (complete remission) and nine tumors decreasing in size by 50% or more (partial remission). The median survival for all the dogs as well as for a subset of 5 dogs with pulmonary metastasis was 96 weeks. For dogs without pulmonary metastasis, the median survival was 127 weeks. This difference was not statistically significant, likely because of the small sample size. The most reliable determinant of outcome was growth rate of the tumor. In dogs with tumors that grew an estimated 5% or less per week, the median survival was 127 weeks. For tumors that increased in size by more than 5% per week, median survival was 44 weeks.

Radioiodide therapy

The appropriateness of ^{131}I treatment for thyroid carcinoma remains controversial. Initially, it was believed that ^{131}I would be effective only for functional thyroid tumors, (ie, dogs that were clinically hyperthyroid as a consequence of excess thyroid hormone produced by their cancer). Nevertheless, a few studies have reported positive outcomes with this modality, irrespective of thyroid hormone status [37–39]. A difficulty in interpreting the results of these studies stems from the variety of dosing schemes, most of which were empiric. Reported doses range from 410 to 7100 MBq (11–191 mCi) [37–39], although the weight of the dog, size of the tumor, and degree of radionuclide uptake have been used to estimate an appropriate dose in some instances. In addition, many dogs received more than one treatment, and the intervals between doses varied widely.

Decrease in tumor size was not a consistent finding after treatment, and many dogs were treated multiple times. Some of the dogs underwent surgery in combination with ^{131}I, although the reported outcomes were not significantly affected by surgery. In two recent studies, a total of 114 dogs yielded similar survival times. In the first study [38], median survival in dogs that received ^{131}I alone was 30 months compared with 34 months in dogs that underwent surgery before receiving [131]I. This difference was not statistically significant, and outcome was not influenced by stage of disease at the time of treatment in this study. In contrast, the second study [37] reported a median survival of 28 months for dogs that had locoregional disease (primary tumor with or without lymph node metastasis) compared with 12 months when distant metastases were present. In both of these studies, 20% to 50% of the dogs were hyperthyroid, although thyroid hormone levels did not predict response to therapy.

The ^{131}I treatments were well tolerated by most dogs. Ablation of normal thyroid tissue was expected and required levothyroxine supplementation in most dogs. Myelosuppression has been recognized as another complication of ^{131}I therapy [37,39]. In most instances, the dogs were asymptomatic and pancytopenia resolved spontaneously. Fatal myelosuppression was observed in 3 of 39 dogs in one study, however, all of which received ^{131}I doses higher than the median dose based on body weight (160 MBq/kg [4.2 mCi/kg]) [37]. None of these dogs was hyperthyroid before treatment.

[131]I also poses technical and practical issues. Most studies relied on pertechnetate scans as a basis for using [131]I. The kinetics of pertechnetate differ from those of ^{131}I, however, in that pertechnetate does not undergo organification. Consequently, it may not accurately predict the uptake and biologic half-life of ^{131}I in tumor-bearing dogs. Reliance on pertechnetate scans may lead to variations in the effective dose of radionuclide in individual patients. Organification of iodine produces maximal accumulation 24 to 72 hours after a dose of ^{131}I is administered, compared with 40 to 60 minutes for pertechnetate [38]. In dogs with hypersecreting tumors, greater organification of ^{131}I should result in higher radionuclide concentrations within the tumor, thus yielding a high effective dose of radiation. A mathematic model for determining the dose of ^{131}I in individual dogs has been reported using a small tracer dose of [131]I [55]. This method is cumbersome, however, and requires additional hospitalization. Nevertheless, tracer ^{131}I studies have revealed a disparity with pertechnetate scans that would likely have clinical implications regarding the effectiveness of [131]I [45].

Another obstacle to ^{131}I treatment is its limited availability because of stringent regulatory requirements regarding use of this radioisotope and the need for lengthy hospital stays in isolation until exposure rates fall to within acceptable limits. This has been reported to be approximately 1 to 2 weeks [37,39].

Chemotherapy

The role of chemotherapy in the management of canine thyroid carcinoma has not been fully elucidated. Only a few studies involving small numbers of dogs with thyroid tumors have been published. Doxorubicin, a first-line chemotherapeutic agent for thyroid carcinoma in human patients, has demonstrated activity against this neoplasm in dogs [40,56]. A study evaluating the efficacy of doxorubicin against a variety of canine neoplasms included 13 dogs with solid follicular carcinomas. Of these, 1 dog had complete remission (defined as complete resolution of all clinically detectable disease) and 2 dogs experienced partial remission (defined as 50% or greater reduction in total tumor burden). The duration of the responses was not reported [56]. In another study of 17 dogs with thyroid carcinoma treated with doxorubicin alone or in combination with cyclophosphamide or vincristine, 4 (44%) of 9 dogs receiving chemotherapy alone achieved partial remission of the primary tumor. Pulmonary metastatic disease seemed to be more refractory to doxorubicin, with only one objective partial response among 5 dogs, although owners of 2 additional dogs reported improvement in their animal's breathing after treatment. Median survival among all 16 dogs was 33 weeks. If gross pulmonary metastasis was present at the time of presentation, median survival was reported to be 16 weeks [40].

The response to mitoxantrone, a chemotherapeutic agent related to doxorubicin, was reported as one partial remission lasting 21 days in 10 dogs with measurable thyroid carcinoma [57]. All these dogs received doses of 4.5 mg/m^2 or less, however, which is less than the currently accepted range of 5.0 to 6.0 mg/m^2 in dogs.

Cisplatin has also been shown to have activity against human and canine thyroid carcinoma, producing objective responses in 7 of 13 dogs [58]. All but one of the responses were partial remissions. The single complete remission was in a dog that did not have palpable disease (after incomplete surgical resection) but had carcinoma cells detected on fine-needle aspiration of the surgical field before chemotherapy. Nevertheless, 8 of the dogs in this study had tumors greater than 5 cm (of which 3 were responders). The median progression-free interval for responders was 252 days. The median overall survival of dogs in this study was 98 days for all dogs and 322.5 days among dogs that responded to cisplatin.

These studies indicate that doxorubicin, cisplatin, and likely mitoxantrone have activity against canine thyroid carcinoma but that the responses may last for months only. As with most solid tumors, chemotherapy alone is not curative for thyroid carcinomas. In general, conventional cytotoxic chemotherapy has its greatest effect on microscopic metastatic disease. Studies evaluating the benefit of chemotherapy in extending progression-free or overall survival in dogs that have undergone definitive therapy for local disease are lacking, however.

Other medical management

Nonsteroidal anti-inflammatory drugs (NSAIDs) have been gaining widespread use for the treatment of certain carcinomas in human and veterinary medicine. Their mechanism of action is to block cyclooxygenase (COX), which has been implicated in tumor progression through a variety of mechanisms, including the induction of VEGF and other components of the angiogenic cascade. Many neoplastic tissues have been shown to overexpress the inducible isoform of the COX-2 enzyme, including human follicular and medullary thyroid carcinomas [54,59,60]. Evidence suggests that this enzyme may play an important role in the progression from benign to malignant thyroid tumors [60] and that increased COX-2 expression may correlate with increased tumor recurrence and death [61]. Moreover, NSAIDs have been shown to inhibit growth of human medullary carcinomas in murine models [62]. Nevertheless, a clinical trial in human patients with metastatic thyroid cancer did not prevent disease progression for 12 months or longer in most patients [63]. Despite inconsistent initial reports, the use of NSAIDS in the treatment of canine thyroid carcinoma warrants further investigation.

Thyroid hormone supplementation has been proposed as a treatment for thyroid tumors. The intent of this therapy is to use intrinsic feedback inhibition of TSH release, because this hormone may act as a growth factor for tumors that retain avid TSH binding sites. To date, no studies have examined the effectiveness of this treatment in inhibiting growth of the primary tumor or metastases in dogs.

MULTIPLE ENDOCRINE NEOPLASIA

MEN describes a well-recognized phenomenon of combinations of endocrine neoplasia in people that is believed to be genetically linked. The tumors involved include parathyroid tumors (usually hyperplasia), pancreatic islet cell tumors, gastrinomas, insulinomas, pituitary tumors, adrenocortical tumors (or hyperplasia), medullary thyroid carcinomas, and thyroid follicular adenomas. The various forms of MEN have stringent criteria for categorization. According to this scheme, there are few reports of MEN among dogs. Dogs with thyroid tumors are at increased risk of developing other primary tumors, however. Among 144 dogs diagnosed with thyroid carcinoma, 45 developed a total of 69 other primary tumors [28]. When multiple neoplasias arise concurrently, the general recommendation is to address the problems most likely to result in death or organ dysfunction or to compromise of quality of life first.

FELINE THYROID TUMORS

Hyperthyroidism is a common disorder of older cats, resulting from abnormal proliferation of thyroid tissue. Adenomatous hyperplasia is most common, although carcinomas may also occur infrequently [3,4,64]. Interestingly, the clinical presentation for malignant tumors may be indistinguishable from that for benign nodules, because both types of masses typically produce excess thyroid hormone. Nevertheless, a large or fixed cervical mass may increase suspicion of carcinoma.

Clinical Presentation, Staging, and Diagnosis

The clinical signs recognized by owners often are referable to hyperthyroidism, including weight loss, polydipsia, hyperactivity, and sometimes anorexia [65].

Occasionally, clinical signs similar to those seen in the dog, such as dysphagia or dyspnea, may result from a large cervical mass impinging on the trachea or esophagus. Physical examination may reveal tachycardia, a palpable cervical mass, cardiac murmur, and an abnormal coat. In addition to elevated T_3 and T_4 levels, routine chemistry profiles often indicate high serum activities of liver enzymes. Occasionally, hypercalcemia may be detected as a consequence of parathyroid hormone–related peptide production [66]. Cardiac evaluation is also indicated, because functional carcinomas are equally likely as adenomas to produce cardiomyopathy [65,67].

Feline thyroid carcinomas in cats tend to be highly metastatic [65,67,68]. In contrast to dogs, regional lymph node metastasis seems to be more common than pulmonary metastasis in cats. Nevertheless, thoracic radiographs or scintigraphy is warranted if a malignant neoplasm is suspected. Radiographs may reveal a military pattern within the lungs [68]. Scintigraphy has the added advantage of identifying ectopic thyroid tissue.

On histologic examination, mixed compact and follicular carcinomas are reported to be the most common form of malignant thyroid tumors in cats, although follicular and papillary forms are seen less commonly [7,65].

Treatment

Although surgical excision may be successful in achieving local control of feline thyroid carcinoma [64], many malignant tumors cannot be fully excised because of extension into the surrounding normal structures. In such cases, ^{131}I is the treatment of choice [65,67]. The cats received doses of ^{131}I ranging from 750 to 1000 MBq (20–30 mCi). Survival times ranged from 10 to 41 months, with a median of approximately 20 months. Although feline thyroid carcinomas have high metastatic potential, the effectiveness of chemotherapy has not been reported. Supportive care may include medications for cardiac dysfunction or hypertension, analgesics, and nutritional support, as indicated.

SUMMARY

The clinical presentation and biologic behavior of thyroid tumors vary widely among dogs, cats, and human beings. Although thyroid tumors in dogs are rare, they are most likely to be malignant. Clinical signs are usually the result of impingement on surrounding structures, and clinical hyperthyroidism is rare. In contrast, hyperthyroidism resulting from benign thyroid proliferation is relatively common among older cats. Malignant tumors are extremely uncommon but have high metastatic potential. Irrespective of the tumor's ability to produce functional thyroid hormone, scintigraphy is often helpful in the diagnosis and staging of thyroid tumors in all three species. Treatment with surgery is a reasonable treatment option for noninvasive tumors. ^{131}I is a well-established treatment for thyroid nodules in cats, but its effectiveness in dogs is controversial. In dogs, external beam radiation therapy has produced more consistent results in affording local tumor control when surgery is not possible.

References

[1] Carling T, Udelsman R. Cancer of the endocrine system. Section 2. Thyroid tumors. In: DeVita VT, Hellman S, Rosenberg SA, editors. Cancer: principles and practice of oncology. 7th edition. Philadelphia: Lippincott Williams & Wilkins; 2004. p. 1727–840.

[2] Mazzaferri EL. Management of a solitary thyroid nodule. N Engl J Med 1993;328:553–9.

[3] Broussard JD, Peterson ME, Fox PR. Changes in clinical and laboratory findings in cats with hyperthyroidism from 1983–1993. J Am Vet Med Assoc 1995;296:302–5.

[4] Peterson ME, Becker DV. Radioiodine treatment of 524 cats with hyperthyroidism. J Am Vet Med Assoc 1995;207:1422–8.

[5] Welches CD, Scavelli TD, Matthiesen DT, et al. Occurrence of problems after three techniques of bilateral thyroidectomy in cats. Vet Surg 1989;18:392–6.

[6] Brodey RS, Kelly DF. Thyroid neoplasms in the dog. A clinicopathologic study of fifty-seven cases. Cancer 1968;22:406–16.

[7] Leav I, Schiller Al, Rijnberk A, et al. Adenomas and carcinomas of the canine and feline thyroid. Am J Pathol 1976;83:61–122.

[8] Brander A, Viikinkoski P, Nickels J, et al. Thyroid gland: US screening in a random adult population. Radiology 1991;181:683–7.

[9] Haley PJ, Hahn FF, Muggeburg BA, et al. Thyroid neoplasms in a colony of beagle dogs. Vet Pathol 1989;26:438–41.

[10] Moley JF. Medullary thyroid cancer. Surg Clin North Am 1995;75:405–20.

[11] Carver JR, Kapatkin A, Pataik AK. A comparison of medullary thyroid carcinoma and thyroid adenocarcinoma in dogs. A retrospective study of 38 cases. Vet Surg 1995;24:315–9.

[12] Patnaik AK, Lieberman PH. Gross, histologic, cytochemical and immunocytochemical study of medullary thyroid carcinoma in sixteen dogs. Vet Pathol 1991;28:223–33.

[13] Ron E, Lubin JH, Shore RE, et al. Thyroid cancer after exposure to external radiation: a pooled analysis of seven studies. Radiat Res 1995;141:259–77.

[14] Hancock SL, Cox RS, McDougall IR. Thyroid diseases after treatment of Hodgkin's disease. N Engl J Med 1991;325:599–605.

[15] Dickman PW, Holm LE, Lundell G, et al. Thyroid cancer risk after thyroid examination with 131I: a population-based cohort study in Sweden. Int J Cancer 2003;106:580–7.

[16] Robbins J, Schneider AB. Thyroid cancer following exposure to radioactive iodine. Rev Endocr Metab Disord 2000;1:197–203.

[17] Benjamin SA, Saunders WJ, Lee AC, et al. Non-neoplastic and neoplastic thyroid disease in beagles irradiated during prenatal and postnatal development. Radiat Res 1997;147:422–30.

[18] Larimore TC, Moley JF. Cancer of the endocrine system. Section 1. Molecular biology of endocrine tumors. In: DeVita VT, Hellman S, Rosenberg SA, editors. Cancer: principles and practice of oncology. 7th edition. Philadelphia: Lippincott Williams & Wilkins; 2004. p. 1727–840.

[19] Benjamin SA, Stephens LC, Hamilton BF, et al. Associations between lymphocytic thyroiditis, hypothyroidism, and thyroid neoplasia in beagles. Vet Pathol 1996;33:486–94.

[20] Soh EY, Sobhi SA, Wong MG, et al. Thyroid-stimulating hormone promotes the secretion of vascular endothelial growth factor in thyroid cancer cell lines. Surgery 1996;120:944–7.

[21] Verschueren CP, Rutteman GR, Vos JH, et al. Thyrotrophin receptors in normal and neoplastic (primary and metastatic) canine thyroid tissue. J Endocrinol 1992;132:461–8.

[22] Suarez HG, du Villard JA, Severino M, et al. Presence of mutations in all three ras genes in human thyroid tumors. Oncogene 1990;5:565–70.

[23] Ito T, Seyama T, Mizuno T, et al. Unique association of p53 mutations with undifferentiated but not with differentiated carcinomas of the thyroid gland. Cancer Res 1992;52:1369–71.

[24] Devilee P, Van Leeuwen IS, Voesten A, et al. The canine p53 gene is subject to somatic mutations in thyroid carcinoma. Anticancer Res 1994;14:2039–46.

[25] Verschueren CP, Rutteman GR, Kuipers-Dijkshoorn NJ, et al. Flow-cytometric DNA ploidy analysis in primary and metastatic canine thyroid carcinomas. Anticancer Res 1991;11:1755–61.

[26] Birchard SJ, Roesel OF. Neoplasia of the thyroid gland in the dogs. A retrospective study of 16 cases. J Am Anim Hosp Assoc 1981;17:369–72.

[27] Harari J, Patterson JS, Rosenthal RC. Clinical and pathologic features of thyroid tumors in 26 dogs. J Am Vet Med Assoc 1986;188:1160–4.

[28] Hayes HM Jr, Fraumeni JF Jr. Canine thyroid neoplasms: epidemiologic features. J Natl Cancer Inst 1975;55:931–4.

[29] Mitchell M, Hurov LI, Troy GC. Canine thyroid carcinomas: clinical occurrence, staging by means of scintiscans, and therapy in 15 cases. Vet Surg 1979;8:112–8.

[30] Forman J, Reed CI. Tumors in dogs. I. Carcinomas of the thyroid gland. Ohio J Sci 1917;17: 177–86.

[31] Kent MS, Griffery SM, Verstraete FJM, et al. Computer-assisted image analysis of neovascularization in thyroid neoplasms from dogs. Am J Vet Res 2002;63:363–9.

[32] Marks SL, Koblik PD, Hornof WJ, et al. ^{99}mTc-pertechnetate imaging of thyroid tumors in dogs: 29 cases (1980–1992). J Am Vet Med Assoc 1994;204:756–60.

[33] Klein MK, Powers BE, Withrow SJ, et al. Treatment of thyroid carcinoma in dogs by surgical resection alone: 20 cases (1981–1989). J Am Vet Med Assoc 1995;206:1007–9.

[34] Sullivan M, Cox F, Pead MJ, et al. Thyroid tumours in the dog. J Small Anim Pract 1987;28: 505–12.

[35] Pack L, Roberts RE, Dawson SD, et al. Definitive radiation therapy for infiltrative thyroid carcinoma in dogs. Vet Radiol Ultrasound 2001;42:471–4.

[36] Brearley MJ, Hayes Am, Murphy S. Hypofractionated radiation therapy for invasive thyroid carcinoma in dogs: a retrospective analysis of survival. J Small Anim Pract 1999;40: 206–10.

[37] Turrel JM, McEntee MC, Burke BP, et al. Sodium I 131 treatment of dogs with nonresectable thyroid tumors: 39 cases (1990–2003). J Am Vet Med Assoc 2006;229:542–8.

[38] Worth AT, Zuber RM, Hockin M. Radioiodide (^{131}I) therapy for the treatment of canine thyroid carcinoma. Aust Vet J 2005;83:208–14.

[39] Adams WH, Walker MA, Daiel GB, et al. Treatment of differentiated thyroid carcinoma in 7 dogs utilizing 131 I. Vet Radiol Ultrasound 1995;36:417–24.

[40] Jeglum KA, Wereat A. Chemotherapy of canine thyroid carcinoma. Compendium of Continuing Education for the Practicing Veterinarian 1983;5:96–8.

[41] Feldman EC, Nelson RW. Canine thyroid tumors and hyperthyroidism. In: Feldman EC, Nelson RW, editors. Canine and feline endocrinology and reproduction. 3rd edition. St. Louis (MO): Saunders; 2004. p. 219–49.

[42] Girard C, Helie P, Odi M. Intrapericardial neoplasia in dogs. J Vet Diagn Invest 1999;11: 73–8.

[43] Ware WA, Merkley DF, Riedesel DH. Intracardiac thyroid tumor in a dog. Diagnosis and surgical removal. J Am Vet Med Assoc 1994;30:20–3.

[44] Stephens LC, Saunders WJ, Jaeke RS. Ectopic thyroid carcinoma with metastases in a beagle dog. Vet Pathol 1982;19:669–75.

[45] Theon AP, Marks SL, Feldman ES, et al. Prognostic factors and patterns of treatment failure in dogs with unresectable differentiated thyroid carcinomas treated with megavoltage irradiation. J Am Vet Med Assoc 2000;216:1775–9.

[46] Verschueren CP, Rutteman GR, van Dijk JE, et al. Evaluation of some prognostic factors in surgically-treated canine thyroid cancer. In: Verschueren CPLJ, editor. Clinicopathological and endocrine aspects of canine thyroid cancer [thesis]. Rijksuniversiteit, Utrecht, Netherlands: 1992. p.11–25.

[47] Slensky KA, Volk SW, Schawarz T, et al. Acute severe hemorrhage secondary to arterial invasion in a dog with thyroid carcinoma. J Am Vet Med Assoc 2003;223:649–53.

[48] Owen LN, editor. TNM classification of tumours in domestic animals. Geneva (IL): World Health Organization; 1980. p. 51–2.

[49] Thompson EJ, Stirtzinger T, Lumsden JH, et al. Fine needle aspiration cytology in the diagnosis of canine thyroid carcinoma. Can Vet J 1980;21:186–8.

[50] Sessions RB, Davidson BJ. Thyroid cancer. Med Clin North Am 1993;77:517–38.
[51] Moore FM, Kledzik GS, Wolf HJ, et al. Thyroglobulin and calcitonin immunoreactivity in canine carcinomas. Vet Pathol 1984;21:168–73.
[52] Leblanc B, Parodi AL, Lagadic M, et al. Immunocytochemistry of canine thyroid tumors. Vet Pathol 1991;28:370–80.
[53] Leblanc B, Paulus G, Andreu M, et al. Immunocytochemistry of thyroid C-cell complexes in dogs. Vet Pathol 1990;27:445–52.
[54] Ito Y, Yoshida H, Nakano K, et al. Cyclooxygenase-2 expression in thyroid neoplasms. Histopathology 2003;42:492–7.
[55] Peterson ME, Kintzer PP, Hurley JR, et al. Radioactive iodine treatment of a functional thyroid carcinoma producing hyperthyroidism in a dog. J Vet Intern Med 1989;3:20–5.
[56] Ogilvie GK, Reynolds HA, Richardson RC, et al. Phase II evaluation of doxorubicin for treatment of various canine neoplasms. J Am Vet Med Assoc 1989;195:1580–3.
[57] Ogilvie GK, Obradovich JE, Elmslie RE, et al. Efficacy of mitoxantrone against various neoplasms in dogs. J Am Vet Med Assoc 1991;198:1618–21.
[58] Fineman LS, Hamilton TA, de Gortari A, et al. Cisplatin chemotherapy for treatment of thyroid carcinoma in 13 cases. J Am Anim Hosp Assoc 1998;34:109–12.
[59] Garcia-Gonzalez M, Abdulkader I, Boquete AV, et al. Cyclooxygenase-2 in normal, hyperplastic and neoplastic follicular cells of the human thyroid gland. Virchows Arch 2005;447:12–7.
[60] Casey MB, Zhang S, Jin L, et al. Expression of cyclooxygenase-2 and thromboxane synthase in non-neoplastic and neoplastic thyroid lesions. Endocr Pathol 2004;15:107–16.
[61] Haynik DM, Prayson RA. Immunohistochemical expression of cyclooxygenase 2 in follicular carcinomas of the thyroid. Arch Pathol Lab Med 2005;129:736–41.
[62] Quidville V, Segond N, Pidoux E, et al. Tumor growth inhibition by indomethacin in a mouse model of human medullary thyroid cancer: implication of cyclooxygenases and 15-hydroxyprotaglandin dehydrogenase. Endocrinology 2004;145:2561–71.
[63] Mrozek E, Kloos RT, Ringel MD, et al. Phase II study of celecoxib in metastatic differentiated thyroid carcinoma. J Clin Endocrinol Metab 2006;91:2201–4.
[64] Naan EC, Kirpensteijn J, Kooistra HS, et al. Results of thyroidectomy in 101 cats with hyperthyroidism. Vet Surg 2006;35:287–93.
[65] Turrel JM, Feldman EC, Nelson RW, et al. Thyroid carcinoma causing hyperthyroidism in cats: 14 cases (1981–1986). J Am Vet Med Assoc 1988;193:359–64.
[66] Bolliger AP, Graham PA, Richard V, et al. Detection of parathyroid hormone-related protein in cats with humoral hypercalcemia of malignancy. Vet Clin Pathol 2002;31:3–8.
[67] Guptill L, Scott-Moncrieff CR, Janovitz EB, et al. Response to high-dose radioactive iodine administration in cats with thyroid carcinoma that had previously undergone surgery. J Am Vet Med Assoc 1995;207:1055–8.
[68] Cook SM, Daniel GB, Walker MA, et al. Radiographic and scintigraphic evidence of focal pulmonary neoplasia in three cats with hyperthyroidism: diagnostic and therapeutic considerations. J Vet Intern Med 1993;7:303–8.

Pharmacologic Management of Feline Hyperthyroidism

Lauren A. Trepanier, DVM, PhD[a,b,*]

[a]Department of Medical Sciences, School of Veterinary Medicine, University of Wisconsin-Madison, 2015 Linden Drive, Madison, WI 53706-1102, USA
[b]Department of Pharmaceutical Sciences, University of Wisconsin-Madison, Rennebohm Hall, Madison, WI 53705-222, USA

Hyperthyroidism is the most common endocrine disorder in cats, with a prevalence of 2% in cats presented to teaching hospitals [1]. Management options include radioiodine therapy, thyroidectomy, or medical treatment with antithyroid drugs, such as methimazole. Radioiodine is considered the treatment of choice for hyperthyroidism, based on its high efficacy and relative lack of complications (Table 1). There are some situations in which methimazole therapy may be preferred over radioiodine, however. Practical considerations, such as lack of a convenient referral center with a radiation license, client fears about radiation or quarantine, or initial cost to the client, may drive the use of methimazole. Methimazole can be used before thyroidectomy to normalize serum thyroxine (T_4) concentrations [2] and reduce the risk of complications, such as tachyarrhythmias, during anesthesia. Methimazole, which is reversible, is similarly indicated in cats with renal insufficiency for long-term therapy or as a "test dose" regimen to determine whether serum T_4 can be safely lowered without causing renal decompensation.

METHIMAZOLE ACTIONS, DOSING, AND EFFICACY

Methimazole blocks thyroid hormone synthesis by inhibiting thyroid peroxidase, the enzyme involved in the oxidation of iodide to iodine, incorporation of iodine into thyroglobulin, and coupling of tyrosine residues to form T_4 and triiodothyronine (T_3). Methimazole does not block the release of preformed thyroid hormone, which explains the delay of 2 to 4 weeks before serum T_4 concentrations fully normalize after beginning treatment in cats [2].

Supported in part by grants from the Winn Feline Foundation and the University of Wisconsin-Madison, School of Veterinary Medicine, Companion Animal Fund.

*Department of Medical Sciences, School of Veterinary Medicine, University of Wisconsin-Madison, 2015 Linden Drive, Madison, WI 53706-1102. E-mail address: latrepanier@svm.vetmed.wisc.edu

0195-5616/07/$ – see front matter
doi:10.1016/j.cvsm.2007.03.004

Table 1
Advantages and disadvantages of major therapies for feline hyperthyroidism

Treatment	Advantages	Disadvantages
Radioiodine	>90% efficacy Single injection Few side effects (rare dysphagia) Curative Effective for ectopic tissue or carcinoma	High initial expense Somewhat limited availability Irreversible
Thyroidectomy	~90% efficacy Curative	High initial expense Anesthetic risks Risk of hypoparathyroidism Risk of recurrent laryngeal nerve damage (uncommon) Irreversible
Methimazole	Low initial expense ~90% efficacy in cats that do not have side effects Reversible	Daily drug administration Drug side effects

Adapted from Trepanier LA. Medical management of hyperthyroidism. Clin Tech Small Anim Pract 2006;21:23.

Methimazole does not decrease goiter size; in fact, goiters may become larger over time despite therapy.

Typical starting doses of methimazole range from 1.25 to 2.5 mg administered twice daily (Table 2). More frequent dosing (every 8 hours) is rarely necessary. A higher dose of 5 mg administered two to three times daily, which was used in original cases of cats with relatively high serum T_4 concentrations [2], is probably not needed for initial therapy of cats with mild to moderate hyperthyroidism and could potentially increase the risk of renal decompensation from a rapid fall in serum T_4. Methimazole is effective in normalizing T_4 in most treated cats, and this effect is dose dependent [2]. Starting doses can be titrated upward if there is an inadequate initial response to lower doses of methimazole over 2 to 4 weeks. In cats that tolerate methimazole without side effects, efficacy is greater than 90% [2–4].

In people, methimazole has a long residence time in the thyroid gland and can exert antithyroid effects for 24 hours or more [5,6] despite a short plasma elimination half-life. Because of this, methimazole can be given once daily in human patients with remission rates that are comparable to those of divided daily dosing [7,8]. In our study of 40 hyperthyroid cats, we found that once-daily dosing (5 mg administered every 24 hours) was less effective than divided dosing (2.5 mg administered every 12 hours), with only 54% of cats euthyroid after 2 weeks of once-daily treatment compared with 87% of cats treated with divided dosing [4]. Therefore, unless clients are absolutely unable to dose more frequently than once daily, divided twice-daily dosing of methimazole is preferred to maximize efficacy. Dosing less frequently than once daily is unlikely to be effective, because serum T_4 concentrations rise to pretreatment hyperthyroid values within 48 hours after discontinuing methimazole [2].

METHIMAZOLE SIDE EFFECTS

Side effects of methimazole have been reported in 18% of treated cats, including simple gastrointestinal upset, blood dyscrasias, facial excoriation, and hepatotoxicity [2]. Positive antinuclear antibodies (ANAs) have been documented in more than 20% of treated cats, with uncertain clinical significance [2]. The risk of positive ANAs increases with the dose and duration of therapy and can be reversed with dose reduction. Positive ANAs were not associated with blood dyscrasias or other adverse clinical events, and no affected cats had lupus-like signs. [2] The cats reported in this large series had relatively high serum T_4 concentrations (with many cats having serum T4 values >20 µg/dL) and were administered methimazole at a dose of 10 to 15 mg/d. The incidence of positive ANAs has not been subsequently evaluated in cats with milder hyperthyroidism treated with lower daily doses of methimazole.

Simple Gastrointestinal Upset

Anorexia, vomiting, and lethargy are seen in approximately 10% of cats treated with methimazole. Simple gastrointestinal upset is most common in the first 4 weeks of treatment and can resolve with a reduction in dose. These signs may be partially attributable to direct gastric irritation from the drug, because transdermal administration of methimazole is associated with significantly fewer gastrointestinal side effects than the oral route [3].

Blood Dyscrasias

Methimazole can lead to neutropenia or thrombocytopenia in 3% to 9% of treated cats [2,3], with aplastic anemia reported rarely [9]. Cats with mild methimazole-induced blood dyscrasias usually recover within a week of drug discontinuation. Continuing methimazole in the face of thrombocytopenia has led to clinically significant hemorrhage, including epistaxis and oral bleeding [2]. Rechallenge with methimazole in one cat with neutropenia led to a recurrence of severe neutropenia within 7 days of readministration [2].

Although the mechanisms for these blood dyscrasias in cats have not been established, methimazole-induced neutropenia in human beings is associated with an arrest of myeloid progenitors in the bone marrow [10,11]. Serum from affected people inhibits normal granulocyte-macrophage (GM) colony-forming units (CFUs) in vitro, suggesting antibody- or cytokine-mediated effects [12]. Studies in human beings have found an association between methimazole-associated neutropenia and the presence of antineutrophil antibodies and certain human leukocyte antigen (HLA) gene mutations, further implicating autoimmune mechanisms [13,14]. Treatment with GM colony-stimulating

Table 2
Drugs useful in the medical management of hyperthyroidism

Drug	Indications	Dose	Side effects	Comments
Methimazole	Hyperthyroid cats with azotemia or for clients declining radioiodine	1.25 to 5 mg per cat twice daily (start at lower end)	Gastrointestinal upset Facial excoriation Blood dyscrasias Hepatopathy	Transdermal route has fewer gastrointestinal side effects
Atenolol	Control of hypertension, tachyarrhythmias, or hyperactivity	3.125 to 6.25 mg per cat twice daily		β_1-selective blocker
Enalapril or benazepril	Control of hypertension	0.5 mg/kg once or twice daily	Lethargy, inappetence	Potential effect of limiting glomerulosclerosis in cats with renal disease, benazepril does not accumulate in renal failure
Amlodipine	Control of moderate to severe hypertension	0.625 mg per cat once daily	Lethargy, inappetence	Drug of choice for severe hypertension
Propylthiouracil	Unclear if useful for cats intolerant of methimazole	25 mg per cat twice daily (empiric)	Hemolytic anemia Thrombocytopenia Bleeding diathesis	
Carbimazole	Prodrug of methimazole	2.5 to 5 mg per cat twice daily	Gastrointestinal upset Facial excoriation Blood dyscrasias Hepatopathy	Not recommended in cats intolerant of methimazole

Drug	Indication	Dosage	Adverse Effects	Mechanism/Comments
Propranolol	Control of tachyarrhythmias or hyperactivity, adjunct control of triiodothyronine in cats intolerant of full doses of methimazole	2.5 to 5 mg per cat three times daily	Bronchoconstriction in cats with prior lower airway disease	Inhibits conversion of thyroxine to triiodothyronine
Potassium iodate (KIO$_3$)	Transient inhibition of thyroid hormone synthesis before thyroidectomy, in cats intolerant of methimazole	21.25 to 42.5 mg per cat three times daily (empiric)	Vomiting, anorexia, bitter taste	Thyroid effects are transient (can pretreat 10 days before surgery, along with propranolol)
Iopanoic acid or calcium ipodate	Adjunct control of triiodothyronine in cats intolerant of methimazole	100 to 200 mg once daily (empiric)		Inhibits conversion of thyroxine to triiodothyronine, effects are transient

Adapted from Trepanier LA. Medical management of hyperthyroidism. Clin Tech Small Anim Pract 2006;21:24.

factor (CSF) has been advocated in human patients [15] but does not seem to hasten recovery in most cases [16]. In cats, methimazole treatment has been associated with red blood cell autoantibodies [2], but the presence of antibodies attributable to platelet or neutrophil antigens has not been evaluated.

Facial Excoriation

Approximately 2% to 3% of cats treated with methimazole develop excoriations of the face and neck [2], leading to characteristic scabbed lesions in front of the pinnae. Generalized erythema and pruritus may also occur. These excoriations are inconsistently responsive to glucocorticoids, and drug discontinuation is usually required [2]. Pruritus has also been reported in human patients treated with methimazole, but the mechanisms for these reactions have not been explored [15].

Hepatotoxicity

Increases in serum alkaline phosphatase (SAP), bilirubin, or alanine aminotransferase (ALT) are observed in approximately 2% of cats treated with methimazole [2,3]; a liver biopsy may show hepatic necrosis and degeneration [2]. Liver enzyme elevations are usually reversible over several weeks after drug discontinuation, although nutritional and fluid support may be required. Rechallenge has led to recurrent hepatopathy [2], and future drug avoidance is generally recommended. Methimazole is associated rarely with cholestatic hepatopathy in people [17]. In rodent models of methimazole hepatotoxicity, an oxidative metabolite has been implicated and toxicity is exacerbated by glutathione depletion [18]. The role of glutathione depletion, or supplementation, in methimazole-associated hepatotoxicity in cats has not been evaluated.

Renal Decompensation

Cats with hyperthyroidism have abnormally high glomerular filtration rates (GFRs), as measured by iohexol clearance or renal scintigraphy [19–21]. Treating hyperthyroidism with methimazole leads to decreases in GFR in most hyperthyroid cats [19]. Similar results have been found in hyperthyroid cats treated with thyroidectomy or radioiodine [22], with 15% to 22% of cats developing new azotemia [20,21]. Although these biochemical changes are generally clinically silent, occasional cats develop signs of illness referable to underlying renal disease [19]. Because methimazole is reversible, it is the preferred approach for initial treatment of hyperthyroid cats with preexisting azotemia to determine whether lowering of serum T_4 leads to unacceptable renal decompensation [22].

Coagulation Abnormalities

In human beings, methimazole is uncommonly associated with hypoprothrombinemia [23]. Methimazole and, to a lesser extent, propylthiouracil (PTU) inhibit vitamin K–dependent clotting factor activation (γ-carboxylation) and epoxide reductase (necessary for vitamin K recycling) at high concentrations [23]. In a study of 20 hyperthyroid cats treated with methimazole, there were no significant changes in prothrombin time or activated partial thromboplastin time, but 1 cat developed a prolonged PIVKA clotting time [24]. No cats had clinically significant bleeding. This suggests a possible but apparently uncommon "warfarin-like" effect of methimazole in cats as seen in people. This may explain why a single methimazole-treated cat (0.3%) in a large case series [2] developed bleeding diathesis without thrombocytopenia. This reaction is rare enough not to warrant routine monitoring but should be considered in any cat presented with hemorrhage that is also being treated with methimazole.

Acquired Myasthenia Gravis

Another apparently rare side effect of methimazole in cats is the development of acquired myasthenia gravis [25]. Neuromuscular weakness, along with positive antibody titers to the acetylcholine receptor, was reported in four cats treated with methimazole for 2 to 4 months. Creatinine kinase was elevated in two cats, and one cat had a biopsy diagnosis of concurrent polymyositis. Cats responded to drug discontinuation or the addition of prednisone to the methimazole treatment regimen. One cat relapsed with reintroduction of the drug. Although this does not seem to be a side effect of methimazole in human patients, hyperthyroidism itself can copresent with myasthenia in people [26]. In one human patient, methimazole therapy was thought to worsen the clinical signs of myasthenia [27].

CLINICAL MONITORING

Based on the spectrum of possible adverse reactions to methimazole, clinical monitoring at 2 to 3 weeks and 4 to 6 weeks of treatment should include a complete blood cell count (CBC), ALT and SAP levels, and blood urea nitrogen (BUN) and creatinine levels, in addition to serum T_4. In a cat with an apparent adverse reaction to methimazole, it is important to differentiate simple gastrointestinal upset (for which a lower dose or a switch to transdermal methimazole may be effective) from blood dyscrasias or hepatopathy, for which methimazole should be discontinued. Therefore, this same workup should also be performed if a cat becomes clinically ill during methimazole treatment.

It is important to measure renal function and T_4 simultaneously during methimazole therapy to determine whether a cat's kidneys can tolerate the level of GFR associated with normal thyroid function. If a cat becomes newly azotemic with clinical signs, the dose of methimazole can be titrated to maintain the serum T_4 in the high normal range, with additional use of drugs to control hypertension and tachyarrhythmias.

TRANSDERMAL METHIMAZOLE

Methimazole is available through custom compounding pharmacies in a transdermal formulation in pluronic lecithin organogel (PLO). PLO acts as a permeation enhancer to allow drug absorption across the stratum corneum. Although methimazole in PLO has been shown to have poor absorption in cats after a single dose [28], chronic dosing in hyperthyroid cats is effective in lowering serum T_4 concentrations [3,29,30]. Methimazole in PLO is applied to the cat's inner pinna, alternating ears with each dose. Owners wear examination gloves or finger cots during administration and are instructed to remove crusted material with a moistened cotton ball before the next dose.

In a randomized trial comparing oral and transdermal methimazole in PLO in hyperthyroid cats (2.5 mg administered every 12 hours), transdermal methimazole had significantly fewer gastrointestinal side effects (4% of cats) compared with oral methimazole (24% of cats) [3]. There were no differences in the incidence of facial excoriation, neutropenia, thrombocytopenia, or hepatotoxicity between routes. Transdermal methimazole was associated with somewhat lower efficacy (only 67% euthyroid by 4 weeks) compared with oral methimazole (82% euthyroid by 4 weeks), however. This may be attributable to lower bioavailability of the transdermal formulation.

Drawbacks of methimazole in PLO include erythema at the dosing site in some cats [3,30], increased formulation costs, and unproven drug stability. A single prescription of methimazole in PLO seems to be effective (anecdotally) for weeks to months, however. The author recommends that serum T_4 values be checked toward the end of a 2-month prescription of the transdermal formulation to confirm that thyroid control persists. Methimazole in PLO should not be refrigerated and should not be used if there is visible separation of its components in the dosing syringe.

BEFORE PERTECHNETATE SCANNING OR RADIOIODINE THERAPY

Because methimazole does not inhibit iodide uptake by the thyroid, concurrent methimazole therapy does not impair technetium 99m Tc-pertechnetate thyroid scanning in hyperthyroid cats and, in fact, may enhance imaging [31,32]. Methimazole does inhibit iodine organification, however, which may decrease the contact time for radioiodine within the thyroid, and therefore affect radioiodine efficacy. Human patients given methimazole up to 4 days before radioiodine show no differences in outcome [33], but administration of methimazole immediately before or after radioiodine has been associated with poorer responses [34,35]. In hyperthyroid cats, retrospective studies have found no association between the time of methimazole discontinuation before radioiodine and long-term radioiodine efficacy [36,37]. There is some evidence to suggest that recent methimazole discontinuation may actually have a short-term rebound effect to enhance radioiodine efficacy in cats [38]. This is consistent with a study in normal cats in which methimazole, when discontinued 4 to 9 days before radioiodine, led to maximally increased radioiodine ^{123}I uptake compared with no methimazole treatment [32]. The 1- to 2-week washout period for methimazole recommended by many radioiodine facilities is based on efficacy data from the largest cases series published [39] but may be longer than necessary. This requires evaluation in a prospective study.

MANAGEMENT OF HYPERTENSION

Hypertension has been reported to be as prevalent as 87% in hyperthyroid cats [40]; however, it is likely that hospital-induced stress falsely elevated readings in this early study. Subsequent surveys of cats with hyperthyroidism report the prevalence of hypertension to be 5% to 22% in hyperthyroid cats [3,4,41], with many cats with hypertension having concurrent azotemia [41].

Normalizing serum T_4 may not significantly control blood pressure in the first weeks of methimazole therapy [4]. Therefore, direct management of moderate to severe hypertension is indicated along with antithyroid treatment. Commonly used antihypertensive agents include amlodipine, beta-blockers, or the angiotensin-converting enzyme (ACE) inhibitors enalapril or benazepril. There have been no clinical trials evaluating the comparative efficacy of these drugs in this setting, however. Beta-blockers, such as atenolol, may be particularly useful if signs of hyperactivity or tachyarrhythmias are present (see Table 2). The calcium channel blocker amlodipine [42] may be particularly effective for severe hypertension [43]. ACE inhibitors have the potential benefit of reducing intraglomerular pressure in patients with renal disease [44]. In cats with overt azotemia, benazepril, which does not accumulate in renal insufficiency [45], has an advantage over enalapril.

In some hyperthyroid cats without initial hypertension, hypertension can actually develop several months after treatment for hyperthyroidism [41], possibly because of unmasking of underlying renal insufficiency Therefore, rechecking cats for hypertension 2 to 3 months after restoration of a euthyroid state is indicated, even if initial blood pressure readings were normal.

OTHER ANTITHYROID DRUG OPTIONS

Propylthiouracil

PTU was the first drug used in the management of hyperthyroid cats in the early 1980s [46]. This drug is less potent than methimazole and required high doses (eg, 50 mg administered every 8 to 12 hours) to normalize serum T_4 concentrations. PTU was associated with a severe adverse reaction syndrome in approximately 8% of hyperthyroid cats, including positive ANAs, Coombs-positive hemolytic anemia, and thrombocytopenia with bleeding diathesis [47]. This syndrome was reproduced experimentally in more than 50% of cats in a research setting [48], with a dose-dependent induction of ANAs that was attributed to a reactive sulfur atom in the drug's structure [49]. A similar atom is also present in methimazole and, unfortunately, is necessary for the antithyroid action of these drugs [50]. Later attempts to recreate this syndrome experimentally in cats were not successful. Researchers hypothesized that taurine deficiency (with associated impaired drug conjugation and elimination) may have exacerbated the side effects of PTU in cats when it was first used [51]. Methimazole and PTU share structural similarities, and cats with blood dyscrasias, hepatopathy, or facial excoriation from methimazole may well have similar adverse reactions to PTU; however, the degree of cross-reactivity between these two antithyroid drugs has not been critically examined in cats.

Carbimazole

Carbimazole is a substituted derivative of methimazole that was developed with expectations of a longer duration of action in human beings [52].

Carbimazole acts primarily as a prodrug of methimazole in people and cats, however [52,53]. Carbimazole is used in the United Kingdom and Australia for cats with hyperthyroidism [54], and there are anecdotal reports that side effects, such as blood dyscrasias, are less common with carbimazole compared with methimazole. Carbimazole is converted efficiently to methimazole, but because carbimazole has a larger molecular weight, a 5-mg dose of carbimazole yields approximately 50% lower methimazole plasma concentrations than does a 5-mg dose of methimazole [53]. There are no good studies comparing the side effect rates of methimazole and carbimazole, and because carbimazole leads to methimazole exposure, its use in cats with adverse reactions to methimazole is probably ill advised.

Beta Blockers

Beta blockers can reduce the "sympathetic overdrive" characteristic of hyperthyroidism, including tachycardia, arrhythmias, hyperactivity, and aggression. Propranolol has the additional potential benefit of reducing the conversion of T_4 to T_3 (see Table 2), an effect that has been demonstrated in cats [55]. As a nonselective beta-blocker, however, propranolol can lead to bronchospasm in cats with a prior history of reactive airway disease [56,57] because of blockade of β_2 receptors in airway smooth muscle. Atenolol, a selective β_1 blocker, is not associated with bronchospasm and is preferred for beta-blockade in cats with a history of cough or bronchial changes on chest radiographs. Propranolol or atenolol is useful for the short-term management of cats intolerant of methimazole for which radioiodine or thyroidectomy is planned [55,58]. Because neither of these treatments normalizes serum T_4 or prevents weight loss, these drugs alone are not appropriate for long-term management of hyperthyroid cats.

Iodine-Containing Agents

Potassium iodine (KI) transiently blocks thyroid hormone synthesis (Wolff-Chaikoff effect), possibly by means of iodination of proteins and transient inhibition of thyroid peroxidase [59]. Potassium iodate (KIO_3) has similar effects but has a longer shelf life and is reported to be less bitter [60]. Iodate has been used successfully in hyperthyroid cats, in combination with propranolol, for preanesthetic normalization of serum T_4 and serum T_3 before thyroidectomy [55]. The protocol used was propranolol at a dose of 2.5 to 5 mg per cat administered three times daily (up to 7.5 mg administered three times daily), titrated to keep heart rate less than 200 beats per minute. In addition, KIO_3 (21.25 to 42.5 mg per cat administered three times daily) was used in the 10 days before surgery. Serum T_4 normalized in 36% of cats treated with this regimen, with serum T_3 normalizing in 89% of cats in which T_3 was elevated before treatment. Gastrointestinal upset from the KIO_3 was common and was significant enough to lead to hepatic lipidosis in some cats.

Iodinated contrast agents, such as ipodate and iopanoic acid, inhibit conversion of T_4 to T_3 [61] and have been advocated for use in hyperthyroid cats that do not tolerate methimazole. The efficacy of ipodate was evaluated in hyperthyroid cats [62] in the form of calcium ipodate at a dose of 100 mg per cat daily, titrated to 200 mg/d as needed. Eight of 12 cats responded with weight gain, decreased serum T_3, and decreased heart rate. Serum T_4 concentrations were unaffected. Ipodate (Oragrafin; iodine, 308 mg, with calcium ipodate, 500 mg) is no longer marketed, but iopanoic acid (Telepaque; iodine, 333 mg, with iopanoic acid, 500 mg) [63] and diatrizoate meglumine (Gastrografin; iodine, 370 mg/mL) have been used anecdotally in hyperthyroid cats at comparable doses. Long-term control may be poor, however, because the effects of these agents are transient in cats and people [62,64].

All iodine-containing agents interfere with thyroid scanning and radioiodine therapy. In human patients, iodinated agents must be discontinued 2 weeks before these procedures [65]. Similar data are not available for cats.

SUMMARY

Methimazole is an effective drug for the treatment of cats with hyperthyroidism. It can be considered the drug of choice in situations in which radioiodine is unavailable or declined by clients or before thyroidectomy to normalize serum T_4 before anesthesia. Methimazole is also indicated over radioiodine in old cats or in cats with serious concurrent medical problems in which the poor likelihood of long-term survival may not justify the cost of radioiodine. Methimazole is useful as a reversible test drug to determine whether cats with preexisting renal insufficiency tolerate the euthyroid state without clinically significant renal decompensation. Significant side effects include dose-dependent gastrointestinal upset and idiosyncratic blood dyscrasias, facial excoriation, or hepatopathy. Significant hypertension should be controlled concurrently with atenolol, amlodipine, or an ACE inhibitor.

References

[1] Edinboro CH, Scott-Moncrieff JC, Janovitz E, et al. Epidemiologic study of relationships between consumption of commercial canned food and risk of hyperthyroidism in cats. J Am Vet Med Assoc 2004;224:879–86.
[2] Peterson ME, Kintzer PP. Methimazole treatment of 262 cats with hyperthyroidism. J Vet Intern Med 1988;2:150–7.
[3] Sartor LL, Trepanier LA, Kroll MM, et al. Efficacy and safety of transdermal methimazole in the treatment of cats with hyperthyroidism. J Vet Intern Med 2004;18:651–5.
[4] Trepanier LA, Hoffman SB, Kroll M, et al. Efficacy and safety of once versus twice daily administration of methimazole in cats with hyperthyroidism. J Am Vet Med Assoc 2003; 222:954–8.
[5] Okuno A, Yano K, Inyaku F, et al. Pharmacokinetics of methimazole in children and adolescents with Graves disease. Acta Endocrinol 1987;115:112–8.
[6] Jansson R, Dahlberg P, Johansson H, et al. Intrathyroidal concentrations of methimazole in patients with Graves disease. J Clin Endocrinol Metab 1983;57:129–32.
[7] Mashio Y, Beniko M, Matsuda A, et al. Treatment of hyperthyroidism with a small single daily dose of methimazole: a prospective long-term follow-up study. Endocr J 1997;44: 553–8.
[8] Shiroozu A, Okamura K, Ikenoue H, et al. Treatment of hyperthyroidism with a small single daily dose of methimazole. J Clin Endocrinol Metab 1986;63:125–8.
[9] Weiss DJ. Aplastic anemia in cats—clinicopathological features and associated disease conditions 1996–2004. J Feline Med Surg 2006;8:203–6.

[10] Meyer-Gessner M, Benker G, Lederbogen S, et al. Antithyroid drug-induced agranulocytosis: clinical experience with ten patients treated at one institution and review of the literature. J Endocrinol Invest 1994;17:29–36.

[11] Stojanovic N, Ruvidic R, Jovcic G, et al. Drug-induced agranulocytosis: bone marrow granulocytic progenitor cells. Biomed Pharmacother 1990;44:181–4.

[12] Douer D, Eisenstein Z. Methimazole-induced agranulocytosis: growth inhibition of myeloid progenitor cells by the patient's serum. Eur J Haematol 1988;40:91–4.

[13] Weitzman SA, Stossel TP. Drug-induced immunological neutropenia. Lancet 1978;1: 1068–72.

[14] Tamai H, Sudo T, Kimura A, et al. Association between the DRB1*08032 histocompatibility antigen and methimazole-induced agranulocytosis in Japanese patients with Graves disease. Ann Intern Med 1996;124:490–4.

[15] Bartalena L, Bogazzi F, Martino E. Adverse effects of thyroid hormone preparations and antithyroid drugs. Drug Saf 1996;15:53–63.

[16] Hirsch D, Luboshitz J, Blum I. Treatment of antithyroid drug-induced agranulocytosis by granulocyte colony-stimulating factor: a case of primum non nocere. Thyroid 1999;9: 1033–5.

[17] Mikhail NE. Methimazole-induced cholestatic jaundice. South Med J 2004;97:178–82.

[18] Mizutani T, Murakami M, Shirai M, et al. Metabolism-dependent hepatotoxicity of methimazole in mice depleted of glutathione. J Appl Toxicol 1999;19:193–8.

[19] Becker TJ, Graves TK, Kruger JM, et al. Effects of methimazole on renal function in cats with hyperthyroidism. J Am Anim Hosp Assoc 2000;36:215–23.

[20] Graves TK, Olivier NB, Nachreiner RF, et al. Changes in renal function associated with treatment of hyperthyroidism in cats. Am J Vet Res 1994;55:1745–9.

[21] Adams WH, Daniel GB, Legendre AM. Investigation of the effects of hyperthyroidism on renal function in the cat. Can J Vet Res 1997;61:53–6.

[22] DiBartola S, Broome M, Stein B, et al. Effect of treatment of hyperthyroidism on renal function in cats. J Am Vet Med Assoc 1996;208:875–8.

[23] Lipsky JJ, Gallego MO. Mechanism of thioamide antithyroid drug associated hypoprothrombinemia. Drug Metabol Drug Interact 1988;6:317–26.

[24] Randolph JF, DeMarco J, Center SA, et al. Prothrombin, activated partial thromboplastin, and proteins induced by vitamin K absence or antagonists clotting times in 20 hyperthyroid cats before and after methimazole treatment. J Vet Intern Med 2000;14:56–9.

[25] Shelton G, Joseph R, Richter K, et al. Acquired myasthenia gravis in hyperthyroid cats on Tapazole therapy. Proceedings of the 15th Annual Forum of the American College of Veterinary Internal Medicine 1997.

[26] Marino M, Ricciardi R, Pinchera A, et al. Mild clinical expression of myasthenia gravis associated with autoimmune thyroid diseases. J Clin Endocrinol Metab 1997;82:438–43.

[27] Kuroda Y, Endo C, Neshige R, et al. Exacerbation of myasthenia gravis shortly after administration of methimazole for hyperthyroidism. Jpn J Med 1991;30:578–81.

[28] Hoffman S, Yoder A, Trepanier L. Bioavailability of transdermal methimazole in a pluronic lecithin organogel (PLO) in healthy cats. J Vet Pharmacol Ther 2002;25:189–93.

[29] Hoffmann G, Marks S, Taboada J, et al. Transdermal methimazole treatment in cats with hyperthyroidism. J Feline Med Surg 2003;5:77–82.

[30] Lecuyer M, Prini S, Dunn ME, et al. Clinical efficacy and safety of transdermal methimazole in the treatment of feline hyperthyroidism. Can Vet J 2006;47:131–5.

[31] Fischetti AJ, DiBartola SP, Chew DJ, et al. Effects of methimazole on thyroid gland uptake of 99mTC-pertechnetate in 19 hyperthyroid cats. Vet Radiol Ultrasound 2005;46:267–72.

[32] Nieckarz JA, Daniel GB. The effect of methimazole on thyroid uptake of pertechnetate and radioiodine in normal cats. Vet Radiol Ultrasound 2001;42:448–57.

[33] Andrade VA, Gross JL, Maia AL. The effect of methimazole pretreatment on the efficacy of radioactive iodine therapy in Graves' hyperthyroidism: one-year follow-up of a prospective, randomized study. J Clin Endocrinol Metab 2001;86:3488–93.

[34] Koroscil TM. Thionamides alter the efficacy of radioiodine treatment in patients with Graves' disease. South Med J 1995;88:831–6.

[35] Marcocci C, Gianchecchi D, Masini I, et al. A reappraisal of the role of methimazole and other factors on the efficacy and outcome of radioiodine therapy of Graves' hyperthyroidism. J Endocrinol Invest 1990;13:513–20.

[36] Chun R, Garrett LD, Sargeant J, et al. Predictors of response to radioiodine therapy in hyperthyroid cats. Vet Radiol Ultrasound 2002;43:587–91.

[37] Forrest L, Baty C, Metcalf M, et al. Feline hyperthyroidism: efficacy of treatment using volumetric analysis for radioiodine dose calculation. Vet Radiol Ultrasound 1996;37:141–5.

[38] Slater MR, Komkov A, Robinson L, et al. Long-term follow-up of hyperthyroid cats treated with iodine-131. Vet Radiol Ultrasound 1994;35:204–9.

[39] Peterson ME, Becker DV. Radioiodine treatment of 524 cats with hyperthyroidism. J Am Vet Med Assoc 1995;207:1422–8.

[40] Kobayashi DL, Peterson ME, Graves TK, et al. Hypertension in cats with chronic renal failure or hyperthyroidism. J Vet Intern Med 1990;4:58–62.

[41] Elliott J. Feline hypertension: diagnosis and management. World Small Animal Veterinary Association (WSAVA) Congress; 2002.

[42] Henik R, Snyder P, Volk L. Treatment of systemic hypertension in cats with amlodipine besylate. J Am Anim Hosp Assoc 1997;33:226–34.

[43] Elliott J, Barber PJ, Syme HM, et al. Feline hypertension: clinical findings and response to antihypertensive treatment in 30 cases. J Small Anim Pract 2001;42:122–9.

[44] Brown SA, Brown CA, Jacobs G, et al. Effects of the angiotensin converting enzyme inhibitor benazepril in cats with induced renal insufficiency. Am J Vet Res 2001;62:375–83.

[45] King JN, Strehlau G, Wernsing J, et al. Effect of renal insufficiency on the pharmacokinetics and pharmacodynamics of benazepril in cats. J Vet Pharmacol Ther 2002;25:371–8.

[46] Peterson ME. Propylthiouracil in the treatment of feline hyperthyroidism. J Am Vet Med Assoc 1981;179:485–7.

[47] Peterson ME, Hurvitz AI, Leib MS, et al. Propylthiouracil-associated hemolytic anemia, thrombocytopenia, and antinuclear antibodies in cats with hyperthyroidism. J Am Vet Med Assoc 1984;184:806–8.

[48] Aucoin DP, Peterson ME, Hurvitz AI, et al. Propylthiouracil-induced immune-mediated disease in the cat. J Pharmacol Exp Ther 1985;234:13–8.

[49] Aucoin DP, Rubin RL, Peterson ME, et al. Dose-dependent induction of anti-native DNA antibodies in cats by propylthiouracil. Arthritis Rheum 1988;31:688–92.

[50] Lindsay RH, Aboul-Enein HY, Morel D, et al. Synthesis and antiperoxidase activity of propylthiouracil derivatives and metabolites. J Pharm Sci 1974;63:1383–6.

[51] Waldhauser L, Uetrecht J. Antibodies to myeloperoxidase in propylthiouracil-induced autoimmune disease in the cat. Toxicology 1996;114:155–62.

[52] Jansson R, Dahlberg PA, Lindstrom B. Comparative bioavailability of carbimazole and methimazole. Int J Clin Pharmacol Ther Toxicol 1983;21:505–10.

[53] Peterson ME, Aucoin DP. Comparison of the disposition of carbimazole and methimazole in clinically normal cats. Res Vet Sci 1993;54:351–5.

[54] Bucknell DG. Feline hyperthyroidism: spectrum of clinical presentations and response to carbimazole therapy. Aust Vet J 2000;78:462–5.

[55] Foster DJ, Thoday KL. Use of propranolol and potassium iodate in the presurgical management of hyperthyroid cats. J Small Anim Pract 1999;40:307–15.

[56] Apperley GH, Daly MJ, Levy GP. Selectivity of beta-adrenoceptor agonists and antagonists on bronchial, skeletal, vascular and cardiac muscle in the anaesthetized cat. Br J Pharmacol 1976;57:235–46.

[57] Plumb D. Veterinary drug handbook. 4th edition. White Bear Lake (MN): PharmaVet Publishing; 2002.

[58] Naan EC, Kirpensteijn J, Kooistra HS, et al. Results of thyroidectomy in 101 cats with hyperthyroidism. Vet Surg 2006;35:287–93.

[59] Markou K, Georgopoulos N, Kyriazopoulou V, et al. Iodine-induced hypothyroidism. Thyroid 2001;11:501–10.

[60] Pahuja DN, Rajan MG, Borkar AV, et al. Potassium iodate and its comparison to potassium iodide as a blocker of 131I uptake by the thyroid in rats. Health Phys 1993;65:545–9.

[61] Fontanilla JC, Schneider AB, Sarne DH. The use of oral radiographic contrast agents in the management of hyperthyroidism. Thyroid 2001;11:561–7.

[62] Murray LA, Peterson ME. Ipodate treatment of hyperthyroidism in cats. J Am Vet Med Assoc 1997;211:63–7.

[63] Bruyette D. Feline hyperthyroidism. World Small Animal Veterinary Association (WSAVA) Congress; 2001.

[64] Martino E, Balzano S, Bartalena L, et al. Therapy of Graves' disease with sodium ipodate is associated with a high recurrence rate of hyperthyroidism. J Endocrinol Invest 1991;14:847–51.

[65] Bal CS, Kumar A, Chandra P. Effect of iopanoic acid on radioiodine therapy of hyperthyroidism: long-term outcome of a randomized controlled trial. J Clin Endocrinol Metab 2005;90:6536–40.

Thyroid Surgery in Dogs and Cats

MaryAnn G. Radlinsky, DVM, MS

Department of Small Animal Medicine and Surgery, College of Veterinary Medicine, University of Georgia, 501 DW Brooks Drive, Athens, GA 30602, USA

INDICATIONS FOR SURGERY

Mass lesions of the thyroid gland are the main indication for surgery of the thyroid in dogs and cats. Masses most often are benign and functional in cats and malignant and nonfunctional in dogs. Hyperthyroidism results in many systemic alterations that are more commonly observed in cats than in dogs. Clinical signs of thyrotoxicosis are usually present in geriatric cats with concurrent palpable mass lesions. Secondary cardiac, central nervous system, and muscular effects of thyroxine (T_4) excess should be considered before surgery [1]. Cats with hyperthyroidism may also develop hypertrophic cardiomyopathy with secondary heart failure. Diminished renal function may not be readily diagnosed because of the increase in glomerular filtration rate secondary to increased T_4 levels [2]. Because of the hyperthyroid state and increased risk for anesthesia, ideally, a euthyroid state is established to decrease the risk of anesthesia and to evaluate renal function before surgery.

Dogs do not usually display signs of hyperthyroidism and usually have malignant, invasive, and highly vascular neoplasms. Clinical signs are associated with the mass or are secondary to invasion or compression of surrounding structures. Ventral cervical swelling, dysphagia, dyspnea, coughing, or altered phonation results from compression or invasion of the esophagus, recurrent laryngeal nerve, or trachea. Signs of hyperthyroidism are rarely present, even if triiodothyronine (T_3) and T_4 are elevated; signs of hypothyroidism may be present in rare cases [3–5]. Medullary thyroid carcinoma may represent up to 36% of all thyroid neoplasms [4]. Rarely, medullary carcinoma of the thyroid contains functional calcitonin parafollicular cells, resulting in clinical signs associated with hypocalcemia.

PREOPERATIVE EVALUATION

History, physical examination, and complete blood work, including thyroid evaluation, lead to the suspicion of thyroid disease in dogs and cats and are discussed elsewhere in this issue. Concurrent or metabolic abnormalities attributable to thyrotoxicosis may be evaluated with a complete blood cell

E-mail address: radlinsk@vet.uga.edu

0195-5616/07/$ – see front matter
doi:10.1016/j.cvsm.2007.04.001

count and biochemical profile. Thoracic radiographs, electrocardiography (ECG), and echocardiography should also be considered in cases with clinical signs of hyperthyroidism. Stabilization with propranolol or atenolol should be considered in patients with a resting heart rate greater than 220 beats per minute to decrease the risk associated with general anesthesia [6]. Preoperative treatment with methimazole in hyperthyroid cats for 2 to 4 weeks may result in a return to a euthyroid state; at that time, renal values should be checked for worsening of blood urea nitrogen, creatinine, phosphorous, and other electrolytes [1,6,7]. Significant increases in renal values warrant medical management of both conditions, because thyroidectomy could result in postoperative renal failure. The use of propranolol and potassium iodate has been suggested before surgery to establish a euthyroid state in cats that do not tolerate methimazole therapy [8].

Preoperative technetium scintigraphy is useful for diagnosis of bilateral disease or hyperfunctioning ectopic thyroid tissue. Radionuclide imaging is important in the diagnosis of feline hyperthyroidism before surgery. The test provides information as to the location of all functional tissue, including ectopic thyroid tissue and functioning metastases [1,6,7]. Failure to identify all hyperfunctional tissue may result in failure of resolution of clinical signs and alterations associated with the condition.

Thyroid masses in the dog are usually nonfunctional, invasive, vascular malignancies. Clinical signs are associated with compression or invasion of the surrounding structures. A complete blood cell count, biochemical profile, and urinalysis are used to evaluate canine patients for concurrent disease; thyroid hormone evaluation can be performed if signs of hyperthyroidism are present. Three-view radiographs of the thorax should be made for evaluation of metastasis, which is common [4,5]. Cervical radiographs may demonstrate displacement of surrounding structures [3]. Functional tumors may also be evaluated by nuclear scintigraphy to evaluate the location of the primary tumor and the possibility of secondary tumors. Uptake of radionuclide may be heterogenous as compared with the normal lobe or salivary glands in dogs with thyroid tumors [5]. Fine-needle aspirates typically yield blood contamination because of the vascular nature of thyroid tumors. One study suggested that avoidance of excessive suction and repositioning of the needle during fine-needle aspiration resulted in a good correlation between the cytologic and histopathologic findings of canine thyroid tumors [9]. Tru-cut biopsy must be carefully considered, because thyroid carcinomas are highly vascular. Open biopsy may be performed if the diagnosis is in question [10]. Open biopsy allows planning of placement of incisional biopsy and direct hemostasis. The invasiveness and vascularity make excision of large thyroid tumors difficult. Freely moveable tumors should be considered for surgical excision; tumors less than 7 cm long may also be considered removable [1]. Clinical signs of laryngeal paralysis and dysphagia warrant caution. Compression or invasion of the recurrent laryngeal nerve, trachea, or esophagus should be differentiated before considering surgery. Such tumors are rarely resectable.

ANATOMY OF THE THYROID GLANDS

The thyroid glands are paired and lie on the lateral aspects of the trachea at the fifth through eighth tracheal rings. The glands are approximately 1 cm long and 3 to 5 mm wide in the cat and may be that size to three times as large in the dog [1]. The glands are closely adhered to the trachea, deep to the sternohyoideus and sternothyroideus muscles [11]. The right thyroid may be located more cranial than the left, at the caudal aspect of the larynx [11]. The right gland is closely associated with the structures of the ipsilateral carotid sheath: the carotid artery, internal jugular vein, and vagosympathetic trunk [11]. The recurrent laryngeal nerves pass dorsal to the thyroid glands. The left thyroid gland is closely associated with the esophagus, which lies dorsolateral to the gland and separates it from the carotid sheath [11].

The thyroid tissue in dogs may include a stromal connection between the two glands, ventral to the trachea [11]. The parathyroid glands are intimately associated with the thyroid tissue [11]. The external parathyroids are generally located on the ventral surface of the cranial aspect of each gland [11]. Internal parathyroid glands are usually located in the parenchyma of the caudal aspect of each thyroid gland [11]. Considerable variation in the location of the parathyroid glands has been reported [1]. Each parathyroid gland is approximately 4 mm in diameter in the cat and 1.5 to 2 times that size in the dog [1].

Blood is supplied to the thyroid and parathyroid glands by the cranial and caudal thyroid arteries [11]. The main blood supply is by way of the cranial artery, which arises from the common carotid. The caudal thyroid artery is a branch of the brachiocephalic artery and is absent in the cat [12]. The major supply to the thyroid and parathyroid glands is the cranial thyroid artery, which also supplies the laryngeal structures [11]. The cranial artery anastomoses with the caudal thyroid artery on the dorsal surface of each gland [11]. Many delicate vessels anastomose across the surface of the thyroid glands and enter its parenchyma by way of septae and trabeculae, forming the rete arteriosum [11]. Arteriovenous anastomoses within the parenchyma have been described [11]. The venous drainage of the thyroid and parathyroid is similar to that of the arterial supply, by way of the cranial and caudal thyroid veins [11]. The cranial vein drains into the internal jugular vein, and the caudal vein enters the brachycephalic vein [11]. Lymphatic drainage is by way of the cranial and caudal deep cervical lymph nodes [11]. Efferent lymphatics reach the venous system by way of the right lymphatic duct and left tracheal duct [11].

The anatomy of the thyroid glands is extremely important when considering surgery of the glands to correct hyperplasia and neoplasia. Adjacent structures (eg, carotid artery, internal jugular vein, vagosympathetic trunk, recurrent laryngeal nerve, esophagus) make the procedure complicated if the lesion is large. Damage to those structures can lead to significant alterations in function. The blood supply of the thyroid gland explains the significant risk of hemorrhage associated with large lesions, especially in canine patients. Lastly, the intimate association of the parathyroid glands and the shared blood supply

explains the risk of hypoparathyroidism leading to hypocalcemia in animals requiring bilateral thyroid gland surgery.

APPROACH TO THE THYROID GLANDS

The patient should be placed in dorsal recumbency with the neck extended
over a small support [1,3,6,7]. Extending the thoracic limbs caudally and cross-
ing the leg ties dorsal to the thorax before securing them to the operating table
reduces the risk of inhibiting thoracic movement and ventilation. The ventral
neck should be clipped and aseptically prepared from the caudal mandible to
and including the cranial thorax. Incise the skin from the larynx to just cranial
to the manubrium. The sphincter colli muscles are likewise incised to expose
the longitudinal fibers of the paired sternohyoideus muscles. Digital pressure
on the midline allows identification of the separation of the right and left muscles, which permits a ventral midline approach to the trachea and surrounding
structures (Fig. 1). The small vein courses through the median raphe may be
ligated or cauterized [1]. If the incision must be extended to the manubrium,
as with caudally displaced thyroid masses, sharply incise the median raphe between the paired sternocephalicus muscles with Metzenbaum scissors. Lateral
retraction of the sternohyoideus muscles allows exploration of the entire length
of the trachea. Take care to examine all structures for involvement with the
affected thyroid gland(s).

Lateral retraction of the more dorsolaterally located sternothyroideus muscles allows for more dorsolateral inspection to identify thyroid glands that
are not immediately identified. The right carotid sheath, esophagus, and recurrent laryngeal nerves should be identified and avoided. Both thyroid glands
and the external parathyroid glands should be evaluated before excision of either thyroid gland. If bilateral thyroidectomy is deemed necessary, identification of the external parathyroid glands is important for preservation of the
parathyroid gland and its blood supply. The branch supplying the parathyroid
gland may be visible on the surface of the thyroid gland. Branches that are not
visible likely originate in the thyroid parenchyma. At least one parathyroid
gland should be preserved if both thyroid glands are to be removed.

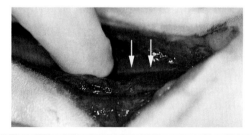

Fig. 1. Dorsal pressure on the ventral aspect of the sternohyoideus musculature exposes the
median raphe (*arrows*) for midline incision.

FELINE THYROIDECTOMY

The blood supply is usually easily identified entering cranially and caudally on a long vascular pedicle (Fig. 2) [1,3,6,7,13]. With unilateral disease leading to hyperthyroidism, the contralateral gland should be atrophied as a result of negative feedback secondary to oversecretion of the hypertrophied or adenomatous gland. Cats rarely have adenocarcinoma rather than benign enlargement of the thyroid [14]. Evaluate both thyroid glands as described to rule out the lack of atrophy and need for bilateral excision. The cat's thyroid glands may be removed by one of a variety of techniques: the extracapsular, intracapsular, and modified extracapsular techniques [6,13]. Care should be taken to avoid trauma to the adjacent structures and to the external parathyroid glands and their blood supply with any of the techniques used.

The extracapsular technique is useful for unilateral disease [6]. The cranial and caudal blood supply to the affected gland is ligated, the external parathyroid is sharply dissected from the thyroid capsule, and the entire thyroid gland is excised with its capsule intact [1,7,13]. Modification of the extracapsular technique was developed to decrease the risk of postoperative hypocalcemia [1,7]. Incise the 2 mm of thyroid capsule adjacent to the external parathyroid gland, being careful to preserve the blood supply to the parathyroid gland [1,7]. Enlarge the incision with fine scissors, and use a moistened cotton-tipped applicator to dissect the thyroid tissue deep to the capsule attached to the external parathyroid gland [1,7]. The blood supply to the parathyroid and a small amount of thyroid parenchyma and capsule remain in place with the external parathyroid gland [1,7]. The caudal continuation of the thyroid artery supplying the parathyroid branch should be ligated or coagulated with fine bipolar cautery forceps [1,7]. The thyroid gland and remaining capsule are dissected and removed after ligation and division of the caudal blood supply to the thyroid gland [1,7].

The intracapsular technique for thyroidectomy involves incision of the thyroid capsule on its ventral surface and dissection and removal of the thyroid parenchyma, leaving the capsule in situ [1,7,13]. Dissect with a moistened cotton-tipped applicator as for the modified extracapsular technique. Because the intracapsular technique has the potential to leave a significant amount of

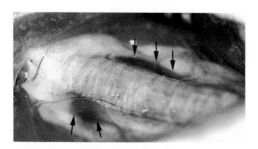

Fig. 2. Normal feline thyroid glands are outlined with arrows.

thyroid parenchyma behind, modification has been described in which the capsule caudal to the parathyroid gland is excised after the thyroid parenchyma has been removed.

Staged procedures have been described for bilateral thyroidectomy in the cat [13]. A period of 3 to 4 weeks between procedures gives time for resolution of transient vascular or parenchymal parathyroid damage [13]. The necessity of two anesthetic episodes is the major drawback of the technique, considering the older age of the patients often affected [13]. Parathyroid autotransplantation has also been described as a treatment for accidental removal of the parathyroid or if complete devascularization occurs during thyroidectomy [15]. The parathyroid gland is cut into small 1-mm pieces and inserted into a small pocket made in the cervical musculature [15]. Revascularization can occur, and resumption of parathyroid function may result, decreasing the severity and time of postoperative hypocalcemia [15].

CANINE THYROIDECTOMY

Canine thyroid tumors should be considered malignant carcinomas, and excision is usually performed by means of the extracapsular technique. Far fewer thyroid mass lesions are diagnosed as benign adenoma (range: 12%–37%) [5,16]. Complete excision with the associated parathyroid gland is often possible, because most thyroid tumors deemed resectable are unilateral, not extremely large, and moveable (Fig. 3) [1,5]. Large immobile tumors or tumors associated with respiratory or gastrointestinal dysfunction are usually considered inoperable [1]. Bilateral thyroid carcinomas or a thyroid tumor that extends across midline may require bilateral thyroidectomy. Care should be taken to preserve the parathyroid glands, or bilateral thyroid and parathyroidectomy may be performed, with preoperative and postoperative attention to calcium homeostasis.

It is not surprising that canine thyroid neoplasms are highly vascular, considering the normal rete arteriosum of the thyroid gland and neovascularization of

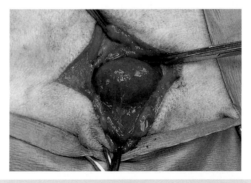

Fig. 3. An encapsulated thyroid carcinoma approached by means of a ventral midline incision.

tumors. After exposing the thyroid glands and evaluating each gland and the associated anatomic structures, carefully dissect the tumor (Fig. 4). A tube in the esophagus may aid in its identification and protection during dissection. Proceed with the dissection from ventral to dorsal; numerous tortuous fragile vessels are encountered. Each should be ligated, or cauterized, being careful not to overestimate the size of vessel that may be cauterized. Significant hemorrhage may necessitate ligation of the common carotid artery and internal jugular vein; unilateral ligation should be well tolerated [1]. Even with excision, tumor cells are likely left behind, because carcinomas tend to invade the supporting fascia within the neck even in moveable tumors. Cervical lymph nodes may be biopsied concurrently for staging.

POSTOPERATIVE MANAGEMENT

The most common complication after bilateral thyroidectomy is hypocalcemia attributable to damage to the parathyroid glands, the blood supply, or inadvertent complete parathyroidectomy. The complication should be anticipated in cats and can occur with any technique used. Extracapsular, intracapsular, and staged intracapsular excisional techniques in cats undergoing bilateral thyroidectomy resulted in 82%, 36%, and 11% rates of postoperative hypocalcemia, respectively, in one study [13]. The single anesthetic and staged intracapsular excisions were not significantly different, however, and were higher than reported in another study, which had a 5% rate of postoperative hypocalcemia after intracapsular thyroidectomy [17]. The modified extracapsular technique resulted in a 23% rate of hypocalcemia in another study [17]. Administration of dihydrotachysterol and calcium immediately after surgery did not reduce the rate of hypocalcemia in 13 of the cats in the study [17].

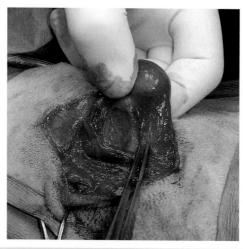

Fig. 4. A small portion of the vascular supply to the carcinoma in Fig. 3 is indicated by the forceps.

Postoperative hypocalcemia generally occurs within 5 days of surgery; the length of time may be related to damage or thrombosis of the parathyroid blood supply if the gland is not removed with the thyroid gland [1,18]. Ionized calcium levels should be monitored for at least 48 hours after surgery [15]. Decreasing values within that time warrant further monitoring for possible signs necessitating intervention [1,3,6,7,18]. Clinical signs of hypocalcemia include anxiety, inappetence, facial pruritus, and twitching and can progress to tetany [1,3,6,7,18]. Feline patients usually show clinical signs when total serum calcium falls to less than 6.5 mg/dL.

Acute management of hypocalcemia in patients showing signs of tetany should consist of intravenous calcium. Calcium gluconate 10% should be administered at a rate of 0.5 to 1.5 mg/kg given over 15 to 20 minutes [1,3,18]. ECG monitoring is recommended during administration, because bradycardia and cardiac arrhythmias can result from intravenous calcium administration. Cats may be placed on a continuous infusion of 10% calcium gluconate (10 mL) in lactated Ringer's solution (250 mL) at 60 mL/kg/d [1,3,18]. Subcutaneous administration of calcium may also be administered, but the solution must be diluted to a ratio of at least 1:1 in 0.9% saline to prevent irritation and necrosis at the injection site [1,3,18]. Six to eight milliliters of the solution should be administered every 6 to 8 hours in cats [1,3,18]. Oral medication can be instituted once the patient is stable and eating. Oral calcium lactate (400–600 mg/kg/d divided) or calcium gluconate (500–750 mg/kg/d divided at least q 12h) and dihydrotachysterol (0.02–0.03 mg/kg/d) can be started [1,3,6,18]. The initial dose of dihydrotachysterol is higher than the maintenance dose and requires 2 to 3 days to take effect. The dose of dihydrotachysterol should be decreased to 0.005 mg/kg/d after the initial 5 to 7 days of therapy [1,3,6,18]. Tapering of the medications after 4 to 10 weeks can be attempted [1,18]. Patients in which parathyroid tissue was not removed may recover parathyroid activity and experience no ill effects from tapering and discontinuing medical therapy. Calcium levels should be monitored at least weekly during the diminution of dihydrotachysterol and calcium supplementation. Patients that fail to regain parathyroid function may require calcium and dihydrotachysterol supplementation for life.

The recurrent laryngeal nerve may also be damaged during thyroidectomy in cats or dogs. The nerve should be identified and protected during the procedure to prevent transection. Neuropraxia may result from retraction during excision of large tumors, especially in dogs. Such damage may be temporary and may not result in significant respiratory compromise if it is unilateral. Change in phonation may be noted when the canine patient barks or the feline patient purrs or vocalizes. Bilateral damage to the recurrent laryngeal nerves may require surgical intervention, which typically consists of unilateral arytenoid lateralization.

Hypothyroidism may occur in any patient undergoing bilateral thyroidectomy. Evaluation of thyroid hormone levels should diagnose the condition, although thyroid supplementation may not be necessary unless clinical signs are apparent.

Postoperative hemorrhage can be severe in dogs. Initial therapy with cool compresses and a cervical bandage may allow tamponade of minor hemorrhage, but compressive bandages must be avoided to permit adequate ventilation. Transfusion therapy and reoperation may be required with significant hemorrhage.

PROGNOSIS

Recurrence of hyperthyroidism in cats undergoing thyroidectomy ranges from 0% to 36% and may take up 2 to 3 years to occur [19]. The lowest rates have been associated with the extracapsular technique (range: 0%–9%) [13,20]. The intracapsular technique resulted in an 8% recurrence in two studies [19,21] and a 22% occurrence in another study [17]. The modifications of the intracapsular technique and extracapsular techniques were associated with recurrence rates of 0% to 5% [13,17] and 4% [17], respectively. The trade-off of postoperative hypercalcemia and recurrence is evident, because the more aggressive the excision, the higher is the rate of hypocalcemia. Cats with thyroid carcinomas that have recurrence of a mass or hyperthyroidism after surgery may respond to high-dose radioactive iodine [22]. Recurrence may be local or caused by a hyperfunctional contralateral or ectopic thyroid. The intracapsular thyroidectomy technique resulted in higher (range: 8%–22%) recurrence as compared with the modified extracapsular technique (4%) [17,21]. The modified intracapsular technique was associated with a recurrence rate of 0% to 22% but was also associated with severe hypocalcemia after surgery in 13% of patients in the study [17].

Complete excision of canine thyroid adenoma results in an excellent outcome. Thyroid adenocarcinomas in the dog treated with surgery alone usually result in recurrence. Complete excision of encapsulated noninvasive carcinomas may result in a 1-to 3-year survival time; however, a survival time of 7 months has also been reported [5,23]. Resection of freely movable thyroid tumors with no evidence of pulmonary metastasis at the time of diagnosis resulted in survival times of 44, 24, and 17 months for solid, follicular, and solid-follicular carcinomas, respectively [24]. Medullary carcinomas may be more frequently resectable because they tended to be less invasive in one study [4]; however, the survival times were not different from those for adenocarcinomas. Eleven of 16 tumors demonstrated vascular or lymphatic invasion, and none had wide margins of normal tissue [4]. Recurrence rates for thyroid carcinomas in the dog average 45% within 2 years [18]. Surgical excision of thyroid malignancies represents an excellent means of cytoreduction of the tumor load in cases that are deemed resectable. Adjuvant chemotherapy or radiation therapy should be considered in each case.

References

[1] Flanders JA. Surgical therapy of the thyroid. Vet Clin North Am Small Anim Pract 1994; 24(3):607–21.

[2] DiBartola SP, Broome MR, Stein BS, et al. Effect of treatment of hyperthyroidism on renal function in cats. J Am Vet Med Assoc 1996;208(6):875–8.

[3] Birchard SJ. Thyroidectomy and parathyroidectomy in the dog and cat. Probl Vet Med 1991;3(2):277–89.

[4] Carver JR, Kapatkin A, Patnaik AK. A comparison of medullary thyroid carcinoma and thyroid adenocarcinoma in dogs: a retrospective study of 38 cases. Vet Surg 1995;24(4): 315–9.

[5] Harari J, Patterson JS, Rosenthal RC. Clinical and pathologic features of thyroid tumors in 26 dogs. J Am Vet Med Assoc 1986;188(10):1160–4.

[6] Flanders JA. Surgical options for the treatment of hyperthyroidism in the cat. J Feline Med Surg 1999;1:127–34.

[7] Padgett S. Feline thyroid surgery. Vet Clin North Am Small Anim Pract 2002;32(4):851–9.

[8] Foster DJ, Thoday KL. Use of propranolol and potassium iodate in the presurgical management of hyperthyroid cats. J Small Anim Pract 1999;40(7):307–15.

[9] Thompson EJ, Stirtzinger T, Lumsden JH, et al. Fine needle aspiration cytology in the diagnosis of canine thyroid carcinoma. Can Vet J 1980;21(6):186–8.

[10] Langenbach A, Anderson MA, Dambach DM, et al. Extraskeletal osteosarcomas in dogs: a retrospective study of 169 cases (1986–1996). J Am Anim Hosp Assoc 1998;34: 113–20.

[11] Hullinger RL. The endocrine system. In: Evans HE, editor. Miller's anatomy of the dog. 3rd edition. Philadelphia: WB Saunders; 1993. p. 559–85.

[12] Nicholas JS, Swingle WW. An experimental and morphological study of the parathyroid glands of the cat. Am J Anat 1925;34:469.

[13] Flanders SA, Harvey HJ. Feline thyroidectomy: a comparison of postoperative hypocalcemia associated with three different surgical techniques. Vet Surg 1987;16(5):362–6.

[14] Turrel JM, Feldman EC, Nelson RW, et al. Thyroid carcinoma causing hyperthyroidism in cats: 14 cases (1981–1986). J Am Vet Med Assoc 1988;193(3):359–64.

[15] Padgett SL, Tobias KM, Leathers CW, et al. Efficacy of parathyroid gland autotransplantation in maintaining serum calcium concentrations after bilateral thyroparathyroidectomy in cats. J Am Anim Hosp Assoc 1998;34(3):219–24.

[16] Leav I, Schiller AL, Rijnberk A, et al. Adenomas and carcinomas of the canine and feline thyroid. Am J Pathol 1976;83(1):61–122.

[17] Welches CD, Scavelli TD, Matthiesen DT, et al. Occurrence of problems after three techniques of bilateral thyroidectomy in cats. Vet Surg 1989;18(5):392–6.

[18] Ehrhart N. Thyroid. In: Slatter D, editor. Textbook of small animal surgery. 3rd edition. Philadelphia: Saunders; 2003. p. 1700–10.

[19] Swalec KM, Birchard SJ. Recurrence of hyperthyroidism after thyroidectomy in cats. J Am Anim Hosp Assoc 1990;26(4):433–7.

[20] Holzworth J, Theran P, Carpenter JL, et al. Hyperthyroidism in the cat: ten cases. J Am Vet Med Assoc 1980;176(4):345–53.

[21] Birchard SJ, Peterson ME, Jacobson A. Surgical treatment of feline hyperthyroidism: results of 85 cases. J Am Anim Hosp Assoc 1984;20(5):705–9.

[22] Guptill L, Scott-Moncrieff CR, Janovitz EB, et al. Response to high-dose radioactive iodine administration in cats with thyroid carcinoma that had previously undergone surgery. J Am Vet Med Assoc 1995;207(8):1055–8.

[23] Kent MS, Griffey SM, Verstraete FJ, et al. Computer-assisted image analysis of neovascularization in thyroid neoplasms from dogs. Am J Vet Res 2002;63(3):363–9.

[24] Klein MK, Powers BE, Withrow SJ, et al. Treatment of thyroid carcinoma in dogs by surgical resection alone: 20 cases (1981–1989). J Am Vet Med Assoc 1995;206(7):1007–9.

ELSEVIER
SAUNDERS

Vet Clin Small Anim 37 (2007) 799–821

VETERINARY CLINICS
SMALL ANIMAL PRACTICE

Nuclear Imaging and Radiation Therapy in Canine and Feline Thyroid Disease

Daniel A. Feeney, DVM, MS*, Kari L. Anderson, DVM

Department of Veterinary Clinical Sciences, College of Veterinary Medicine, University of Minnesota, 1352 Boyd Avenue, St. Paul, MN 55108, USA

Thyroid disorders are not uncommon in the veterinary patient. Hyperthyroidism is currently the most commonly diagnosed endocrine disorder in middle-aged and geriatric cats [1–3]. The reported incidence of canine hypothyroidism ranges from 0.2% to 0.8% [4,5]. Thyroid neoplasia accounts for 1.2% to 4% of all canine neoplasms [6,7] and approximately 10% to 15% of all head and neck tumors in the dog [1]. Because of the variety of thyroid diseases, the clinician must have an understanding of the diagnostic and treatment options available. This article explores the role of nuclear imaging and radiation therapy in clinical management of thyroid disorders.

DILEMMAS IN THYROID DISEASE ASSESSMENT

Various diagnostic tests, each possessing advantages and disadvantages, are available to aid the clinician in the diagnosis of thyroid disease. Nuclear imaging can be important in assessing thyroid disease because its strength is the ability to provide physiologic and morphologic information that cannot be provided by any other single diagnostic procedure. Although clinical history, physical examination, and routine laboratory tests are generally reliable in making the diagnosis of certain thyroid diseases, the test results may not always provide the entire clinical picture. For example, cats with mild hyperthyroidism may have normal serum thyroxine (T_4) and triiodothyronine (T_3) [8] or fluctuations of serum T_4 and T_3 between normal and abnormal [9], cats with concurrent nonthyroidal illness may have normal T_4 [2,10], cats with nonthyroidal illness can have high serum free T_4 [8,11], and dogs with thyroid tumors generally do not have increased serum T_4 [6,12]. Additionally, these tests are unable to distinguish unilateral from bilateral involvement, differentiate between benign and malignant thyroid disorders, or identify hyperfunctioning ectopic or metastatic thyroid tissue. Other imaging modalities, such as ultrasound [13–15] and CT [16,17], have been used in veterinary patients to examine

*Corresponding author. E-mail address: feene001@umn.edu (D.A. Feeney).

0195-5616/07/$ – see front matter
doi:10.1016/j.cvsm.2007.03.005

the thyroid gland. Although these modalities can provide thyroid volume and morphologic information, including determining invasiveness, and can guide sampling, they are unable to provide functional information and may not identify ectopic thyroid tissue or metastatic disease.

A thyroid radionuclide scan is a simple, noninvasive, reasonably priced procedure that provides a visual display of functional thyroid tissue after injection of a radiotracer concentrated by thyroid tissue. The scintigram can provide valuable information regarding anatomy and function that is integral in the diagnosis and management of thyroid disease.

Nuclear imaging procedures are generally limited to academic institutions and larger referral practices because of the specialized training and licensing needed to implement and maintain a program. Individuals and institutions are granted a radioactive materials license by the state in which they practice (an "agreement state") or by the Nuclear Regulatory Commission. Generally, demonstrated training in nuclear medicine procedures and radiation safety as well as proven experience is required to obtain a radioactive materials license. As part of the nuclear medicine program, various types of documentation are required, and audits by the granting agency occur approximately annually.

RADIONUCLIDE THYROID IMAGING

Equipment

Specialized equipment is needed for nuclear diagnostic imaging. The equipment consists of a gamma camera (scintillation camera) and collimator, which detect the γ-radiation emitted from the patient after injection of the radioisotope. Within the camera, the γ-radiation is converted to light and then to electrical energy, which is amplified within photomultiplier tubes. Specialized circuitry determines coordinates and intensity of the radiation. This information is then used by the interfaced computer to assign information in a matrix to form an image. The computer acquisition and processing software capabilities include the ability to make qualitative and quantitative assessments of the studies. Although new gamma cameras and computers are expensive, more affordable good-quality used and refurbished equipment is available.

Radiotracer

The most commonly used imaging agent is the radioisotope technetium-99m as pertechnetate ($^{99m}TcO_4^-$). Pertechnetate is a transitional metal that imitates the halogens and acts in a similar fashion as iodine, actively trapped and concentrated but not organified or incorporated into thyroid hormone by the thyroid gland. Pertechnetate also concentrates in the salivary glands, gastric mucosa, choroid plexus, and sweat glands. Pertechnetate is uniquely suited to nuclear imaging because it possesses the ideal imaging characteristics for a radioisotope, including virtually no β-emission and moderately low γ-emission (140 keV) efficiently collimated by the gamma camera. One important characteristic of pertechnetate is its short half-life of 6.01 hours; thus, the patient is not radioactive for long, and the potential for environmental contamination is limited. Pertechnetate is also readily available and relatively inexpensive. Importantly, prior administration of antithyroid drugs, such as methimazole, does not interfere with the uptake of pertechnetate by the thyroid, because these drugs do not affect the trapping mechanism of the thyroid pump [18]. The trapping of pertechnetate is competitive with iodine, however, and recent administration of iodinated contrast material or ingestion of excess administered or dietary iodine may interfere with uptake by the thyroid for weeks [19]. Thyroid hormone supplementation also reduces uptake by the thyroid gland.

Other radioisotopes used in thyroid imaging include iodine-123 (^{123}I) and iodine-131 (^{131}I). ^{123}I and ^{131}I are trapped by the thyroid lobe and are also organified by the thyroid lobe. The long half-life (8.06 days) and β-particle emissions by ^{131}I as well as relatively high γ-ray emissions (364 keV) not suited to collimation by the gamma camera, resulting in inferior images, are disadvantages to the use of this radiotracer. Although ^{123}I is more ideally suited for imaging with the gamma camera (159-keV energy photons), has a shorter half-life (13.3 hours), and lacks β-particle emissions, the radiotracer is less available and more expensive. The radioiodine radiotracers also result in a higher radiation dose to the thyroid. Finally, imaging with radioiodine is delayed until 4 and 24 hours, in comparison to imaging at 20 minutes after pertechnetate administration. In contrast to pertechnetate studies, prior administration of antithyroid drugs may adversely affect radioiodine studies. Studies performed with pertechnetate and radioiodine typically yield concordant localization and identical scintigraphic distribution [19].

Indications

The indications for thyroid imaging are varied and may include the following [6,12,18,20–27]:

1. Evaluation of the functional status of the thyroid glands
2. Determination of unilateral or bilateral thyroid lobe involvement
3. Detection and localization of ectopic thyroid tissue
4. Differentiation between benign and malignant thyroid disease
5. Determination of thyroid gland size for radiation therapy calculations
6. Determination of thyroid or nonthyroid origin of cervical mass
7. Detection of functional metastasis
8. Evaluation of the efficacy of therapy
9. Evaluation for residual tissue after thyroidectomy
10. Differentiation between hypothyroidism and euthyroid sick syndrome
11. Differentiation between primary, secondary, and tertiary hypothyroidism
12. Differentiation between thyroid dysgenesis and inherited iodination defects

Procedure

The procedure itself is simple and straightforward. The imaging protocol is well described in the veterinary literature [13,21,28]. Because the patient must lie still for image acquisition, sedation or general anesthesia may be necessary to acquire quality images. Opposite lateral and ventral images of the cervical region and thorax are obtained 20 to 60 minutes after intravenous injection of pertechnetate at a dose of 1 to 4 mCi (37–148 MBq) using a low-energy, general purpose, parallel-hole collimator. Images can be obtained using timed acquisition or a count acquisition. A ventral image of the thyroid using a pinhole collimator can provide important information regarding unilateral versus bilateral disease as well as improved spatial resolution of the thyroid lobe morphology that may aid with discrimination between benign and malignant disease [29,30]. The trade-off for the improved resolution and magnified view of the area is a longer image acquisition time.

Image Interpretation and Analysis: Qualitative Analysis

Image interpretation is by visual inspection and quantitative analysis. The images should be assessed for location of uptake relative to the thyroid gland. A normal study should have good visualization of both lobes of the thyroid gland as discrete ovoid areas of radioactivity symmetric in position and size in the midcervical region on the ventral image; [18,31] the thyroid lobes should be superimposed on the lateral images. Normal uptake should also be present in the salivary glands and gastric mucosa, and some patients have additional uptake in the nasal, oral, and pharyngeal areas [28]. Blood pool activity should be seen in the thorax and mediastinum (heart and vessels), and soft tissue activity should outline the patient. Visually, the uptake in the thyroid lobes and the salivary glands should be similar. Figs. 1 and 2 depict normal uptake in the thyroid and salivary glands in the cat and dog, respectively.

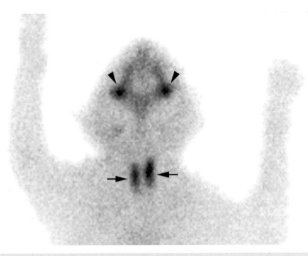

Fig. 1. Normal feline thyroid scan. This ventral image was acquired 20 minutes after intravenous injection of pertechnetate. Note the uniform uptake by both thyroid lobes (*arrows*). The intensity of the uptake is similar to the intensity of the uptake in the zygomatic/molar salivary tissue (*arrowheads*). (*Courtesy of* Gregory Daniel, DVM, MS, Knoxville, TN.)

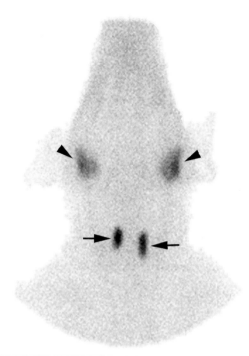

Fig. 2. Normal canine thyroid scan. This ventral image was acquired 20 minutes after intravenous injection of pertechnetate. Note the uniform uptake by both thyroid lobes (*arrows*). The intensity of the uptake is slightly more than the intensity of the uptake in the parotid salivary tissue (*arrowheads*). (*Courtesy of* Gregory Daniel, DVM, MS, Knoxville, TN.)

Image Interpretation and Analysis: Quantitative Analysis

For quantitative analysis, the thyroid-to-salivary (TS) ratio is the most commonly used parameter to determine functional status of the thyroid gland. Of all methods evaluated for quantifying thyroid function (percent uptake of pertechnetate by the thyroid, TS ratio, and rate of thyroid uptake), the simplest method, the TS ratio, had the strongest correlation with serum T_4 in cats [32]. Computer software is used to draw regions of interest around each thyroid lobe. Regions of interest are also drawn around the zygomatic/molar salivary glands in the cat or the parotid salivary glands in the dog. The TS ratio is determined by dividing the mean count density within the thyroid gland (both lobes summed) region by the mean count density within the salivary gland (both glands summed) region. The normal TS ratio that has been reported in the largest population of normal cats ranges from 0.48 to 1.66 (95% prediction interval) [33]. Other studies have reported TS ratios in smaller younger populations of cats ranging from 0.56 to 1.07 [28,32,34]. It has been shown that healthy cats treated with methimazole for 21 days have significant radiotracer uptake in the thyroid lobes [35], thus potentially yielding a false-positive result; however, 30 days of methimazole treatment in hyperthyroid cats did not alter pertechnetate uptake by the thyroid gland [36]. Historically, a few studies in dogs have reported a TS ratio of approximately 1.0 [12,22,31,37,38]. In a quantitative study, the TS ratio ranged from 0.9 to 2.2 at 20 minutes and from 0.8 to 2.4 at 1 hour [39] after injection in 13 normal beagles. Fig. 3 depicts the regions of interest drawn for quantitative analysis.

Feline Hyperthyroidism

The most common use for veterinary thyroid imaging is in the assessment of feline hyperthyroidism. The utility of thyroid imaging is in the determination of unilateral versus bilateral disease for surgical planning. Additionally, ectopic hyperfunctioning tissue located anywhere from the base of the tongue to the base of the heart can be identified. The cause of feline hyperthyroidism in most cases is adenomatous hyperplasia, functional thyroid adenoma, or multinodular adenomatous tumors [23]. Seventy-one percent to 77% of cats have bilateral thyroid uptake, and 23% to 29% have unilateral thyroid uptake [18,40,41]. A range from 9% to 21% of cases have ectopic uptake [20,40]. It has also been suggested that thyroid imaging can be used to determine malignancy, although malignant feline hyperthyroidism occurs in less than 3% of all hyperthyroid cats [18,20,42]. In these cases, nuclear imaging can be used to evaluate for metastasis as well. It has been reported that 70% of identified cases have metastasis [42].

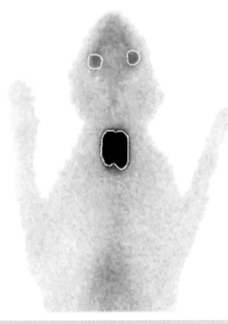

Fig. 3. Quantitative analysis of thyroid uptake of pertechnetate in a cat. Regions of interest are drawn around the thyroid and zygomatic/salivary tissue. A ratio of the count density of the thyroid to the salivary tissue is calculated for quantification of thyroid function. The calculated TS ratio in this cat with bilateral hyperthyroidism is 4.9.

Uniform increased uptake with smooth and regular margins is seen with thyroid adenomatous hyperplasia. The hyperplastic functioning tissue should suppress the normal tissue; therefore, in unilateral hyperthyroidism, the contralateral lobe should not be visible on a scan. If the contralateral lobe is identified, the diagnosis of bilateral disease is made. In bilateral involvement, the lobes may be similar in uptake, size, and location or they may be unequal in uptake and size, with the larger more intense lobe often migrating caudally toward the thoracic inlet. Nodular areas of uptake can be seen with hyperfunctioning thyroid adenomas or multinodular adenomatous tumors. In malignancy, the lobe may be distorted, activity may extend beyond the expected confines of the lobe, the thyroid gland may show hot and cold regions or multiple foci of uptake, and uptake may extend caudally toward or into the thoracic inlet [43]. Findings of multiple masses in the cervical region, masses extending into the thoracic inlet/cranial mediastinum, or lung uptake are more likely to represent malignancy [42]. In cases such as these, a surgical biopsy should be performed for confirmation and therapeutic planning. Figs. 4 through 7 show examples of the various patterns of uptake in hyperthyroid cats.

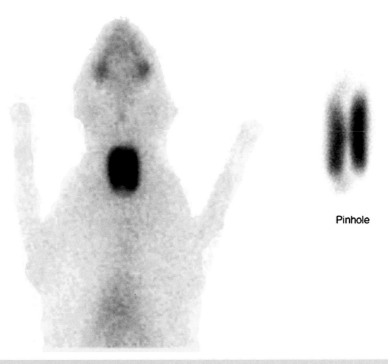

Pinhole

Fig. 4. Thyroid scan from a hyperthyroid cat. These ventral and pinhole images were acquired 20 minutes after intravenous injection of pertechnetate. There is increased uptake by both thyroid lobes in this cat with bilateral thyroid disease.

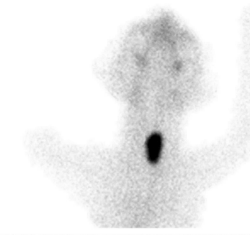

Fig. 5. Thyroid scan from a hyperthyroid cat. This ventral image was acquired 20 minutes after intravenous injection of pertechnetate. There is marked increased uptake by the left thyroid lobe. Note the suppression of the contralateral lobe in this cat with unilateral thyroid disease. (*Courtesy of* Gregory Daniel, DVM, MS, Knoxville, TN.)

Canine Thyroid Tumors

In comparison to the cat, the use of scintigraphy to evaluate canine thyroid diseases has generally been limited to the imaging of thyroid neoplasms and the diagnostic workup for canine cervical masses. In these patients, scintigraphy

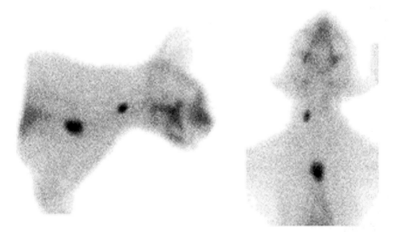

Fig. 6. Thyroid scan from a hyperthyroid cat. These ventral and right lateral images were acquired 20 minutes after intravenous injection of pertechnetate. There is increased uptake by the right thyroid lobe. In addition, there is a focal area of uptake seen in the region of the cranial mediastinum that represents ectopic hyperfunctional thyroid tissue. (*Courtesy of* Gregory Daniel, DVM, MS, Knoxville, TN.)

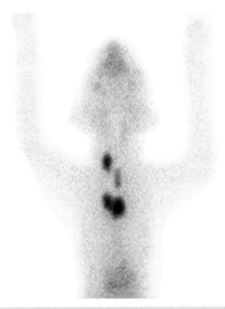

Fig. 7. Thyroid scan from a hyperthyroid cat with thyroid carcinoma. This ventral image was acquired 20 minutes after intravenous injection of pertechnetate. Note the irregular distribution of uptake with numerous areas of disorganized uptake outside the confines of the left and right thyroid lobes. (*Courtesy of* Gregory Daniel, DVM, MS, Knoxville, TN.)

is useful for diagnosis of thyroid involvement, staging of ectopic tissue and distant metastasis, determining functional status of nonneoplastic and neoplastic tissue [6,12,22], and follow-up evaluation of therapy. The image is inspected to determine if the mass is of thyroid or nonthyroid origin. If the mass is of nonthyroid origin, both thyroid lobes should appear uniform in activity and of similar size. If the mass is of thyroid origin, two patterns of uptake have been described: well-circumscribed homogeneous radionuclide uptake and poorly circumscribed heterogeneous radionuclide uptake [12,24]. Dogs with the first pattern of uptake undergoing surgical therapy had a greater likelihood for complete surgical resection. Margins may be irregular, with uptake beyond the margin indicating local extension [6,22]. One or both thyroid lobes may be involved. Many investigators have documented distant metastasis using scintigraphy [6,22,26,44], and focal areas of uptake within the thorax or in unusual areas of the cervical region are interpreted as highly suspicious for metastatic disease [12]. Fig. 8 shows an example of canine thyroid carcinoma. Most canine thyroid tumors are nonfunctional from a physiologic standpoint (do not cause elevated serum T_4), and it has been suggested that up to 30% of dogs with detectable thyroid tumors may actually be hypothyroid [24]. Fortunately, most tumors still have variable increased radiotracer uptake allowing scintigraphic evaluation because they retain the ability to trap and organify radioiodine (functional from a nuclear imaging standpoint) [22].

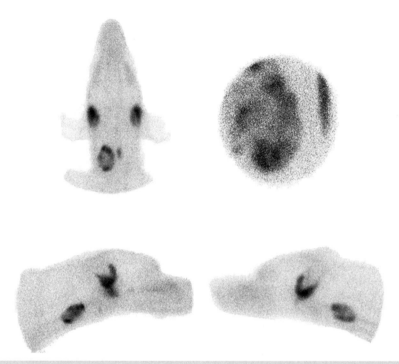

Fig. 8. Thyroid scan from a dog with thyroid carcinoma. These ventral, ventral pinhole, and lateral images were acquired 20 minutes after intravenous injection of pertechnetate. Note the disorganized pattern of uptake in the enlarged right thyroid lobe. This tumor is considered functional from a nuclear imaging standpoint but is not producing excess thyroid hormone, because there is minimal suppression of the contralateral thyroid lobe. (*Courtesy of* Gregory Daniel, DVM, MS, Knoxville, TN.)

Canine Hypothyroidism

Another potential application of thyroid scintigraphy in dogs is to aid in evaluation of hypothyroidism. In cases of equivocal diagnostic tests in which hypothyroidism is suspected, quantitative scintigraphy may be able to differentiate the normal patient from dogs with mild thyroid dysfunction [39]. It has been stated that dogs with true hypothyroidism typically show diminished radionuclide thyroid uptake, whereas dogs with nonthyroidal illness are typically normal [38,45]. Thyroid scintigraphy can also differentiate thyroid agenesis from iodination defects in puppies with congenital hypothyroidism [46]. Scintigrams in thyroid agenesis show minimal radionuclide uptake in the thyroid, whereas scintigrams in iodination defects show large thyroid lobes with normal or increased TS ratios.

Posttreatment Evaluation

Scintigraphy can be useful to re-evaluate after treatment for thyroid carcinoma. With complete excision of the tumor, no radionuclide localization should be demonstrated in the tumor bed or in any remaining normal thyroid [22]. After high-dose radioiodine treatment, ^{131}I imaging may be necessary to demonstrate metastatic tissue not demonstrated by pertechnetate imaging [47]. It is likely that the amount of functional tissue is sufficiently small or its uptake is so low that it is obscured by adjacent soft tissue structures in pertechnetate imaging, whereas thyroid tissue has greater uptake of ^{131}I and delayed imaging also allows for greater soft tissue clearance.

RADIATION SAFETY IN NUCLEAR IMAGING

Special radiation safety precautions must be followed for nuclear medicine studies, because the patient is radioactive during and after the procedure. Not only does the patient emit γ-rays after injection, but the radioisotopes used for thyroid imaging are eliminated mainly through the urine; however, because activity localizes in the salivary glands, the saliva may also be radioactive. Personnel working with the patient and the radionuclide should always wear a laboratory coat and disposable gloves to prevent contamination to their bodies and should be monitored for radiation exposure with a film badge, thermoluminescent dosimeter (TLD) badge, or pocket dosimeter. Personnel should follow the universal radiation safety concept of keeping the radiation exposure as low as reasonably achievable (ALARA). This is achieved by minimizing the time spent exposed to the radiation source (the radionuclide and the radioactive patient); maximizing the distance from the radiation source; and, when possible, placing protective shielding (eg, lead, cement walls) between the radiation source and the person.

Regulations differ depending on the agency licensing the facility; however, most facilities require confinement of the patient for some time after the procedure. The release criteria are variable, but the patient is generally able to be released when the radiation emitted has reached a level that poses no radiation safety threat to the general public. At the authors' institution, the patient can be released when the radioactivity measured at the surface of the patient does not exceed 2 mR/h, which results in less than a 24-hour stay in isolation. After release, the patient is still emitting a low level of radiation; clients are counseled to limit contact with the pet, washing their hands well after contact with the pet and waste, and are instructed how to handle the minimally radioactive urine for another 36 hours (the specifics vary depending on the issuer of the radioactive materials license). The overall dose of radiation that the patient is exposed to for a thyroid scan is minimal. In the authors' experience, adverse side effects have not been seen.

DILEMMAS IN THYROID DISEASE TREATMENT

There two primary considerations in the treatment determination of potential thyroid disease. One is the diagnosis that includes applicable staging in the scenario of potential malignancy. This is discussed elsewhere in this article. The other is the medical condition of the patient and the physiologic side effects of thyroid treatment, particularly renal function. These are addressed elsewhere [1,9,45,48–60]. Although benign hypothyroidism, particularly in dogs, is not part of this discussion, there are numerous considerations and caveats there as well [46]. This discussion focuses on thyroid malignancies in dogs and cats and benign hyperthyroidism in cats. Malignancy must be considered in euthyroid or hyperthyroid disease in dogs and cats. As already mentioned, previous reports indicate that thyroid malignancies account for between 1% and 4% of canine malignancies [61]. In addition, canine malignant thyroid disease is more common than benign thyroid disease based on antemortem assessments [6,61–65], but they are approximately equal when postmortem sampling is undertaken [66]. Most canine thyroid malignancies do not result in hypothyroid or hyperthyroid states [6,64,67–69]. Canine hyperthyroidism, regardless of the cause, is quite uncommon [64,67]. By comparison, benign hyperthyroidism in aged cats is not an uncommon occurrence, although the actual incidence of the disease is unknown [64,69]. Approximately 1% to 2% of hyperthyroid cats have an underlying carcinoma [42,67]. Most feline hyperthyroidism is attributable to benign hyperplasia, and at least 70% of such cases are attributable to bilateral disease [18,59].

With that as background, the approach to any ionizing radiation–based treatment for thyroid disease is obviously species dependent. In addition, the routine necessary local/regional and distant disease staging is different between these species. Dogs have a high probability of locally invasive thyroid malignancies as well as the worrisome, although varied, likelihood of metastatic disease [63,67,68]. This varies depending on the canine thyroid carcinoma subtypes, which are simplistically defined here as follicular carcinoma or adenocarcinoma and medullary carcinoma, although more detailed and sophisticated descriptions exist [70]. Based on limited data, the medullary variety are considered more resectable than the follicular variety [70], although 1-year postsurgical survival is actually a bit better for the follicular carcinomas or adenocarcinomas (1-year survival rate of 45%) than for the medullary carcinomas (1-year survival rate of 30%) [70]. Some authors believe that the correct approach to canine malignancies is to surgically resect when plausible and that more than half are resectable [69–72]. The authors support that belief and recommend detailed local staging, including ultrasonographic and CT imaging, as well as practical systemic staging, including thoracic and abdominal radiographic and abdominal ultrasonographic imaging. Another dilemma in dogs, however, is the likelihood of occult regional disease, which may be amenable to adjuvant external beam radiotherapy, and the likelihood of distant metastases, many of which have no iodine trapping capacity, rendering radioiodine therapy of dubious value [44]. Despite this hypothesis, survival well beyond 1 year has been reported for dogs and cats with thyroid malignancies after radioiodine therapy [22,73–75]. Therapeutic considerations are further complicated by the option for coarse fractionation in dose ranges lower than those considered potentially curative for disease not amenable to any kind of worthwhile surgical debulking [76]. The limited reports available on external beam radiotherapy for primary treatment of canine thyroid carcinoma have demonstrated reasonable 1-year survival results (>50%) and provide some reasonable option for residual or unresectable local or regional disease as well [69,76–78]. The limited reports on radioiodine therapy for canine thyroid carcinoma offer a different potentially systemic approach but with the limitation that the more anaplastic the primary tumor or its metastatic sites are, the less effective radioiodine therapy is likely to be [44]. Similarly, the limited reports on systemic chemotherapy for canine thyroid malignancies did not engender confidence in the authors regarding their applicability for anything other than adjuvant status [69,79–83].

Cats have a low probability of locally invasive disease with thyroid malignancies, but the possibility of metastatic and ectopic thyroid malignancies cannot be ignored [42,73]. Radioiodine therapy, antithyroid drug therapy, and surgical resection are currently the mainstays for the management of benign hyperthyroid disease in the cat [20,84–101]. As with the dog, staging is an issue, but the overall odds of broad-spectrum metastatic disease are much lower [67,73]. The relevance of radionuclide scintigraphy in the management of feline hyperthyroid disease has been discussed previously in this article but continues to be debated [18,29,31–33,35,37,102–105]. The argument for semiquantitative scintigraphy is the refinement of radioiodine dose, the detection of ectopic thyroid tissue, and possibly the detection of an unsuspected metastatic focus for occult differentiated carcinomas. The argument against semiquantitative scintigraphy is that the outcome of routine hyperthyroid treatment adjusted based on scintigraphy compared with just an empiric dose of radioiodine modified for (total T_4) and body size is not practically different in cats but that the costs for treatment are quite different. Similarly, the use of scintigraphy to differentiate unilateral from bilateral disease in benign feline hyperthyroidism to facilitate the surgical decision has been changed based on two factors. First, the parathyroid-sparing bilateral thyroidectomy has reduced the concern about postoperative hypoparathyroidism [101]. Second, there is the possibility that what was seemingly unilateral disease at scintigraphy is potentially occult bilateral disease, effectively limiting the utility of unilateral thyroidectomy for long-term management of benign feline hyperthyroidism [106]. Therefore, the options for treatment of feline benign hyperthyroidism are basically antithyroid drugs, unilateral thyroidectomy, parathyroid-sparing bilateral thyroidectomy, and radioiodine therapy. Obviously, surgical resection has the associated procedural and anesthetic risks, the possibility of hypoparathyroidism and hypothyroidism for bilateral techniques, and the complexity involved with surgically addressing ectopic hyperfunctioning tissue [20,86–89,98,101].

From the authors' perspective, ethanol injection for the treatment of feline benign hyperthyroidism seems to have merit approximately equal to that of surgery, including the facts that precision requires vigorous chemical restraint, there are procedural risks, including laryngeal paralysis, and there is a significant learning curve [107–109]. Antithyroid drugs, such as methimazole and related compounds, when tolerated, are a cost-effective but often temporary solution [84,85,90–97,99,100]. Furthermore, although antithyroid medications may control the clinical manifestations of hyperthyroidism, they do not stop the progression of the disease at the level of the thyroid gland [1].

Radioiodine, however, has a different set of issues, including radioisotope licensure; the safety of personnel handling the radioiodine and the radioactive cats; the environmental contamination issues in the treatment facilities as well as in the cat's home; the documentation of receipt, administration, and monitoring of the radioiodine; and the admittedly low possibility of posttreatment hypothyroidism [110,111]. It is the authors' contention that aggressive and expensive staging for feline hyperthyroidism as a routine procedure cannot be justified by the outcome improvements. The authors' approach is that only if there is something unusual about the cat at presentation, such as a large thyroid mass, additional regional masses or suspected lymphadenopathy, or sustained tachycardia greater than 220 beats per minute (bpm), is anything indicated beyond routine hematologic and biochemical analyses and survey radiographic screening for masses anywhere, lung nodules, heart failure, or renal size. For those unusual cases, scintigraphy, regional ultrasonography, and echocardiography are considered on a case-by-case basis. Systemic chemotherapy for feline thyroid malignancies has been inadequately addressed, presumably because of the low occurrence rates of malignancy in the feline thyroid glands and the response to radioiodine therapy.

RADIATION THERAPY OF THYROID DISEASE
Thyroid Conditions Amenable to Radiation Therapy
In the authors' practice, radioiodine therapy is the primary method of managing benign feline hyperthyroidism. Generally, the modal dose is an empiric dose of 1.48×10^8 Bq (4 mCi), which is adjusted within the range between 3 and 6 mCi based on the radiologist's judgment about the cat's body weight (total T_4) and the presence of documented thyroid nodules. Because of the authors' limited expectation of feline carcinoma as the cause for feline hyperthyroidism, they treat for benign hyperthyroidism. When the progress at subsequent assessment is not as expected, a more aggressive radioiodine approach is undertaken, usually with doses several orders of magnitude higher. As mentioned in the preceding section, if there are circumstances at examination interpreted to be more complex (eg, possible carcinoma), more extensive screening, including scintigraphy, ultrasonography, and even CT, may be used. Because of the conflicting issues on the limited uptake of radioiodine in undifferentiated malignant thyroid tissue, the report of reasonable survival with radioiodine therapy for canine thyroid carcinoma, and the noteworthy radiation safety issues, the authors do not use it [22,44,67,73,74,110,111]. Their hesitancy is based more on the radiation safety aspects than on the efficacy aspects, however. Available literature suggests that radioiodine treatment for carcinoma in dogs or cats requires higher doses than benign disease [22,44,73,74]. The result is the magnification of the safety, licensing, and environmental contamination issues previously defined for benign disease treatment. There is a role for external beam radiotherapy in canine thyroid carcinoma that may

be the sole mode of treatment, particularly if surgical removal is not an option, or it may be adjuvant to surgery for local or regional disease control [76–78]. Available information, although limited, indicates that median survival times in excess of 1 year after treatment are not unusual [76,78].

Radioiodine Therapy

The authors have used the oral, intravenous, and subcutaneous routes for radioiodine administration in cats. They are currently using the subcutaneous route, as described by other authors [41,112–125]. All routes seem to be effective; thus, the choice of route should be based on available facilities and approved policies as well as on the primary concern for minimizing the exposure and potential contamination of involved personnel as well as the owners when the cat is dismissed. In general, the authors recommend withdrawal from antithyroid drugs for 7 to 10 days before radioiodine treatment to ensure maximum uptake. There may even be a rebound effect after discontinuance of methimazole that may facilitate radioiodine uptake [35]. The authors acknowledge that others have suggested a withdrawal period from antithyroid drugs may be potentially advantageous or unnecessary before radioiodine therapy [113,126,127]. Nevertheless, they prefer to limit the variables in treatment and mandate withdrawal, except in extenuating medical circumstances.

The outcome after radioiodine therapy for feline hyperthyroidism is surprisingly predictable, although nominal variations have been reported. In general, approximately 90% of cats become euthyroid, less than 5% require retreatment because of continued hyperthyroidism, less than 5% become permanently biochemically hypothyroid (total T_4), and even fewer become clinically ill as a result of their "biochemical" hypothyroidism [126]. Because of the limited morbidity and reasonable success of radioiodine therapy, the authors do not routinely perform surgical resection or ethanol injection for benign feline hyperthyroidism. Although a decrease in renal function after radioiodine therapy has been described [128–130], the authors have experienced only limited problems, perhaps because of precise screening and judicious clinical judgment. Similarly, although significant cardiac abnormalities are possible, they are becoming less frequent [131–138]. If the cat is sufficiently ill to require more than twice-daily medical management (eg, subcutaneous fluids, antibiotics, cardiac-related pharmaceutics), it is not treated with radioiodine in the authors' facility. This decision was made based on a combination of cost, personnel radiation exposure, and experience-based outcomes. Collaborative research with an off-site colleague who uses radioiodine to treat cats afflicted with a broader spectrum of thyroid-related and nonthyroid disease, however, has led the authors to believe that the problems are generally manageable and the alternatives are limited (Ralph C. Weichselbaum, DVM, PhD, personal communication, 2002). Obviously, that may not be a universally accepted approach. As radiologists, the authors do not make the decision about antithyroid drug therapy, although based on personal communication as well as on the literature, they believe that it is a practical and cost-effective management tool [90–97,99,100].

Perhaps the most debatable issues surrounding radioiodine therapy for benign feline hyperthyroidism are the acceptable γ-radiation emissions from the cat at dismissal; the interpretation of state and, where applicable, federal guidelines for radiation exposure to members of the general public (usually the family) from these cats; environmental contamination attributable to these cats' evacuation and grooming habits; and the acceptable length and cost of isolation of these cats in a managed treatment facility [110,139–142]. Information about these topics can be found in the literature as mentioned previously and on the World Wide Web [143]. The authors have chosen to limit dismissal of radioiodine-treated benign hyperthyroid cats to that point at which their surface and urine emissions are sufficiently low to meet the strictest interpretation of the Nuclear Regulatory Commission regulations [144,145]. Basically, these are surface exposure at the thyroid as measured by a calibrated Geiger-Mueller instrument at less than 2 mR/h surface over the thyroid glands [110,111]. In the authors' facility, radioiodine-contaminated materials, such as cat litter, cage paper, or miscellaneous utensils, are held in isolation until they are equal to background γ-levels. Obviously, interpretations of available radioisotope safety guidelines vary, and that is reflected in the isolation times at various facilities. The authors' goal is a safe environment, unrestricted dismissal, and comfortable cats, however. Currently, the authors' isolation time ranges between 10 and 14 days depending on surface and urine emissions. Most cats actually gain weight during the isolation phase, and owner acceptance is reasonable.

External Beam Radiotherapy

Because of the judgment against radioiodine therapy for canine thyroid carcinoma, the authors rely heavily on the staging methods defined previously. These include surgery where applicable, some customized combination of external beam radiotherapy (full course or coarse fractionation), and an oncologist's decision about adjuvant chemotherapy. Each treatment is based on the balance of efficacy, complications, and cost. For full-course therapy, the authors typically use a minimum tumor dose of 48 to 54 Gy delivered in 16 to 18 daily weekday fractions. Available literature offers some data-based insight (48 Gy, 12 fractions, and nonprogression rate of 80% at 1 year and 72% at 3 years) [77,78]. For those dogs with unresectable thyroid carcinoma, particularly if there are defined systemic metastases, the authors consider a hypofractionated protocol as an acceptable and reasonable cost approach to improving quality of life temporarily [76]. For the hypofractionated approach, the authors typically use a minimum tumor dose of 24 to 30 Gy delivered in 8 to 10 Gy fractions on a 0-, 7-, and 21-day schedule. Available literature on this topic is limited but offers some cautious encouragement for survival in excess of 1 year [76]. The authors' approach is based on Co^{60} γ-irradiation and is not applicable to orthovoltage protocols. The availability of veterinary-specific treatment facilities has been discussed elsewhere [146]. The role of radioiodine or external beam radiation therapy in human thyroid neoplasia is controversial beyond basic surgery, with or without postoperative adjuvant radioiodine treatment of well-differentiated thyroid carcinoma [147]. By comparison, the human data on and approach to poorly differentiated thyroid adenocarcinoma and medullary thyroid carcinoma are quite variable without a statistically clear difference in the approaches [147]. There may be some advantage to postoperative external beam radiotherapy and chemotherapy, however, but survival is still quite poor. The authors have little to add other than that they carefully balance the radiation tolerance of regional tissues, the potential effects of previous surgery, and the concomitant or sequential effects of adjuvant chemotherapy, if applicable, when prescribing external beam doses. Available data on chemotherapy for canine thyroid carcinoma are limited, but chemotherapy has some promise in selected situations [79,83].

References

[1] Mooney C. Hyperthyroidism. In: Ettinger SJ, Feldman EC, editors. Textbook of veterinary internal medicine. 6th edition. Philadelphia: Elsevier Saunders; 2005. p. 1544–60.

[2] McLoughlin MA, DiBartola SP, Birchard SJ, et al. Influence of systemic nonthyroidal illness on serum concentration of thyroxine in hyperthyroid cats. J Am Anim Hosp Assoc 1993;29: 227–34.

[3] Gerber H, Peter H, Ferguson DC, et al. Etiopathology of feline toxic nodular goiter. Vet Clin North Am Small Anim Pract 1994;24:541–65.

[4] Panciera DL. Hypothyroidism in dogs: 66 cases (1987–1992). J Am Vet Med Assoc 1994;204:761–7.

[5] Dixon RM, Reid SW, Mooney CT. Epidemiological, clinical, haematological and biochemical characteristics of canine hypothyroidism. Vet Rec 1999;145(17):481–7.

[6] Harari J, Patterson JS, Rosenthal RC. Clinical and pathologic features of thyroid tumors in 26 dogs. J Am Vet Med Assoc 1986;188:1160–4.

[7] Page RL. Tumors of the endocrine system. In: Withrow SJ, MacEwen EG, editors. Small animal clinical oncology. 6th edition. Philadelphia: WB Saunders Company; 2001. p. 418–44.

[8] Peterson ME, Melian C, Nichols R. Measurement of serum concentrations of free thyroxine, total thyroxine, and total triiodothyronine in cats with hyperthyroidism and cats with nonthyroidal disease. J Am Vet Med Assoc 2001;218:529–36.

[9] Peterson ME, Graves TK, Cavanagh I. Serum thyroid hormone concentrations fluctuate in cats with hyperthyroidism. J Vet Intern Med 1987;1:142–6.

[10] Peterson ME, Gamble DA. Effect of nonthyroidal illness on serum thyroxine concentrations in cats: 494 cases (1988). J Am Vet Med Assoc 1990;197:1203–8.

[11] Mooney CT, Little CJL, Macrae AW. Effect of illness not associated with the thyroid gland on serum total and free thyroxine concentrations in cats. J Am Vet Med Assoc 1996;208: 2004–8.

[12] Marks SL, Koblik PD, Hornof WJ, et al. 99mTc-pertechnetate imaging of thyroid tumors in dogs: 29 cases (1980–1992). J Am Vet Med Assoc 1994;204:756–60.

[13] Wisner ER, Theon AP, Nyland TG, et al. Ultrasonographic examination of the thyroid gland of hyperthyroid cats: comparison to 99mTcO4– scintigraphy. Vet Radiol Ultrasound 1994;35:53–8.

[14] Wisner ER, Nyland TG, Mattoon JS. Ultrasonographic examination of cervical masses in the dog and cat. Vet Radiol Ultrasound 1994;35:310–5.

[15] Brömel C, Pollard RE, Kass PH, et al. Ultrasonographic evaluation of the thyroid gland in healthy, hypothyroid, and euthyroid golden retrievers with nonthyroidal illness. J Vet Intern Med 2005;19:499–506.

[16] Drost WT, Mattoon JS, Samii VF, et al. Computed tomographic densitometry of normal feline thyroid glands. Vet Radiol Ultrasound 2004;45(2):112–6.

[17] Drost WT, Mattoon JS, Weisbrode SE. Use of helical computed tomography for measurement of thyroid glands in clinically normal cats. Am J Vet Res 2006;67(3):467–71.

[18] Peterson ME, Becker DV. Radionuclide imaging of 135 cats with hyperthyroidism. Vet Radiol Ultrasound 1984;25:23–7.

[19] Thrall JH, Ziessman HA. Endocrine system. In: Thrall JH, editor. Nuclear medicine: the requisites. 2nd edition. St. Louis (MO): Mosby Inc; 2001. p. 363–87.

[20] Naan EC, Kirpensteijn J, Kooistra HS, et al. Results of thyroidectomy in 101 cats with hyperthyroidism. Vet Surg 2006;35:287–93.

[21] Daniel GB, Brawner WR. Thyroid scintigraphy. In: Daniel GB, Berry CR, editors. Textbook of veterinary nuclear medicine. 2nd edition. American College of Veterinary Radiology; 2006. p. 181–98.

[22] Adams WH, Walker MA, Daniel GB, et al. Treatment of undifferentiated thyroid carcinoma in 7 dogs with I-131. Vet Radiol Ultrasound 1995;36:417–24.

[23] Feldman EC, Nelson RW. Feline hyperthyroidism (thyrotoxicosis). In: Feldman EC, Nelson RW, editors. Canine and feline endocrinology and reproduction. 3rd edition. St. Louis (MO): WB Saunders Company; 2004. p. 152–218.

[24] Feldman EC, Nelson RW. Canine thyroid tumors and hyperthyroidism. In: Feldman EC, Nelson RW, editors. Canine and feline endocrinology and reproduction. 3rd edition. St. Louis (MO): WB Saunders; 2004. p. 219–49.

[25] Greco DS, Feldman EC, Peterson ME, et al. Congenital hypothyroid dwarfism in a family of giant schnauzers. J Vet Intern Med 1991;5(5):306–7.

[26] Mitchell M, Hurov L, Troy GC. Canine thyroid carcinomas: clinical occurrence, staging by means of scintiscans, and therapy of 15 cases. Vet Surg 1979;8:112–8.

[27] Broome MR. Thyroid scintigraphy in hyperthyroidism. Clin Tech Small Anim Pract 2006;21:10–6.

[28] Beck KA, Hornof WJ, Feldman EC. The normal feline thyroid: technetium of pertechnetate imaging and determination of thyroid to salivary gland ratios in 10 normal cats. Vet Radiol Ultrasound 1985;26:35–8.

[29] Mooney CT, Thoday KL, Nicoll JJ, et al. Qualitative and quantitative thyroid imaging in feline hyperthyroidism using technetium-99m as pertechnetate. Vet Radiol Ultrasound 1992;33:313–20.

[30] Young K, Daniel GB, Bahr A. Application of the pin-hole collimator in small animal nuclear scintigraphy: a review. Vet Radiol Ultrasound 1997;38(2):83–93.

[31] Kintzer PP, Peterson ME. Thyroid scintigraphy in small animals. Semin Vet Med Surg (Small Anim) 1991;6:131–9.

[32] Daniel GB, Sharp DS, Nieckarz JA, et al. Quantitative thyroid scintigraphy as a predictor of serum thyroxin concentration in normal and hyperthyroid cats. Vet Radiol Ultrasound 2002;43:374–82.

[33] Henrikson TD, Armbrust LJ, Hoskinson JJ, et al. Thyroid to salivary ratios determined by technetium-99m pertechnetate imaging in thirty-two euthyroid cats. Vet Radiol Ultrasound 2005;46:521–3.

[34] Lambrechts N, Jordaan MM, Pilloy WJ, et al. Thyroidal radioisotope uptake in euthyroid cats: a comparison between 131I and 99mTcO4. J S Afr Vet Assoc 1997;68:35–9.

[35] Nieckarz JA, Daniel GB. The effect of methimazole on thyroid uptake of pertechnetate and radioiodine in normal cats. Vet Radiol Ultrasound 2001;42:448–57.

[36] Fischetti AJ, Drost WT, DiBartola SP, et al. Effects of methimazole on thyroid gland uptake of 99mTC-pertechnetate in 19 hyperthyroid cats. [Erratum appears in Vet Radiol Ultrasound. 2005 jul-aug;46(4):355 note: Drost, william tod [added]]. Vet Radiol Ultrasound 2005;46:267–72.

[37] Branam JE, Leighton RL, Hornof WJ. Radioisotope imaging for the evaluation of thyroid neoplasia and hypothyroidism in a dog. J Am Vet Med Assoc 1982;180:1077–9.

[38] Hall IA, Campbell KL, Chambers MD, et al. Effect of trimethoprim/sulfamethoxazole on thyroid function in dogs with pyoderma. J Am Vet Med Assoc 1993;202:1959–62.

[39] Adams WH, Daniel GB, Petersen MG, et al. Quantitative 99m-Tc-pertechnetate thyroid scintigraphy in normal beagles. Vet Radiol Ultrasound 1997;38(4):323–8.

[40] Forrest LJ, Baty CJ, Metcalf MR, et al. Feline hyperthyroidism: efficacy of treatment using volumetric analysis for radioiodine dose calculation. Vet Radiol Ultrasound 1996;37(2): 141–5.

[41] Milner RJ, Channell CD, Levy JK, et al. Survival times for cats with hyperthyroidism treated with iodine 131, methimazole, or both: 167 cases (1996–2003). J Am Vet Med Assoc 2006;228:559–63.

[42] Turrel JM, Feldman EC, Nelson RW, et al. Thyroid carcinoma causing hyperthyroidism in cats: 14 cases (1981–1986). J Am Vet Med Assoc 1988;193:359–64.

[43] Cook SM, Daniel GB, Walker MA, et al. Radiographic and scintigraphic evidence of focal pulmonary neoplasia in three cats with hyperthyroidism: diagnostic and therapeutic considerations. J Vet Intern Med 1993;7:303–8.

[44] Peterson ME, Kintzer PP, Hurley JR, et al. Radioactive iodine treatment of a functional thyroid carcinoma producing hyperthyroidism in a dog. J Vet Intern Med 1989;3:20–5.

[45] Peterson ME, Ferguson DC. Thyroid diseases. In: Ettinger SJ, editor. Textbook of veterinary internal medicine. 3rd edition. Philadelphia: WB Saunders Company; 1989. p. 1632–74.

[46] Catherine J, Scott-Moncrieff R, Guptill-Yoran L. Hypothyroidism. In: Ettinger SJ, Feldman EC, editors. Textbook of veterinary internal medicine. 6th edition. Philadelphia: WB Saunders Company; 2005. p. 1535–44.

[47] Broome MR, Donner GS. The insensitivity of 99mTc pertechnetate for detecting metastases of a functional thyroid carcinoma in a dog. Vet Radiol Ultrasound 1993;34:118–24.

[48] Broome MR, Feldman EC, Turrel JM. Serial determination of thyroxine concentrations in hyperthyroid cats. J Am Vet Med Assoc 1988;192:49–51.

[49] Broussard JD, Peterson ME, Fox PR. Changes in clinical and laboratory findings in cats with hyperthyroidism from 1983–1993. J Am Vet Med Assoc 1995;206:302–5.

[50] Bucknell DG. Feline hyperthyroidism: spectrum of clinical presentations and response to carbimazole therapy. Aust Vet J 2000;78:462–5.

[51] Ferguson DC, Peterson ME, Nachreiner RF. Serum free and total iodothyronine concentrations in normal cats and cats with hyperthyroidism. J Vet Intern Med 1989;3:121.

[52] Graves TK, Peterson ME. Diagnostic tests for feline hyperthyroidism. Vet Clin North Am Small Anim Pract 1994;24:567–76.

[53] Graves TK, Peterson ME. Diagnosis of occult hyperthyroidism in cats. Probl Vet Med 1990;2:683–92.

[54] Holzworth J, Theran P, Carpenter JL, et al. Hyperthyroidism in the cat: ten cases. J Am Vet Med Assoc 1980;176:345–53.

[55] Kintzer PP. Considerations in the treatment of feline hyperthyroidism. Vet Clin North Am Small Anim Pract 1994;24:577–85.

[56] Meric SM. Diagnosis and management of feline hyperthyroidism. Compendium on Continuing Education for the Practicing Veterinarian 1989;11:1053.

[57] Mooney CT. Pathogenesis of feline hyperthyroidism. J Feline Med Surg 2002;4:167–9.

[58] Mooney CT. Feline hyperthyroidism. Diagnostics and therapeutics. Vet Clin North Am Small Anim Pract 2001;31:963–83.

[59] Peterson ME, Kintzer PP, Cavanagh PG, et al. Feline hyperthyroidism: pretreatment clinical and laboratory evaluation of 131 cases. J Am Vet Med Assoc 1983;183: 103–10.

[60] Thoday KL, Mooney CT. Historical, clinical and laboratory features of 126 hyperthyroid cats. Vet Rec 1992;131:257–64.

[61] Scarlett JM. Epidemiology of thyroid diseases of dogs and cats. Vet Clin North Am Small Anim Pract 1994;24:477–86.

[62] Birchard SJ, Roesel OF. Neoplasia of the thyroid gland in the dog: a retrospective study of 16 cases. J Am Anim Hosp Assoc 1981;17:369–72.

[63] Leav I, Schiller AL, Rijnberk A, et al. Adenomas and carcinomas of the canine and feline thyroid. Am J Pathol 1976;83:61–122.

[64] Orsher RJ, Eigenmann JE. Endocrine tumors. Vet Clin North Am Small Anim Pract 1985;15:643–58.

[65] Sullivan M, Cox F, Pead MJ, et al. Thyroid tumours in the dog. J Small Anim Pract 1987;28:505–12.

[66] Brodey RS, Kelly DF. Thyroid neoplasms in the dog. A clinicopathologic study of fifty-seven cases. Cancer 1968;22:406–16.

[67] Lurye JC, Behrend EN. Endocrine tumors. Vet Clin North Am Small Anim Pract 2001;31:1083–110.

[68] Susaneck SJ. Thyroid tumors in the dog. Compendium on Continuing Education for the Practicing Veterinarian 1983;5:35–42.

[69] Withrow SJ, MacEwen EG. Small animal clinical oncology. 3rd edition. Philadelphia: WB Saunders Co; 2001. p. 423–30.

[70] Carver JR, Kapatkin A, Patnaik AK. A comparison of medullary thyroid carcinoma and thyroid adenocarcinoma in dogs: a retrospective study of 38 cases. Vet Surg 1995;24:315–9.

[71] Klein MK, Powers BE, Withrow SJ, et al. Treatment of thyroid carcinoma in dogs by surgical resection alone: 20 cases (1981–1989). J Am Vet Med Assoc 1995;206:1007–9.

[72] Lantz GC, Salisbury SK. Surgical excision of ectopic thyroid carcinoma involving the base of the tongue in dogs: three cases (1980–1987). J Am Vet Med Assoc 1989;195:1606–8.

[73] Guptill L, Scott-Moncrieff JCR, Janovitz EB, et al. Response to high-dose radioactive iodine administration in cats with thyroid carcinoma that had previously undergone surgery. J Am Vet Med Assoc 1995;207:1055–8.

[74] Turrel JM, McEntee MC, Burke BP, et al: Sodium iodide I 131 treatment of dogs with non-resectable thyroid tumors: 39 cases (1990–2003). J Am Vet Assoc 2006;229:542–8.

[75] Worth AJ, Zuber RM, Hocking M. Radioiodide (131I) therapy for the treatment of canine thyroid carcinoma. Aust Vet J 2005;83:208–14.

[76] Brearley MJ, Hayes AM, Murphy S. Hypofractionated radiation therapy for invasive thyroid carcinoma in dogs: a retrospective analysis of survival. J Small Anim Pract 1999;40:206–10.

[77] Pack L, Roberts RE, Dawson SD, et al. Definitive radiation therapy for infiltrative thyroid carcinoma in dogs. Vet Radiol Ultrasound 2001;42:471–4.

[78] Theon AP, Marks SL, Feldman ES, et al. Prognostic factors and patterns of treatment failure in dogs with unresectable differentiated thyroid carcinomas treated with megavoltage irradiation [see comment]. J Am Vet Med Assoc 2000;216:1775–9.

[79] Fineman LS, Hamilton TA, de Gortari A, et al. Cisplatin chemotherapy for treatment of thyroid carcinoma in dogs: 13 cases. J Am Anim Hosp Assoc 1998;34:109–12.

[80] Jeglum KA, Whereat A. Chemotherapy of canine thyroid carcinoma. Compendium on Continuing Education for the Practicing Veterinarian 1983;5:96–8.

[81] Knapp DW, Richardson RC, Bonney PL, et al. Cisplatin therapy in 41 dogs with malignant tumors. J Vet Intern Med 1988;2:41–6.

[82] Ogilvie GK, Obradovich JE, Elmslie RE, et al. Efficacy of mitoxantrone against various neoplasms in dogs. J Am Vet Med Assoc 1991;198:1618–21.

[83] Ogilvie GK, Reynolds HA, Richardson RC, et al. Phase II evaluation of doxorubicin for treatment of various canine neoplasms. J Am Vet Med Assoc 1989;195:1580–3.

[84] Becker TJ, Graves TK, Kruger JM, et al. Effects of methimazole on renal function in cats with hyperthyroidism. J Am Anim Hosp Assoc 2000;36:215–23.

[85] Behrend EN. Medical therapy of feline hyperthyroidism. Compendium on Continuing Education for the Practicing Veterinarian 1999;21:235–44.

[86] Birchard SJ, Peterson ME, Jacobson A. Surgical treatment of feline hyperthyroidism: results of 85 cases. J Am Anim Hosp Assoc 1984;20:705–9.

[87] Flanders JA, Harvey HJ, Erb HN. Feline thyroidectomy. A comparison of postoperative hypocalcemia associated with three different surgical techniques. Vet Surg 1987;16:362–6.

[88] Flanders JA. Surgical options for the treatment of hyperthyroidism in the cat. J Feline Med Surg 1999;1:127–34.

[89] Flanders JA. Surgical therapy of the thyroid. Vet Clin North Am Small Anim Pract 1994;24: 607–21.

[90] Mooney C. Decision making in the treatment for hyperthyroidism in cats. In Pract 1996;18: 150–6.

[91] Mooney CT, Thoday KL, Doxey DL. Carbimazole therapy of feline hyperthyroidism. J Small Anim Pract 1992;33:228–35.

[92] Murray LA, Peterson ME. Ipodate treatment of hyperthyroidism in cats. J Am Vet Med Assoc 1997;211:63–7.

[93] Peterson ME. Propylthiouracil in the treatment of feline hyperthyroidism. J Am Vet Med Assoc 1981;179:485–7.

[94] Peterson ME, Aucoin DP. Comparison of the disposition of carbimazole and methimazole in clinically normal cats. Res Vet Sci 1993;54:351–5.

[95] Peterson ME, Aucoin DP, Davis CA, et al. Altered disposition of propylthiouracil in cats with hyperthyroidism. Res Vet Sci 1988;45:1–3.

[96] Peterson ME, Hurvitz AI, Leib MS, et al. Propylthiouracil-associated hemolytic anaemia, thrombocytopenia, and antinuclear antibodies in cats with hyperthyroidism. J Am Vet Med Assoc 1984;184:806–8.

[97] Peterson ME, Kinzer PP, Hurvitz AI. Methimazole treatment of 262 cats with hyperthyroidism. J Vet Intern Med 1988;2:150–7.

[98] Salisbury SK. Hyperthyroidism in cats. Compendium on Continuing Education for the Practicing Veterinarian 1991;13:1399–403.

[99] Trepanier LA. The use of antithyroid drugs in the medical management of feline hyperthyroidism. Probl Vet Med 1990;2:668–82.

[100] Trepanier LA, Peterson ME, Aucoin DP. Pharmacokinetics of methimazole in normal cats and cats with hyperthyroidism. Res Vet Sci 1991;50:69–74.

[101] Welches CD, Scavelli TD, Matthiesen DT, et al. Occurrence of problems after three techniques of bilateral thyroidectomy in cats. Vet Surg 1989;18:392–6.

[102] Kintzer PP, Peterson ME. Nuclear medicine of the thyroid gland. Scintigraphy and radioiodine therapy. Vet Clin North Am Small Anim Pract 1994;24:587–605.

[103] Nap AM, Pollak YW, van den Brom WE, et al. Quantitative aspects of thyroid scintigraphy with pertechnetate (99mTcO4−) in cats. J Vet Intern Med 1994;8:302–3.

[104] Nykamp SG, Dykes NL, Zarfoss MK, et al. Association of the risk of development of hypothyroidism after iodine 131 treatment with the pretreatment pattern of sodium pertechnetate Tc 99m uptake in the thyroid gland in cats with hyperthyroidism: 165 cases (1990–2002). J Am Vet Med Assoc 2005;226:1671–5.

[105] Page RB, Scrivani PV, Dykes NL, et al. Accuracy of increased thyroid activity during pertechnetate scintigraphy by subcutaneous injection for diagnosing hyperthyroidism in cats. Vet Radiol Ultrasound 2006;47:206–11.

[106] Swalec KM, Birchard SJ. Recurrence of hyperthyroidism after thyroidectomy in cats. J Am Anim Hosp Assoc 1990;26:433–7.

[107] Goldstein RE, Long C, Swift NC, et al. Percutaneous ethanol injection for treatment of unilateral hyperplastic thyroid nodules in cats. J Am Vet Med Assoc 2001;218:1298–302.

[108] Wells AL, Long CD, Hornof WJ, et al. Use of percutaneous ethanol injection for treatment of bilateral hyperplastic thyroid nodules in cats. J Am Vet Med Assoc 2001;218:1293–7.

[109] Mallery KF, Pollard RE, Nelson RW, et al. Percutaneous ultrasound-guided radiofrequency heat ablation for treatment of hyperthyroidism in cats. J Am Vet Med Assoc 2003;223: 1602–7.

[110] Feeney DA, Jessen CR, Weichselbaum RC, et al. Relationship between orally administered dose, surface emission rate for gamma radiation, and urine radioactivity in radioiodine-treated hyperthyroid cats. Am J Vet Res 2003;64:1242–7.

[111] Weichselbaum RC, Feeney DA, Jessen CR. Evaluation of relationships between pretreatment patient variables and duration of isolation for radioiodine-treated hyperthyroid cats. Am J Vet Res 2003;64:425–7.

[112] Bauer R, Puille M, Spillmann T, et al. Radioiodine therapy in cats. Tierarztliche Praxis. Ausgabe K, Kleintiere/Heimtiere 2000;28:295–303.

[113] Chambers M, Hightower D, Tveter D. Treatment of feline hyperthyroidism with radioactive iodine. Southwestern Veterinarian 1987;38:37–42.

[114] Chun R, Garrett LD, Sargeant J, et al. Predictors of response to radioiodine therapy in hyperthyroid cats. Vet Radiol Ultrasound 2002;43:587–91.

[115] Craig A, Zuber M, Allan GS. A prospective study of 66 cases of feline hyperthyroidism treated with a fixed dose of intravenous I-131. Australian Veterinary Practitioner 1993;23:2–6.

[116] GunnMoore DA, Galloway PE, Godfrey A, et al. The use of subcutaneous administration of radio-iodine for the treatment of feline hyperthyroidism—a study of nine cases. Feline Pract 1995;23:13–5.

[117] Klausner JS, Johnston GR, Feeney DA, et al. Results of radioactive iodine therapy in 23 cats with hyperthyroidism. Minnesota Journal of Veterinary Medicine 1987;27:28–32.

[118] Malik R, Lamb WA, Church DB. Treatment of feline hyperthyroidism using orally administered radioiodine: a study of 40 consecutive cases. Aust Vet J 1993;70:218–9.

[119] Meric SM, Rubin SI. Serum thyroxine concentrations following fixed dose radioactive iodine treatment in hyperthyroid cats. J Am Vet Med Assoc 1990;197:621–3.

[120] Meric SM, Hawkins EC, Washabau RJ, et al. Serum thyroxine concentrations after radioactive iodine therapy in cats with hyperthyroidism. J Am Vet Med Assoc 1986;188:1038–40.

[121] Mooney CT. Radioactive iodine therapy for feline hyperthyroidism: efficacy and administration routes. J Small Anim Pract 1994;35:289–94.

[122] Peterson ME, Becker DV. Radioiodine treatment of 524 cats with hyperthyroidism. J Am Vet Med Assoc 1995;207:1422–8.

[123] Slater MR, Komkov A, Robinson LE, et al. Long-term follow up of hyperthyroid cats treated with iodine-131. Vet Radiol Ultrasound 1994;35:204–9.

[124] Theon AP, VAn Vechtan MK, Feldman E. Prospective randomized comparison of intravenous versus subcutaneous administration of radioiodine for treatment of hyperthyroidism in cats. Am J Vet Res 1994;55:1734–8.

[125] Turrel JM, Feldman EC, Hays M, et al. Radioactive iodine therapy in cats with hyperthyroidism. J Am Vet Med Assoc 1984;184:554–9.

[126] Peterson ME. Radioiodine treatment of hyperthyroidism. Clin Tech Small Anim Pract 2006;21:34–9.

[127] Trepanier LA. Medical management of hyperthyroidism. Clin Tech Small Anim Pract 2006;21:22–38.

[128] Adams WH, Daniel GB, Legendre AM, et al. Changes in renal function in cats following treatment of hyperthyroidism using I^{131}. Vet Radiol Ultrasound 1997;38:231–8.

[129] DiBartola SP, Broome MR, Stein BS, et al. Effect of treatment of hyperthyroidism on renal function in cats. J Am Vet Med Assoc 1996;208:875–8.

[130] Stiles J, Polzin DJ, Bistner SI. The prevalence of retinopathy in cats with systemic hypertension and chronic renal failure of hyperthyroidism. J Am Vet Med Assoc 1994;30:564–72.

[131] Bond BR, Fox PR, Peterson ME, et al. Echocardiographic findings in 103 cats with hyperthyroidism. J Am Vet Med Assoc 1988;192:1546–9.

[132] Fox PR, Peterson ME, Broussard JD. Electrocardiographic and radiographic changes in cats with hyperthyroidism: comparison of populations evaluated during 1992–1993 vs. 1979–1982. J Am Anim Hosp Assoc 1999;35:27–31.

[133] Graves TK, Olivier NB, Nachreiner RF, et al. Changes in renal function associated with treatment of hyperthyroidism in cats. Am J Vet Res 1994;55:1745–9.

[134] Jacobs G, Hutson C, Dougherty J, et al. Congestive heart failure associated with hyperthyroidism in cats. J Am Vet Med Assoc 1986;188:52–6.

[135] Liu SK, Peterson ME, Fox PR. Hypertrophic cardiomyopathy and hyperthyroidism in the cat. J Am Vet Med Assoc 1984;185:52–7.

[136] Moise NS, Dietze AE, Mezza LE, et al. Echocardiography, electrocardiography, and radiography of cats with dilatation cardiomyopathy, hypertrophic cardiomyopathy, and hyperthyroidism. Am J Vet Res 1986;47:1476–86.

[137] Moise NS, Dietze AE. Echocardiographic, electrocardiographic and radiographic detection of cardiomegaly in hyperthyroid cats. Am J Vet Res 1986;47:1487–94.

[138] Weichselbaum RC, Feeney DA, Jessen CR. Relationship between selected echocardiographic variables before and after radioiodine treatment in 91 hyperthyroid cats. Vet Radiol Ultrasound 2005;46:506–13.

[139] Berg GE, Michanek AM, Holmberg EC, et al. Iodine-131 treatment of hyperthyroidism: significance of effective half-life measurements. J Nucl Med 1996;37:228–32.

[140] Ibis E, Wilson CR, Collier BE, et al. Iodine-131 contamination from thyroid cancer patients. J Nucl Med 1992;33:2110–5.

[141] Mathieu I, Caussin J, Smeesters P, et al. Recommended restrictions after Iodine-131 therapy: measured doses in family members. Health Phys 1999;76:129–36.

[142] Ponto JA, Ponta LL, Bricker JA. Evaluation of external monitoring versus urine assay for determining post-therapy body retention of I-131. Health Phys 1987;52::891–921

[143] Klein M. Iodine found in trash delivery. Available at: http://www.nyjournal.com/. [original publication 5/23/01]. Accessed January 23, 2002.

[144] Code of Federal Regulations, Title 10–Energy, Subpart D—Radiation Dose Limits for Individual Members of the Public, Subsection 20.1301a. US Nuclear Regulatory Commission. Code of Federal Regulations. Title 10. Part 20. Subpart D: radiation dose limits for individual members of the public. Dose limits for individual members of the public. Washington, DC: US Nuclear Regulatory Commission, 1997; 20:1301a.

[145] Code of Federal Regulations, Title 10, Subpart J—Precautionary Procedures, Subsection 20.1905. US Nuclear Regulatory Commission. Code of Federal Regulations. Title 10. Part 20. Subpart J: precautionary procedures. Exemptions to labeling requirements. Washington, DC: US Nuclear Regulatory Commission, 1995; 20:1905.

[146] LaRue SM, Gillete EL. Radiation therapy. In: Withrow SJ, MacEwen EG, editors. Small animal oncology. 3rd edition. Philadelphia: WB Saunders; 2001. p. 119–37.

[147] Carling T, Udelsman R. Thyroid tumors. In: DeVita VT, Hellman S, Rosenberg SA, editors. Cancer: principles and practice of oncology. 7th edition. Philadelphia: Lippincott Williams and Wilkins; 2005. p. 1502–20.

INDEX

Note: Page numbers of article titles are in **boldface** type.

0195-5616/07/$ – see front matter
doi:10.1016/S0195-5616(07)00077-0